Natural
Stomach
Care

Natural Stomach Care

Treating and Preventing Digestive Disorders
Using the Best of Eastern and
Western Healing Therapies

ANIL MINOCHA, M.D.,
AND DAVID CARROLL

AVERY
a member of Penguin Group (USA) Inc.
New York

Most Avery books are available at special quantity discounts for bulk purchase for sales promotions, premiums, fund-raising, and educational needs. Special books or book excerpts also can be created to fit specific needs. For details, write Penguin Group (USA) Inc. Special Markets, 375 Hudson Street, New York, NY 10014.

a member of
Penguin Group (USA) Inc.
375 Hudson Street
New York, NY 10014
www.penguin.com

Library of Congress Cataloging-in-Publication Data

Minocha, Anil.
Natural stomach care : treating and preventing digestive disorders using the
best of Eastern and Western healing therapies / Anil Minocha and David Carroll.
p.   cm.
Includes index.
ISBN 1-58333-159-X
1. Indigestion—Alternative treatment.   2. Gastrointestinal system—Diseases—
Alternative treatment.   3. Naturopathy.   I. Carroll, David, date.   II. Title.
RC827.M566   2003   2003043727
616.3'069—dc21

Printed in the United States of America
1   3   5   7   9   10   8   6   4   2

contents

Natural Stomach Care

chapter one

An Introduction to Your Digestive Health

There is an aphorism that you will find repeated throughout medical texts in both Eastern and Western scientific literature. It dates back to the time of Hippocrates, and probably before. What it tells us speaks volumes about the human constitution and about the digestive system in particular. This aphorism tells us that *all sickness and all health begin in the stomach.*

Sounds profound, doesn't it? Significant. But what does it really mean? It means that the food we eat every day, as well as the refinement process it undergoes in our digestive tract, ends up nourishing every cell in our bodies and keeps our bodies fit and strong. If this food is of inferior quality, or if it is not properly processed and assimilated by the many organs involved—including the stomach, liver, pancreas, gallbladder, large intestine, and small intestine—we soon weaken and grow sick. When our digestion fails, the rest of us fails too.

Food, in other words, is our fuel, and the digestive system is the engine that burns this fuel, distributes the energy it produces, and gets rid of its wastes. Without a finely tuned synergy between food and its internal processing, troubles develop, and sickness soon follows.

Currently, Americans suffer from more than forty types of gastrointestinal disorders, many of which are lumped together under a single generic heading: indigestion.

These disorders run the gamut of seriousness from ordinary belly discomfort, to chronic digestive disorders, to life-threatening disease. Gastritis, heartburn, irritable bowel syndrome, diverticulosis, colitis, Crohn's disease, and cancer, plus an array of other illnesses are all related to digestive tract malfunction. All take their toll on more than 50 million Americans a year.

Diseases caused by digestive malfunction do not afflict only the gastrointestinal tract. A number of maladies begin in the gut, and then end up causing symptoms in parts of the body that are seemingly unrelated to the digestive process itself. Familiar ailments in this category include headaches, sinus pressure, joint pains, bad breath, hemorrhoids, fevers, skin rashes, allergies, asthma, fungus infections, gum and tooth problems, fatigue, hepatitis, arthritis, kidney stones, depression, anxiety, and more.

The number of gut-related disorders in the United States is presently on the rise and is increasing at alarming speeds. By the year 2010, digestion-related disease will be the *number-one cause* of missed days in the workplace and the primary reason that people visit physicians.

In short, health indeed begins in the stomach, and clearly a well-working gut leads to a healthy mind in a healthy body.

ALTERNATE WAYS OF HEALING

Over the past decades, conventional Western medicine has developed an amazingly extensive collection of chemical medications and surgical procedures to treat digestive tract disorders. These medications do just what their name implies—medicate. They bring relief in a number of gratifying ways, marvelously stemming the tide of human pain and disease. The world would be an unimaginably tragic and ailing place without them.

However, while conventional medicines help us in so many ways, they do nothing to *prevent* digestive problems from occurring, and in many instances they palliate our symptoms rather than cure them. What's more, preventive strategies for avoiding stomach- and bowel-related disorders are rarely offered as options in a physician's office, and they are almost never taught to fledgling doctors in medical schools.

Since it is estimated that 25 to 50 percent of all digestion-related ailments can be prevented and/or modified by proper eating, exercise, natural medicines, and lifestyle modifications, these are troubling facts. Also troubling is the fact that many powerful complementary and nutritional therapies for indigestion are not included in the conventional medical canon, and are rarely offered by physicians to patients as part of the healing programs.

And yet, despite these omissions, as the many medical professionals who now practice complementary medicine well know, there are a vast number of natural remedies available today that dramatically relieve common digestive disorders and sometimes cure them. The problem is, medical doctors rarely tell their patients about these remedies.

LEARNING TO FEEL WELL AGAIN

My name is Anil Minocha, M.D., and I practice gastroenterology, the branch of medical science that specializes in treatment of the stomach, intestines, and related digestive organs.

During the two decades since my graduation from medical school, I have performed clinical work on a wide range of digestion-related diseases, and I have become familiar with a number of therapies, both modern and traditional, for healing disorders of the gut.

In my years of working with patients, it has become evident to me that for serious digestive ailments, prescription medications and, at times, surgery are the best tools for restoring health. For lesser and chronic unrelenting digestive disorders, however, and certainly for preventive techniques, there are two natural alternatives that do the job equally and sometimes better than conventional medicine. These alternatives are:

3

1. Proper eating and nutrition
2. Natural medicines and therapies

I'll start out by giving you a brief overview of how the digestive tract works, then I'll tell you ways in which proper eating, the first alternative, assures a sound and healthy digestive system. I will also provide you with some of the interesting nutritionally oriented folk wisdom I have learned along the way, both here in the West and in my native India.

While these remedies are not clinically proven, and, to date, there has been little controlled scientific testing done on them to establish their effectiveness, I have found that many of these simple solutions to complex digestive problems often work—sometimes with gratifying speed and effectiveness. I include them in this book not only because they are natural and helpful, but also because they have often saved my day.

The remaining chapters in this book feature various natural healing modalities that are designed to treat specific digestive ailments such as constipation, diarrhea, heartburn, gas, and many others. While these techniques, in my experience, are effective and powerful, they are all in a way secondary to our eating habits themselves. That is, a vast majority of these remedies would be unnecessary if patients would eat properly to begin with.

Therefore, even as we study and apply different natural therapies throughout the book, we continue to refer back to diet and nutrition as *the most powerful* of all healing tools for the gut. When all is said and done, eating right is helpful for just about *anything* that ails us—and, most of all, for compromised digestion.

Sound nutrition is the number one prerequisite for digestive wellness. On this point, most health-care professionals agree. On a parallel track, a well-working digestive system is needed to digest food properly and to extract the nutrients that our bodies require. Good nutrition demands a healthy digestive system, and a sound digestive system requires good nutrition.

Let's start by reviewing the mechanics of human digestion and learning how this process works from the moment we eat a morsel of food to the moment the residues from this morsel are eliminated.

THE HUMAN DIGESTIVE SYSTEM

The human digestive system is a complex and many-sectioned biological mechanism designed to break down foods into small, easily absorbable particles, and to eliminate the unusable remains.

In the process, food remnants are chemically transformed: carbohydrates are turned into small sugar molecules, proteins into small peptides and amino acids, and fats into fatty acids and glycerol. These substances are absorbed into the cells lining the intestine, processed again, and transferred into the blood and lymphatic system for transport. They are then used as building blocks and energy-producing fuel for the entire body.

The process of digestion begins in the mouth, at the top end of the 30-foot-long alimentary canal. It continues down through the esophagus, stomach, small and large intestines, ending finally at the rectum where wastes from digestive action are voided through the anal canal. The movement of food from the mouth to the rectum can take up to two to three days or more, depending on the efficiency and vitality of the organs processing it.

The meat, bread, salad, and potatoes we eat every day are too gross in their present form to serve us nutritionally. Before the body can make use of these foodstuffs, they must first be broken down on a biochemical and molecular level until they are small enough and refined enough to be absorbed for transport to the rest of the body. This process of refinement begins in the mouth.

The Mouth

The moment we take a bite of food, salivary glands in the mouth secrete enzymes that break down complex sugars and starches into simple sugars. As the food literally starts to melt in our mouth, our teeth chop and grind even more until the food forms a coarse bolus (ball) that is soft and pulpy enough to pass easily down the esophagus. While some of this food may be gulped, depending on chewing habits, a majority of it reaches the esophagus already well smoothed.

The Esophagus

The tongue and the swallowing muscles in the throat now push the bolus of food into the esophagus, a tube of muscle that is about 25 centimeters long. It starts at the bottom of the throat and ends at the stomach. The lower end of the esophagus is capped with a ring of muscle known as the lower esophageal sphincter. This ring opens when it senses pressure from food, then closes once the food has passed through. As the bolus of food makes its way down the esophagus, the esophagus contracts rhythmically, moving the food quickly along and into the stomach.

The Stomach

The stomach is a large, J-shaped organ banded with three layers of internal muscle that form the stomach wall. Once food arrives in this "furnace," the process of digestion swings into high gear. First, the enzyme pepsin starts to break down proteins. It is aided in the process by secretions of hydrochloric acid (HCl), which increase the pepsin's effectiveness and kill potentially harmful bacteria. Though HCl is a powerfully acidic liquid, acidic enough to eat away human flesh, the mucous lining of the stomach wall is constructed in such a remarkably resilient way that it resists all corrosion.

As the stomach fills up, it rhythmically relaxes and contracts, mixing the food, breaking it down into 1- and 2-millimeter particles, and saturating it with gastric fluids. After two, three, or more hours of this intense churning, the food is finally broken down into a blended mixture known as chyme. A ring of muscle in the stomach known as the pyloric sphincter then opens on an as-needed basis, accepting this thick liquid and sending portions of it into the small intestine.

The Small Intestine

Once in the small intestine, the chyme continues its journey through the alimentary canal helped along by peristaltic action produced by muscle contractions.

Further enzymatic breakdown takes place now, assisted by secretions from the pancreas and from fat-digesting bile sent to it by the gallbladder and liver. The first part, a short, curved section of the intestines known as the duodenum, converts the aggregations of fats, proteins, and carbohydrates that are included in most of the meals we eat into easily assimilated substances. These three nutrients—fats, proteins, and carbohydrates—compose the three major nutrient groups needed by the body to sustain life.

Eventually, substances in the intestines decompose to the point where they are molecularly small enough to absorb into the intestinal cells and be reprocessed for eventual transport by the blood and lymphatic system. These absorbed nutrients are then used by the body as building blocks and fuel to sustain the life of the organism. Meanwhile, all undigested leftovers of food pass into the large intestine for final processing and disposal.

The Large Intestine or Colon

By the time food residues reach the large intestine, the work of digestion and absorption is almost, but not quite, complete. It is now the job of the beneficial bacteria that line the colon to feed on these waste materials and to convert some of them to useful nutrients for absorption.

First, wastes in the colon are moved by peristalsis upward through a section known as the ascending colon. Then, they are passed horizontally across the transverse colon. Next, they move downward into the descending colon. Finally, as they near the end of the alimentary canal, they take a sharp turn along the sigmoid flexure and pass on into the rectum for disposal.

While moving through these various sections of the large intestine, the friendly flora that make their home along the colon wall, besides converting waste matter into feces, produce enzymes that perform a last bit of digestion, breaking down stubborn particles of fiber and vegetable matter. All this time, the colon continues to absorb water and electrolytes.

Finally, the long and remarkable task of digestion and absorption complete, the remaining indigestible residues are passed through the rectum

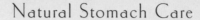

and out in the form of feces. Job complete. A job well done results in a healthy digestive system in a healthy body. However, the job can not be optimal without healthy nutrients fed into this digestive system. In the next chapter we review some powerful strategies for accomplishing this goal.

chapter two

Power Nutrition:
Eating to Prevent Digestive
Problems, Eating to Heal Them

Given the complex and finely tuned workings of the body's internal food-processing plant, it is clear that the successful completion of nutrient breakdown and assimilation depends to a large degree on the type of food the gut is called upon to digest.

Here is where the direct relationship between food and digestive health comes most into play. The higher the quality of foods we eat and the more balanced our meals, the more likely our digestive tract and body metabolism are to turn this food into high-octane energy.

Remember, the foods we ingest on an everyday basis include about 100,000 chemicals, only 300 of which have any dietary value, and only 45 of which can be identified as essential nutrients. We are what we eat. Or, as computer experts are fond of saying, "quality in, quality out; garbage in, garbage out."

However, before we can understand what balanced eating really consists of and before we can apply this information to our own digestive needs, we need to become familiar with the fundamentals of nutrition itself. As it so happens, these fundamentals begin and end with the three nutrients groups that make up our meals—carbohydrates, proteins, and fats—supplemented by vitamins and minerals. All three of these groups are essential for human health and for maximum nutrition, and all three should be included in any power nutrition regimen.

The following is a thumbnail description of each of these nutrient groups.

Carbohydrates

Because they provide a lavish source of calories and energy, carbohydrates are often referred to as "the fuel of life." Despite their importance in the nutritive process, however, many people equate carbohydrates with sweets or junk fare, and dismiss them as foods that "make you fat."

While it is true that carbohydrates may, at times, be part of a junk meal, especially meals served at fast-food restaurants, this is not the carbohydrate's fault. Or, to put it a more scientific way, there are two types of carbohydrates:

1. Processed carbohydrates
2. Natural carbohydrates

The processed kind are carbohydrate-based foods that are denatured during preparation and cooking in various ways. They may, for example, be fried in low-quality oils, denuded of their nutrient-rich skins and coverings, mixed with animal fats, tampered with via sweetening, over-salted, or preserved. You know the drill. The results? Largely low-quality calories—foodless foods.

Natural carbohydrates, on the other hand, are carbohydrates that remain unprocessed and au naturel. They consist of fresh vegetables, fresh fruits, and fresh grains as nature made them. These include vegetables such as carrots, celery, beets, turnips, lettuce, radishes, beans, peas, tomatoes, and potatoes; grains such as rice, barley, corn, millet, and wheat; and fruits such as apples, pears, mangoes, bananas, and grapes. Fresh vegetables, grains, and fruits are all carbohydrates and are the stuff of power nutrition.

Relatively simple in molecular construction, carbohydrate structure takes three basic forms: monosaccharides (single sugars), disaccharides (double sugars), and polysaccharides (complex sugars, also known as starches). During the digestive process, all three of these structures are broken down to fundamental body sugars such as glucose, which are then processed in the liver and sent out to power our machine.

Found in many sweet vegetables and fruits such as celery, cucumbers, lettuce, beets, apples, grapes, berries, and pears—and, of course, in regular commercial sugars like fructose and sucrose—the single and double sugars found in carbohydrates break down in an extremely rapid way and can be transformed into quick fuel, which is one reason why people turn to candy bars or soft drinks when they need instant energy. The jolt received from the single and double sugars, however, is short lived and tends to burn itself out like a shooting star. Soon, eaters need a second hit of this quick-energy sugar source, and a third after that, ad infinitum.

Complex carbohydrate sugars or starches, on the other hand, the kind found in bananas, for instance, or in potatoes, pasta, and grains, digest more slowly and distribute their energy benefits in a more measured way. Beginning the digestive journey in the mouth where they are acted upon by the salivary enzyme amylase, starches enter the small intestine via the stomach and are further broken down by pancreatic enzymes. The glucose extracted from this interaction is then transported to the liver where it is turned into glycogen, stored, and sent out to various cells of the body on an as-needed basis.

The result of starch's slower digestive speed is that a person's blood-sugar level is kept in a desired range sustained for hours at a time, as opposed to the blood-sugar rush and consequent drop experienced with simple sugars. This is one reason why a meal heavy in starches keeps the appetite at bay longer than a meal consisting of the simple sugars found in, say, cherry pie, lettuce, and cola.

Human beings require a certain number of carbohydrates in their diet every day. This is because certain body tissue (such as the brain) can only use the glucose-based calories that carbohydrates provide. When this sugar is not available, the body tries, out of desperation, to convert non-carbohydrate foods into glucose, quickly causing a harmful increase of acid production in the tissue known as *ketosis*.

To maintain health and prevent malnutrition, the average person needs approximately 400 to 600 carbohydrate-produced calories every day. Or, to phrase it more directly, 40 to 60 percent of our total daily calorie intake should be derived from natural carbohydrates. Drop below this level and ketosis sets in. Stay above this level and good health reigns.

PROTEINS

We require a daily dose of protein, not just because protein produces energy, but because it is the basic building block of living cells and because it helps manufacture a majority of the soft and hard tissue that forms our bodies.

The heart, kidneys, liver, and even the eyes, for example, are made up of mostly protein. The same is true for hair, skin, tendons, nerves, hormones, digestive enzymes, amino acids, and genes—all are protein based. Little wonder that the word "protein" is derived from the Greek linguistic root meaning "primary" or "first."

Protein is one of the largest and most complex of all molecular structures in nature. To give you an idea of its enormous mass, a particularly large protein molecule compares in size to a typical carbohydrate molecule as the sun compares to the earth.

Without an adequate supply of protein we would die. Or, at best, we would grow very sick. Prolonged protein deficiency causes anemia, mental retardation, blindness, kidney disease, ulcers, and compromised immunological response. Sometimes it is fatal. Foods that are rich in high-quality protein include meat, fish, milk, butter, cheese (especially cottage cheese), and eggs. Certain vegetables such as potatoes, peas, peanuts, and cooked greens also furnish protein, though in far less quantity and quality than meat and dairy products, and (with a few exceptions) minus the vitamin B_{12} reserves found in eggs and meat.

Protein from animal sources supplies a "complete" protein; that is, a protein that contains all nine essential amino acids required for human metabolism. Not so with vegetables and fruits, which provide a limited but diverse selection of these essential aminos. They are, therefore, labeled "incomplete" proteins.

Moreover, within the body's busy building and repairing factory, protein is the substance that heals wounds, constructs new protoplasm, distributes body water, and manufactures hormones and antibodies. Many enzymes are also produced from its end products. For example, secretin, the hormone that acts as the intermediary between the intestine and the pancreas during digestion, is a protein derivative. Hemoglobin itself, the stuff of the blood, is also protein based.

Protein, in short, is the very stuff and staff of life, and should be a fundamental part of everyone's diet. While carbohydrates power our machines, protein builds them up, maintains them, and keeps them running.

FATS

Though fat is the least important nutrient of the carbohydrate-protein-fat trio, it is nonetheless a required food, and a misunderstood one as well. To begin, there is an important distinction to be made between *body fat* and *dietary fat*. These two forms of fat are often confused.

Body fat is the hard, adipose tissue that covers us like an insulator and serves to store our food and energy reserves.

Dietary fat is a basic nutrient group common to both animal and plant foods. It is found in meats such as pork, beef, chicken, and fish; in eggs; and in dairy products such as butter. Dietary fat is also found, though in smaller quantities, in nuts, seeds, fruits, vegetables, and grains. At the same time, many vegetables do include a surprisingly high amount of dietary fat. Olive oil, for instance, is 100 percent fat. Peanut butter is 50 percent fat, cashew nuts are 47 percent fat, avocados are 15 percent fat, olives are 7 to 10 percent fat, and soybeans are 6 to 18 percent fat.

Digestion wise, dietary fat serves to transport fat-soluble vitamins such as vitamins A, D, and E to different cells in the body. Without an adequate amount of these fatty acids in the bloodstream, these vitamins never reach their destination, and severe deficiencies result. For this reason alone, fat is a prerequisite in the diet. Lack of the essential fatty acids found in dietary fat can likewise lead to hair loss, dermatitis and other skin problems, and a slowdown in general healing.

Finally, fat is a principal source of physical energy, a high-burning combination of hydrogen and carbon that provides us with twice the amount of energy, ounce for ounce, than a protein or a carbohydrate. For this reason, fats help quench the appetite, usually for a period of time that outlasts both carbohydrates and protein. This is one reason why fast-food chains load their foods with so many fats. Not only do fats taste good, but they also fill the hunger spot for hours at a time.

Yet herein lies the danger. Fat digests mostly in the intestines (rather than in the stomach), where it makes enzyme secretion sluggish, and takes its time moving through the intestines. If you use a large amount of fatty substances in food preparation, as in frying, these substances blend with the foods being cooked, and slow down the eater's digestion accordingly. For this reason, and because excess fats harm the cardiovascular system, we are cautioned to keep fat consumption to 30 percent or less of our daily diet.

Fat is chemically made up of three fatty acids joined to a glycerol molecule. There are two kinds of fatty acids—saturated and unsaturated. With the exception of palm oil and coconut oil, saturated fats are solid at room temperature, and are derived from animal sources. Unsaturated fats are more common in fish and plants; they are liquid at room temperature and they lower bad cholesterol. Unsaturated fatty acids are further classified into polyunsaturated or monounsaturated. Polyunsaturated are omega-3 and omega-6 fatty acids. Vegetable oils such as corn oil and sunflower oil are rich in omega-6 fatty acids like linoleic acid, of which the body requires approximately 5 g per day. Omega-3 fatty acids are abundant in tuna, swordfish, and salmon. Consumption of fish at least once a month has been shown to lower blood pressure and decrease heart attack. Monounsaturated fats as in canola oil and olive oil contain oleic acid.

Transfatty acids are unsaturated fatty acids bound to hydrogen; this form is used to prolong the shelf life of junk foods such as cookies and chips. Unlike unsaturated fats, transfatty acids increase the risk of cardiac disease. Fat consumption in the diet may be equally divided among saturated, polyunsaturated, and monounsaturated fats.

We know that dietary fat is in most of the foods we eat and that it is a vital human nutrient. But we know also that only small amounts of fat, perhaps as little as two to three tablespoons or six to eight teaspoons per day of butter or olive oil, are necessary. Emphasis should be on unsaturated vegetable oils (peanut, rapeseed, canola, safflower, and sesame). Use fewer nuts, avocados, and olives, and less coconut oil or palm oil, lard, and bacon fat. In general, if a food has more then 3 g of fat per 100 calories, it has more than the recommended 30-percent intake of fat calories.

PUTTING IT ALL TOGETHER

The question remains: What, in fact, are the *right* foods to put into our system? What types of food are most likely to treat our digestive tract with the care and respect it demands and deserves and, at the same time, deliver the nutritive clout needed to maximize energy?

Though experts have argued this question for centuries, it can be said that, from the standpoint of digestive health in the twenty-first century, there are two basic types of diets worth considering:

1. The Preventive Diet—a diet that prevents digestive disorders
2. The Healing Diet—a diet that helps heal digestive disorders

If, for example, you are constitutionally fortunate enough to possess a strong and disease-free gut, and if you want to keep it this way, the Preventive Diet is the way to go. The Preventive Diet presented below is gentle on your digestive system and, at the same time, keeps all those processing organs finely tuned and in a state of grateful health.

If, on the other hand, you suffer from any of the common problems that beset the digestive tract—constipation, gastritis, diarrhea, bloating, gas, and so on—then the Healing Diet is best for your needs. Both diets are covered in the following sections. Take your pick.

THE PREVENTIVE DIET

The first thing you will notice about the Preventive Diet is that it is *not* necessarily vegetarian. Meat is kept at a minimum here, but it is not outlawed entirely. While meat is slow to digest, its nutritive value far offsets its ponderous movement through the gut. The strategy is to eat meat in limited amounts.

Eggs are also included in this diet despite the fact that they are high in cholesterol. Again, the nutrition is worth the game. When using eggs in recipes, it is better to use two egg whites rather than one whole egg.

The dietary philosophy adopted in the Preventive Diet, in other words, is that animal food is generally good for the health of the gut—*but* with the following caveats:

1. That the meat and eggs be organic, if possible
2. That the meat be fresh and lean
3. That the meat be served in small amounts

Of course, if you happen to dislike meat or wish to avoid it on whatever grounds, simply compensate by eating more protein-rich vegetables (soybeans, almonds, dry beans, peanuts, and peas) and more dairy products (especially milk, yogurt, and cheese).

Here's how the Prevention Diet works:

1. **The Preventive Diet includes approximately 35 percent grains.**

    Stick mostly with whole grains if you can—high-fiber whole-grain bread, whole-grain cereals, unpolished rice, barley, millet, and rye. Two out of your three daily meals should include grains.

2. **Approximately 40 percent of your diet should include high-fiber vegetables (including legumes) and high-fiber fruits.**

Here we mean *fresh* fruits and *fresh* vegetables, not canned or frozen. Vegetables should predominate—for example, 70 percent vegetables and 30 percent fruits, with an emphasis on the high-fiber varieties. (For a list of high-fiber fruits and vegetables, see the table on page 331 in Chapter 16.)

Certain foods, though perhaps okay in the fiber department, should also be avoided. For example, French fries should be eliminated from the diet entirely (fourteen French fries carry 11 g of fat and 225 calories), and iceberg lettuce is best replaced, or at least supplemented, with more robust greens such as ruby red lettuce, endive, cabbage, bok choy, and escarole. Oranges and tomatoes are fine, but are better when eaten in the company of similarly nutritious fruits and vegetables such as apples, pears, papayas, mangoes, bananas, carrots, broccoli, cauliflower, Brussels sprouts, spinach, yams, radishes, cucumbers, parsley, celery, and root vegetables like turnips, beets, and parsnips.

3. **Approximately 15 percent of your diet should include eggs, oils, and meats.**

Eggs are relatively easy to digest, and the quality of the protein they deliver is high, providing a complete range of amino acids. Use fresh organic eggs if possible.

Avoid inexpensive cooking and salad oils. As far as salad and cooking oils are concerned, it is worth paying a few extra dollars for quality products. Quality oils taste better and are better for you.

When shopping for meats, look for fresh, lean cuts, preferably those sold at a butcher's counter. Today, many butcher shops and supermarkets carry organic lamb, chicken, beef, turkey, and pork, all of which come minus the preservatives and antibiotics. If you can find them and can afford them, these meats are vastly superior to the treated kinds.

4. Approximately 10 percent of your diet should include dairy products.

Of this 10 percent, a majority should include live-culture dairy products such as yogurt and buttermilk. Low-fat, 1-percent, or 2-percent milk is a healthy choice except for infants who require whole milk. Go very easy on the butter though, and avoid heavy cream.

5. Avoid certain foods.

The no-no list includes junk foods of all kinds, plus super-rich foods, super-spicy foods, sugared desserts and confections, carbonated drinks (carbonated mineral waters with juice make a great substitute), chocolate, and artificial sweeteners.

Highly preserved and processed foods such as hot dogs, lunch meats, sausage, and the like are best eaten in minute quantities, if at all. Commercial salted snacks such as potato chips, popcorn, peanuts, and crackers, besides taxing the digestion, are cooked in the lowest quality vat oils, and are saturated with preservatives. Instead of the artificial varieties, pop your own organic popcorn, buy unsalted nuts and cover them with a healthy salt substitute, and/or eat whole-grain organic crackers. If you are partial to crunchy snacks, there are many nut, raisin, and seed mixtures available at health-food stores that fill you up, satisfy your urge to crunch, and treat your stomach kindly.

The Healing Diet

The following diet is designed for people who may not have received a diagnosis of a particular stomach or bowel ailment, but who have what is sometimes called "delicate belly," and who are often bothered by generalized digestive troubles such as bloating, gas, heartburn, inflamed stomach or intestinal lining, and acid reflux.

This diet is designed to do what its name implies: keep irritating foods away from an already irritated or inflamed gut, and help the digestive system restore itself to health. While it is not necessarily best for every type of gut ailment—see the individual headings and chapters for specifics—it affords an excellent eating plan for people who suffer from the many persistent irritations that eating can bring.

The first thing you will notice about the Healing Diet is that it recommends certain foods that are excluded from most health-oriented diets—foods such as refined white bread, beef, and canned and cooked vegetables. Meanwhile, certain traditional "health foods" that are on everyone's good-eating list such as whole-wheat breads, whole-grain cereals, bran, and fresh, raw vegetables are discouraged.

The reason behind these exclusions and inclusions is simple—foods that in a healthy person are passed through the gastrointestinal tract with ease can, in persons suffering from a sensitive belly, trigger a host of problems including hyperacidity, gas, bloating, constipation, irritation of the gastrointestinal tract, and more. Moreover, the fact that certain healthy foods are discouraged from this diet does not mean that they are discouraged forever, only that they should be avoided until the patient's digestive system improves. Once healing takes place and the gut starts to behave itself better, most discouraged foods can be eaten again, though often in moderation.

Here is the Healing Diet. It is recommended that you stay within the guidelines of each food group, and that you follow this regimen for at least a month and preferably two to three months.

1. **Dairy Products**
   RECOMMENDED
   Cottage cheese
   Farmer cheese
   Mild cheeses such as cheddar, mozzarella, American,
       and Muenster
   Low-fat milk, non-fat dry milk, or skim milk (one glass a day,
       assuming you are lactose tolerant)
   Yogurt

STAY AWAY FROM

Rich and spicy cheeses

Commercial cheese spreads

Cheeses made with seeds or vegetable matter (such as onions, peppercorns, and garlic)

2. Meat and Fish

RECOMMENDED

Fresh lean beef, veal, and lamb

Fresh chicken and turkey

Organ meats like liver

Ocean- and freshwater fish

STAY AWAY FROM

Fish sticks and commercially processed fish products

Hot dogs, lunch meats, and sausages

Pork

Heavily salted and smoked meats such as jerky

Salted and smoked fish such as anchovies, sardines, herring, smoked salmon, and lox

Fried meats and fish

Fish and meats packed in oil

3. Cereals and Grains

RECOMMENDED

Soft, refined hot breakfast cereals such as cream of wheat, oats, and rice

Strained oatmeal

Grits

Dried flake cereals such as cornflakes

Spaghetti, noodles, and macaroni (without tomato sauce)

White or brown rice

STAY AWAY FROM

Bran cereals

Cereals with nuts, seeds, and dried fruits

Unstrained oatmeal

Corn or potato chips

Popcorn

4. Breads

RECOMMENDED

White breads (French and Italian)

White-flour bagels

Rolls, muffins, cornbread, melba toast, zwieback, and matzoth

STAY AWAY FROM

Whole-wheat breads (refined whole wheat is acceptable in small
portions)

Pumpernickel

Whole-wheat bagels, and bagels covered with poppy seeds,
caraway seeds, and so on

Rye bread

Bread made with seeds or vegetable chunks

Highly salty and spiced crackers (especially whole-wheat
crackers)

5. Eggs

RECOMMENDED

Hard-boiled, soft-boiled, scrambled, or poached eggs

Omelets

Chopped egg

STAY AWAY FROM

Eggs cooked or fried in animal fat (if using butter or butter
substitute, use small amounts)

Raw egg

6. Fruits

RECOMMENDED

Bananas

Avocados

Papaya

Applesauce

Canned or cooked fruits including apples, apricots, cherries, guavas, melon, peaches, pears, and plums

STAY AWAY FROM

Fresh fruits with seeds, such as grapes

All dried fruits, especially dried fruits with many seeds, such as figs

Berries of any kind

Citrus and acid-making fruits including grapefruits, lemons, limes, oranges, and pineapple

7. Vegetables

RECOMMENDED

Canned or cooked vegetables of any kind except tomatoes (see below)

Salad greens

STAY AWAY FROM

Raw vegetables of any kind

Fried vegetables of any kind

Sauerkraut or cabbage dishes, such as coleslaw

Corn

Tomatoes (Actually a fruit, tomatoes are often listed as vegetables. Tomatoes should be avoided by anyone with complaints of "excess acidity," intestinal inflammation, or "nervous gut.")

8. **Vegetable Starch Group**

RECOMMENDED

Potatoes without skins

Sweet potatoes and yams without skins

STAY AWAY FROM

French fries, hash browns, fried potato sticks, and the like

Potato salad

Pastas filled with spicy or acidic stuffing, such as lasagna and
ravioli

Wild rice

9. **Beverages**

RECOMMENDED

Tap water (preferably filtered) and noncarbonated mineral water

Coffee substitutes such as Postum or Morning Thunder

Herbal teas, especially green tea

Apricot, peach, papaya, and pear nectar

Milk (in moderation)

STAY AWAY FROM

Citrus, grapefruit, and spiced vegetable juices, such as V8

Coffee and black tea (including the decaffeinated kinds)

Cola drinks

Alcoholic drinks

Carbonated beverages

Chocolate milk and cocoa

10. **Other Foods**

RECOMMENDED

Salt (in moderation)

Finely ground and chopped leaf herbs such as sage, thyme, and
mint parsley (remove from diet immediately if not tolerated)

STAY AWAY FROM

Seeds and nuts

Spicy condiments and sauces such as barbecue sauce, soy sauce,
and Worcestershire sauce

Jams and preserves with seeds

Rich cream sauces

Pickled and vinegar-based foods and sauces

Horseradish

Hot spices such as chili, paprika, cloves, and pepper

All caffeinated products

Aspirin and ibuprofen

Chewing gum

FIFTEEN POWER FOODS THAT HELP JUST ABOUT EVERYTHING DIGESTIVE

Dietitians, nutritionists, and gastroenterologists all have their favorite list of tasty, healthy, and digestible foods they recommend, and here's mine. I have learned that the following foods are packed with nutritional goodies, provide medicinal benefits, and are richly endowed by nature to promote sound and healthy digestion. These foods are delicious as well. Here's the list:

1. **Yogurt**—There is an entire chapter in this book extolling yogurt's virtues. Take a look at Chapter 7. I recommend this food above all others, not just for improving digestion but for promoting overall wellness of the entire body.

2. **Rice**—Rice is the miracle food par excellence. While unrefined rice comes loaded with fiber, it is extremely gentle on the gut and is the perfect food when you are suffering from diarrhea, nausea, or sour belly. Rice is also a specific for constipation, and when bouts of diarrhea present themselves, drinking the water the rice is boiled in really helps. In fact, whenever digestive problems strike, plain rice is usually the most nutritious and healing of all grains.

3. **Tofu**—Rich in protein and vitamins, tofu is a delicious and ubiquitous meat substitute. It is also reputed to contain a number of anticarcinogenic nutrients. Most people easily digest tofu (except those who are allergic to soy). It goes well in just about any stew, soup, or salad.

4. **Dandelion greens**—A great source of vitamin C, dandelion greens are a traditional blood purifier and digestive aid. Add them to any mixed green salad for a slightly bitter, nutty taste.

5. **Sunflower seeds**—Sunflower seeds have plenty of protein, as well as phosphorus, potassium, and omega-6 fatty acids. Purchase the fresh-hulled varieties from natural food stores where they are usually sold directly from help-yourself dispensers. For added taste, roast the seeds and sprinkle them on salads or cereal with wheat germ and bran.

6. **Sea vegetables**—Sea vegetables such as hijiki, nori, arami, wakame, dulse, and kombu come loaded with almost the entire spectrum of mineral elements needed for human nutrition. They also contain almost all major vitamins, including B vitamins such as niacin, thiamine, riboflavin, and pantothenic acid, all of which aid digestion and calm the nerves. Sea vegetables contain vitamin B_{12}, the vitamin most needed by vegetarians. (Vitamin B_{12} is mainly found in eggs, meat and dairy, or fortified soy products.) You can purchase sea vegetables at health-food stores and Asian groceries.

7. **Miso**—A fermented soybean paste that is especially popular in Japan, miso contains B vitamins (including the elusive vitamin B_{12}). It is easily digested, making miso soup a perfect food for compromised stomachs. Since miso includes powerful digestive agents such as lactic acid bacteria, fermentation molds, and enzymes, its action in the bowels also helps break down foods in a fast and efficient way. Hatcho miso is highest in protein and is generally considered the most nutritious of the many types of miso.

8. **Flaxseed oil**—Flaxseeds and flaxseed oil have many medicinal uses, including strengthening the immune system, regulating blood pressure, and stabilizing cholesterol. Both the oil and the

seeds are also believed to have anticarcinogenic qualities. Flaxseed oil likewise helps lubricate the intestines and increases the ease of bowel movements. It is often prescribed for constipation as well as for diarrhea and irritable bowel syndrome. Or sprinkle the seeds over your breakfast cereal or grind in a blender for use on salads and baked potatoes.

9. **Tempeh**—A staple food in Indonesia for many centuries, tempeh is a soybean product that is just beginning to gain popularity in the West. It tastes something like tofu, yet has its own rich flavor plus its own array of nutrients. Because of its high-protein content and some vitamin B_{12}, tempeh makes an excellent meat substitute. Unlike tofu, it causes very little intestinal gas. It also makes an excellent food for convalescents and for people with weak digestive systems.

10. **Papayas**—Papayas are among the most nutritious of all fruits. Papaya extract is sold at health-food stores and is taken by many people for its healing and stimulating qualities. Both the meat and the juice of the papaya are excellent for digestion problems. Indeed, if you suffer from a bloated, queasy feeling after eating a large meal, eat a papaya and see how quickly the discomfort subsides. Papaya is also one of the most delicious of tropical fruits, and one of the most decorative and colorful when cut into slices and added to fruit salads.

11. **Garlic**—Hippocrates, the father of modern medicine, prescribed garlic for a host of ailments ranging from infections to indigestion. In Chinese medicine, garlic is used to combat worm infestation, infectious diarrhea, chronic cough, asthma, pneumonia, indigestion, intestinal gas, and skin rashes. Likewise, Ayurvedic doctors use it for colds, asthma, heart disease, high blood pressure, arthritis, and nervous conditions of all kinds.

In Japan, Dr. Kyo and colleagues, as reported in *Phytomedicine* (1999), showed that aged garlic extract is useful for combating psychological stress. Dr. Balasenthil and colleagues, as reported in *Nutrition and Cancer* (2001), report that certain constituents of garlic prevent tumor formation in animals by enhancing antioxidant production. Dr. Wang, in an article in the Chinese medical journal *Wei Sheng Yan Jiu* (1998), praises the protective effects of garlic against alcohol in the liver. Employing a double-blind, placebo-controlled study, Dr. Josling in the United Kingdom reports in *Advanced Therapy* (2001) that garlic helps prevent attacks of the common cold virus. Many other positive clinical findings on garlic have been reported. Moral: eat more garlic. Add it to your salads, cook with it, prepare recipes that contain it, and/or eat two or three raw cloves daily with a piece of bread or a spoonful of yogurt. Keep in mind, however, that the type of garlic you eat matters. For example, wild garlic has a greater effect on reducing blood pressure and blood cholesterol than the commercially grown kind.

12. **Turmeric**—In India, turmeric is used in practically every curry recipe, not only to add a cheerful orange color to the food but for its medicinal and detoxifying properties as well. Turmeric's antiseptic and antitoxin properties are believed to do their good work without altering the healthy balance of intestinal flora (in contrast to antibiotics). There is also a great deal of excitement about its potential role in retarding Alzheimer's disease. In paste form, turmeric is used for healing acne, skin disease, and insect bites. Inhaling its smoke is said to stop hiccups and to revive a person who has fainted.

13. **Bananas**—Bananas are highly effective in people with diarrhea, helping tilt the balance in the colon in favor of helpful, "friendly" bacteria. Bananas are also well tolerated, even by persons with food allergies, and they contain enough potassium to make them helpful for people who take diuretics. Dr. Lohsoonthorn and Dr. Danvivia, as reported in the *Asian Pacific Journal of Public Health* (1995), claim that eating bananas on a regular basis lowers the risk of developing cancer by half. Bananas are also believed to help prevent stroke.

14. **Basil**—The holy basil or tulsi plant is worshipped across the entire subcontinent of India. It is renowned for its antiinfection and sooth-

ing properties, and is widely prescribed for coughs, colds, indigestion, diarrhea, arthritis, colic, stress, and food poisoning. Dr. V. Vats and colleagues, as reported in the *Journal of Ethnopharmacology* (2002), found that basil regularizes blood glucose levels in normal as well as diabetic rats. Dr. S. Singh, in the *Indian Journal of Experimental Biology* (1999), tells us that the fixed oil of basil possesses significant antiulcer properties, especially the type of ulcers produced by aspirin and alcohol abuse. Dr. M. Ilori from Nigeria, in the *Journal of Diarrheal Disease Research* (1996), similarly shows that extracts of basil are effective against diarrhea-causing bacteria such as Aeromonas, Escherichia coli, Salmonella, and Shigella.

Basil is a stress-buster too. Dr. R. Archana and Dr. A. Namasivayam studied the effect of basil on noise-induced changes in white blood cell functions in rats. Reporting their findings in the journal *Ethnopharmacology* (2000), they state that pretreatment with the basil extract brings back stress-altered values to normal levels and helps calm patients down.

Dr. T. K. Maity and colleagues studied the effect of basil root extract on swimming performance in mice. Reporting in the journal *Phytotherapy Research* (2000), they state that extracts of basil increase endurance and swimming time, suggesting that basil acts as a stimulant and antistress mechanism on the central nervous system. Reporting their findings in the journal *Plant Foods Human Nutrition* (1997), Dr. Rai and colleagues assert that basil leaf powder fed to rats results in a significant reduction in fasting blood sugar, total cholesterol, triglyceride, and total lipid levels, thus supporting its traditionally claimed role as an aid in diabetes and heart disease. Dr. M. K. Asha and colleagues, writing in the journal *Fitoterapia* (2001), report that basil oil generates a potent antiparasitic effect throughout the entire gut.

As if all of the above is not enough, basil leaves appear to have an aphrodisiac affect, and have been used as such for centuries. Adding taste clout as well as medicinal properties, basil can be added to a number of dishes including soups, pasta, salads, and meat recipes. Or it can be taken separately as a tea once or twice a day.

15. **Sage**—Sage leaves contain antioxidants and antiinflammatory properties, and are especially useful for relieving menopausal symptoms. Dr. V. De Leo studied the effects of sage leaves on menopausal symptoms in thirty women. His findings, reported in the journal *Minerva Ginecology* (1998), show that sage combined with alfalfa eliminated hot flashes and night sweating in two-thirds of test subjects. Use sage as a seasoning in your recipes, or take it straight as a daily tea. When burned as an incense, it purifies the air and helps sharpen concentration.

EATING FOR DIGESTIVE HEALTH THE AYURVEDIC WAY

From the point of view of Ayurvedic medicine, longevity is directly related to the health of the gut and consequently to what you eat every day of your life.

Knowledge of Ayurvedic medicine has served billions of people over thousands of years. While few scientific studies are available in the West to confirm its claims, traditional writings relate that many of the legendary sages who practiced these methods lived long and productive lives, and certainly millions of Indians who followed suit would agree; Ayurveda has been keeping people healthy and curing their ills in India for millennia. Why not give it a try? Identify your "dosha" as outlined below, and lead a life in harmony with it.

According to Ayurvedic philosophy, all of nature is composed of five basic phases or states of matter: air (gases, the atmosphere), fire (electricity, atomic energy, fire), water (all things in a fluid state), earth (all things in a solid state), and ether or empty space. Since these elements are universal, they are active in the workings of the human body, which, like every living organism, is part of the natural order.

Air, for example, represents the human heart and lungs, both of which depend on oxygen for their workings. Earth is represented by the skeletal structure, the hair, and the skin. Water is represented by all bodily fluids. Fire is equivalent to metabolism and the digestive system, while space or ether represents the "empty" parts of the body such as the abdominal cavity and the mouth.

These five phases continually interact with one another within a person's body, and are constantly striving to reach a state of balance, and hence good health. When we eat poorly, or when we otherwise misuse our digestive systems, this balance is thrown off and things go wrong.

Right nutrition is therefore a critical element in maintaining human health. It is so critical that Ayurvedic practice has worked out a nutritional typology, matching certain kinds of foods to certain types of human constitutional types. Underlying this typology is the belief in three basic forms of human energy, known as the *doshas*. Each one of us, Ayurveda teaches, is made up of various combinations and permutations of the five phases, leading to a dosha.

For example, a person with a predominance of the element air in his or her constitution is known as a Vata type. That is his or her dosha. A person with a preponderance of earth and water is known as a Kapha type. And a person with a balance of fire and water is known as a Pitta type.

All human beings have all three of these doshas in their physical and mental makeup. One, however, usually predominates. No one dosha is healthier than the other. Only when the eating habits and lifestyles conflict with the dosha does sickness result.

Each of these three human prototypes, the Vata, Kapha, and Pitta type, in turn have (1) distinct physical and mental weaknesses and strengths according to their type, (2) distinct diseases they are likely to develop because of their type, and (3) distinct varieties of foods that prevent these ailments or encourage their development. Generally speaking, it takes a skilled Ayurvedic practitioner to determine a person's dosha and to make a firm diagnosis. Here is an overview to get you started.

Vata Types

Psychologically, Vata types tend to be worriers. They are anxious, restless, and mentally acute. They are quick in their movements, both in thought and action. They can be unreliable, flighty, oversexed, and changeable, but also energetic, brilliant, and often spiritually minded.

Vata-dominant types are often tall and thin with an angular, bony athletic build and an inclination toward dry skin and thin hair. They tend to sleep poorly and are prone to gut ailments such as gas, colitis, diverticulitis, and especially acid reflux. They are also likely to experience back problems, bone and joint conditions, irregular heartbeats, nervous disorders, and depression.

To combat these constitutional weaknesses, Vata types are encouraged to include plenty of sour, sweet, and salty foods in their daily menu; to eat small, frequent, well-cooked meals; to drink plenty of water; and to avoid raw foods.

Foods that benefit Vata types include rice, wheat, oats, mangoes, bananas, soaked raisins, papayas, honeydew melon, peaches, carrots, green beans, avocados, squash and zucchini, lentils, cucumbers, beets, artichokes, pine nuts, anise, basil, mint, nutmeg, milk, cooked garlic, and cooked onions. Foods with a tendency to disturb the physical balance of Vatas include large heavy meals, cranberries, pomegranates, dried fruits, and too many raw vegetables.

Pitta Types

Pitta types are ruled by fire and water. They are strong-willed, competitive, aggressive, and determined, much like the "Type A" personality of Western medicine. They also tend to be broad-minded, creative, open to new ideas, and highly intelligent, but they sometimes also tend to be angry, fussy, and judgmental. Physically, they are of medium build with smooth skin and a tendency to sweat profusely.

Pitta types are especially prone to ailments of the gut. They frequently suffer from indigestion, heartburn, Crohn's disease, ulcerative colitis, and ulcers, as well as migraine headaches, hypertension, and skin rashes. Mentally, they are often impulsive, argumentative, and high-strung. Their tendency to be workaholics tires them out, and they must learn to pace their activities and to take time off.

Nutritionally, Pitta types are advised to avoid hot and spicy foods, and are encouraged to eat foods that are sweet, bitter, and astringent. Especially recommended are rice, wheat, lentils, asparagus, zucchini, cauliflower, cucumbers, squash, bean sprouts, broccoli, green beans, apricots, melons, peaches, sweet apples, dates, pears, coconut milk, basil, coriander, cumin, saffron, cardamom, cilantro, turmeric, and well-soaked almonds.

In general, Pitta types easily digest most vegetables and are wise to eat as many of them as possible. Foods to avoid include grapes, pineapple, plums, tomatoes, most nuts, and too much sugar, alcohol, and caffeine.

Kapha Types

Kaphas tend to be content, calm, easygoing, and relaxed. They can also be slow, indecisive, and materialistic. Physically, they are on the heavy side, and overweight is often a problem. Kaphas have oily skin; a short, stout body; and a stable, sometimes majestic, gait. They are intelligent in the ways of the world but sometimes slow to absorb new information and data. They love both hot and cold weather, but avoid humidity and are most comfortable in a dry environment.

In their personal relationships, Kaphas may be clinging and possessive. Physically, they frequently develop ailments that involve the production of excess mucus, such as asthma, emphysema, and sinus problems. They also have a tendency toward diabetes, constipation, diarrhea, and sleep and snoring disorders.

Kaphas should avoid eating too many sweets and salty snacks. Pungent and astringent foods are all recommended. Foods agreeable to the Kapha include rice, barley, apples, apricots, pears, mangoes, most lentils, black beans, pinto beans, soaked almonds, most fresh vegetables, mint, mustard greens, garlic, and ginger. Kaphas are advised to go easy on wheat bread, oranges, grapefruits, tomatoes, red meat, red kidney beans, milk, oil, and carbonated beverages.

Although meat products in general are not recommended as part of the Ayurvedic diet, chicken and turkey are tolerated by all three types.

FURTHER EATING SUGGESTIONS FOR POWER NUTRITION AND DIGESTIVE HEALTH

- Avoid fatty meats and fats in general. Keep your consumption of dietary fat to no more than 30 percent of your overall diet.
- Avoid drinking too much liquid with your meals. Liquids thin out enzymes in the saliva and digestive juices, and are counterproductive to good digestion.
- Avoid overeating, even if you are dining on highly digestible foods. Overeating is a primary cause of heartburn, stomach acid, and acid reflux. And, of course, obesity can lead to its own myriad of problems. Moderation is best.
- Avoid lying down immediately after eating. When stretched out, you are more likely to experience heartburn and reflux acid than when standing up or moving about. Some people take a relaxed walk immediately after eating dinner to help the food digest more smoothly.
- If you suffer from chronic acid reflux, try eating five or six small meals a day rather than three large ones. When the digestive system takes in smaller meals, it tends to reflux less acid.
- If your esophagus becomes inflamed from too much acid reflux, try chewing your food more thoroughly. Avoid acidic foods such as oranges, grapefruits, and tomatoes. Eat small, frequent meals.
- You can bolster the Preventive Diet and the Healing Diet featured earlier by taking high-quality multivitamin supplements. Vitamins that are especially helpful for digestive health include vitamins A, B complex, C, and E.

- In many cultures, mealtime is thought of as a sacred event, a special moment of the day when we break bread with our loved ones and share our lives. These cultures know that if you improve the quality of your eating environment, you improve the quality of your digestion as well.

   Next time you eat a meal, for example, sit at a community table rather than in front of the TV set. Play dinner music. Set a beautiful table. Use attractive plates and glasses. Serve the food in an appealing way. Discuss lively topics. Laugh, share, and enjoy. As people have known for centuries, the *way* we eat is almost as important as what we eat.

- Finally, if you are suffering from digestive problems of any kind, remember that nutrition invariably plays a part in the healing process. The watchword here is "patience." Easy does it. Improved eating helps digestion—of this there is no doubt. But it may take time. An old adage tells us that "what takes a long time to come, stays a long time as well."

If you have lived on a diet of fatty foods and junk foods for long periods of time, if your lifestyle pushes the envelope, if you drink heavily and smoke heavily, and if you have ignored the distress signals that your stomach has been sending you over the years, it may take a while to set things straight. But remember: eventually things *will* improve. Stick with your new eating plan, improve your digestive ways and means, and the results will come. Perhaps sooner than you think.

SAMPLE RECIPES FOR COMMON AILMENTS OF THE GUT

What about specific recipes for specific gut ailments? To get you started in this area, and to give you an idea of how certain foods help certain problems of the gut, I am including a sampling of tasty and easily prepared recipes, each of which is geared to help a specific digestive disorder.

   Note that since these recipes are ailment-specific, a few of the discouraged foods listed in the diets discussed earlier may be included, while certain recommended foods may be omitted. The reason for these additions and subtractions is that each digestive problem requires its own treatment, and each comes with it own nutritional needs. What causes one disease can cure another.

❧ Cumin Rice and Spinach ❧

This rice dish is excellent for constipation.

2 cups brown rice

3 onions, sliced

3 cloves garlic, pressed

1 cup peeled, sliced carrots

2½ cups chopped spinach

½ teaspoon cumin seeds

2 tablespoons butter or butter
   substitute

1 chicken bouillon cube

½ teaspoon salt

Pepper to taste

¼ cup water

1. Cook the rice according to package directions.
2. Sauté the onions, garlic, carrots, spinach, and cumin seeds in butter or butter substitute until browned.
3. Add the cooked rice, bouillon cube, salt, and pepper to water. Cook over medium heat until fluffy and slightly moist. Serve.

Serves four.

❧ Oatmeal Pancakes ❧

These high-fiber pancakes are excellent for constipation and diverticulosis. They also help lower blood cholesterol levels.

1 cup oat flakes or rolled oats

2 cups low-fat milk

1½ cups whole-grain flour

1 teaspoon baking powder

2 tablespoons honey

2 egg whites, beaten

¼ cup margarine or other butter
   substitute

High-quality maple syrup or
   honey

1. Soak the oat flakes in milk overnight. If you use commercial rolled oats, soaking is unnecessary.
2. Mix the flour, baking powder, and honey into the oat-and-milk mixture. Add the egg whites and butter substitute.
3. Spoon out small pancakes onto a lightly greased griddle. Set at medium-high heat. Cook pancakes on one side until bubbles appear on the surface, then turn. (Try to turn each pancake only once.)
4. Cover with high-quality maple syrup or honey, and serve.

Serves four.

❧ Basil Salmon and Sun-Dried Tomatoes ❧

This dish helps reduce gas, lowers cholesterol, and adds high amounts of omega-3 fatty acids to the diet, which in turn improves overall digestive (as well as cardiovascular) health.

2 teaspoons extra-virgin olive oil

4 five-ounce fresh salmon fillets

2 tablespoons finely minced olives

4 cloves garlic, minced

½ teaspoon basil

½ teaspoon fennel

10 sun-dried tomatoes, finely chopped

Salt and pepper to taste

1. Preheat the oven to 350°F. Coat a baking pan with olive oil. Dip the salmon fillets in the oil on both sides.
2. Cover the salmon fillets with the olives, garlic, basil, fennel, and sun-dried tomatoes. Add salt and pepper to taste.
3. Bake for ten to twelve minutes.
4. Serve with grits or polenta, a cooked vegetable, and a fresh garden salad.

Serves four.

✤ Blue Cheese Capellini ✤

This pasta dish is good for taming acid reflux and acid stomach.

3 tablespoons water	½ cup walnuts
¼ cup virgin olive oil	1 cup crumbled Roquefort
¼ cup honey	cheese
½ teaspoon oregano	1 cup finely minced parsley
1 pound capellini pasta	Salt and pepper to taste

1. Mix together the water, olive oil, honey, and oregano in a small bowl. Set aside.
2. Cook the capellini according to package directions until al dente. Drain and transfer to a bowl.
3. Pour the oil-and-honey mixture over the pasta and mix. Top with walnuts, cheese, and parsley. Add salt and pepper to taste.
4. Serve with whole-wheat Italian bread.

Serves eight.

✤ Mushroom Risotto ✤

This mushroom dish is good for taming acid reflux and acid stomach.
Shiitake mushrooms are believed to be anticarcinogenic.

6 cups chicken stock	3 tablespoons virgin olive oil
1½ cups dried shiitake	1 cup Italian arborio rice
mushrooms	¼ cup grated Parmesan cheese
2 cloves garlic, minced	½ cup minced parsley
½ teaspoon oregano	Salt and pepper to taste

1. Pour the chicken stock into a bowl and add mushrooms. Allow the mushrooms to soak for at least an hour. Remove the mushrooms and set aside the broth.

2. Sauté the mushrooms, garlic, and oregano in oil until brown. Set aside.

3. Bring the broth to a boil in a saucepan and add the rice. Reduce the heat immediately, and allow the rice to simmer, stirring occasionally, for ten minutes.

4. Add the mushrooms, garlic, oregano, and oil to the rice. Simmer the mixture until the rice is moist and fluffy. Remove from heat and transfer to a bowl.

5. Sprinkle cheese and parsley over the rice. Add salt and pepper to taste, and serve.

Serves four.

❧ Indian Almond Rice Pudding ❧

This pudding is a bland, healing food for people with diarrhea.

½ cup basmati rice

1 cup water

¼ cup natural sugar

¼ teaspoon salt

3 cups almond milk*

¼ cup raisins

¼ teaspoon almond extract

*Almond milk can be found at some health-food stores and most Indian grocery stores.

1. Combine the rice and water in a saucepan. Boil for five minutes, then drain off the remaining water.

2. Place the rice in a saucepan and add the sugar, salt, and almond milk. Bring the mixture to a boil, and reduce to a simmer. Cook uncovered for approximately thirty minutes, stirring frequently.

3. Add the raisins and cook another five to ten minutes until the rice is light and fluffy. Remove from heat, add almond extract, and serve.

Serves four.

❧ Rice Congee ❧

This recipe is specifically designed to help people suffering from diarrhea and nausea. It has been used for this purpose in India and China for thousands of years.

½ cup brown rice

6 cups chicken broth

8 ounces sliced chicken breasts*

2 cups water

2 tablespoons fresh grated ginger

Salt to taste

¼ cup shredded scallions

1 tablespoon virgin olive oil

¼ cup cilantro

*People with extreme cases of diarrhea or nausea may wish to omit the chicken and simply eat the congee.

1. Combine the rice and chicken broth in a saucepan and bring to a boil. Lower the heat and simmer for several hours until the rice reaches the consistency of cream of wheat. (The rice has now become congee.)
2. While the rice is cooking, boil the chicken breasts in water for forty-five minutes. When chicken is finished cooking, slice into bite-sized pieces and set aside.
3. Sauté the ginger, salt, and scallions in oil until slightly brown. Add the sautéed mixture and the chicken pieces to the rice congee. Garnish with cilantro leaves. Serve.

Serves four.

❧ Carob Shake ❧

This shake is especially good for people suffering from irritable bowel syndrome.

2 bananas

4 egg whites

½ cup rice milk or vanilla soy milk

4 tablespoons carob powder

1. Place all of the ingredients into a blender and purée until the mixture reaches the consistency of a smoothie.
2. Serve.

Serves two.

✤ Miso Soup ✤

This is a great natural remedy for queasy stomach, indigestion, constipation, and sluggish bowels.

1 quart water

1 onion, sliced

3 tablespoons miso

Sea vegetables such as hijiki, arami, or dulse

1. Place water and onion in a pot and bring to a boil, then reduce to a simmer.
2. Place miso in a separate bowl with a small amount of hot water. Mash miso with a wooden spoon until it is thoroughly dissolved.
3. Add the miso and sea vegetables to the water and boil for ten minutes. Serve.

Serves four.

Digestion and nutrition are intertwined and interact with diverse systems of the body. Following the right path is essential for health, vitality, and longevity. But what is right and what is wrong? Just because thy neighbor said so doesn't make it correct. In the next chapter, we review and dispel some of the commonly held misconceptions about our digestive systems.

chapter three

The Myth List:
Forty Misconceptions
That Could Be Dangerous
to Your Digestive Health

In my practice as a gastroenterologist, I constantly encounter a number of long-held, deep-rooted convictions on the part of patients that sound wonderfully official but are totally incorrect. These matters pertain to health in general, and to matters of eating, digesting, eliminating, and gastrointestinal disease in particular. Many of my patients insist on the accuracy of these convictions *despite* the fact that these ideas have been discredited for decades.

For many years, I wondered why so many bright people could be so misinformed on such important subjects. Then one day it struck me: it is not my patients who are at fault. *I am the one who is out of step.* There is no reason, I realized, why my patients, or anyone else for that matter, should know all the latest scientific truths about digestion.

Why?

Because no one has told them. And because they cannot learn these facts by talking to their equally misinformed friends or by watching four-minute sound bites on the nightly news. And because the amount of new knowledge that appears in medical journals and texts every week is so overwhelming that it is practically impossible for anyone, professional and layman alike, to keep up. As a result, many people, health-care professionals included, continue to cling to medical ideas that have long since fallen out of favor.

After coming to this realization, I understood that the only way my patients were going to be brought up to speed concerning the all-important subject of their own digestion is if doctors tell them. And so I started putting together a collection of what I now refer to as the "Myth List."

Before we move on to the chapters that deal with specific ailments and specific healing modalities, I would like to present this list for your careful reading and edification. In a nutshell, it provides a catalogue of the forty most common misconceptions, bits of hearsay, potentially dangerous pieces of information, and downright nonsense that people have come to believe about the working of their own gut. All of us through the years, including myself, have subscribed to certain of these myths. Nothing to be ashamed of here. At the same time, knowledge is power, and in some instances, knowledge can save your life—if not your life, then at least a lot of wasted time and a good deal of trouble. Moreover, many of the points touched on in the description of the myths below also supplement information in the chapters that follow, as well as serve as a kind of preamble to the subjects to come.

So before we go any further, let us dispel some die-hard digestive fairy tales, get to the digestive facts, and separate the digestive myths from the digestive truths.

MYTH 1: ALL DIETARY FIBER IS THE SAME, AND ALL DIETARY FIBER IS GOOD FOR YOU

Vegetable fiber is touted by just about everyone, and rightly so. Its powers to prevent constipation, reduce cholesterol, and boost digestive efficiency are legendary. Yet, in the rush to embrace its many benefits, people sometimes overlook the following facts:

1. Not all fiber is the same.
2. Some forms of fiber can trigger unpleasant side effects.
3. Eating too much fiber can plug up the gut rather than clean it out.

Let's have a look at each of these concerns.

Not All Fiber Is the Same

There are two basic types of fiber found in fruits and vegetables: non-soluble fiber and soluble fiber.

Non-Soluble Fiber

The most common forms of non-soluble fiber are cellulose, lignin, and a close cousin of cellulose called hemicellulose. Since human beings do not have the necessary enzymes to digest any of these substances, non-soluble fibers pass through the gut without being broken down. On the way, they stimulate peristalsis, add water to stools, and puff up the size of stools, increasing the speed at which wastes move through the gastrointestinal tract.

Soluble Fiber

Soluble fibers such as pectin are found in vegetables, fruit, and commercially produced laxatives. Soluble fibers are viscous. They bind water, and they generate a laxative effect on the bowels, increasing osmotic pressure and swelling the bulk of the feces. In addition, the bacterial fermentation caused by soluble fiber produces substances that exert a laxative action on the bowels. Metamucil and Konsyl, both of which contain psyllium, and FiberCon, which contains calcium polycarbophil, are examples of commercially available soluble fibers. Based on my experience and the literature, I believe that Isabgol, a form of psyllium widely used in India, Europe, and the United States, provides the most gratifying results in this category.

Some Forms of Fiber Can Trigger Unpleasant Side Effects

Bacteria in the colon, generating annoyingly large quantities of intestinal gas, quickly act upon many soluble fibers. Fortunately, the bowel adapts to this problem, and in a few days, intestinal gas levels usually return to normal. More seriously, certain high-fiber foods like bran occasionally worsen symptoms of spastic colon such as diarrhea.

What's more, fiber can bind to nutrients such as calcium, iron, and zinc. This binding decreases the absorption of these important minerals in our bodies, and reduces their nutritive value. Be aware also that some types of fibers bind to medicinal drugs (such as digoxin), slowing the drug's absorption into the bloodstream and sometimes preventing its action from occurring entirely.

Finally, in a few cases, certain plant gum fibers trigger allergic reactions, causing shortness of breath and difficulty swallowing. On very rare occasions, these reactions are severe and even life threatening. People with allergies tend to be especially sensitive to psyllium husks, a common ingredient used in natural laxatives.

Eating Too Much Fiber Can Plug Up the Gut Rather Than Clean It Out

When exceedingly large amounts of fiber are ingested without adequate fluid to wash them down, feces in the intestinal tract may clump and compact. The result is obstructed bowels. This condition tends to occur among disabled individuals, persons with neurological problems, and bedridden patients in nursing homes.

Be vigilant about drinking plenty of water when taking natural commercial laxatives such as Metamucil and FiberCon. If taken in excessive quantity and not washed down with enough water, they can compact and cause bowel obstruction. Be sure to follow all directions on the label. *Caution*: Such laxatives should be taken with caution by people who are on fluid restriction.

Last, let it be said that the above scenarios are mentioned as simple precautionary alerts, not as dire warnings. In general, fiber is a powerful natural laxative and a significant boon to just about everyone who suffers from occasional irregularity. In an overwhelming majority of cases, its benefits far outweigh its risks.

Myth 2: Diarrhea and Loose Bowels Are the Same

Though most laymen (and some medical professionals) do not realize it, diarrhea and loose bowels are not necessarily the same condition. The very term itself, "diarrhea," is an imprecise one, and can mean different things to different people. The earliest definition, "too rapid evacuation of too fluid stools," is still quoted today. Yet, while patients tend to describe diarrhea in terms of fluidity, physicians also refer to the *weight and quantity of a stool*. For example, about 20 percent of patients may have loose stools. But if the total weight of these stools is normal, then technically speaking the condition is not diarrhea.

Overall, the rule of thumb is that if a person's twenty-four-hour stool output exceeds 200 g, he or she is said to have clinical diarrhea. Many medical professionals also include frequency, fluidity, and volume of stool output in their definition.

Myth 3: Modern Antibiotics No Longer Cause Harmful Side Effects

Old-line antibiotics once caused side effects like diarrhea, many people will tell you, but today's improved varieties no longer trigger these problems. If only it were so.

The truth is that, like their predecessors, modern antibiotics kill much of the helpful digestive bacteria in the bowels, which means that diarrhea is still a fairly common side effect of these medications. Frequently, the problem is mild and self-limiting. Most of us are familiar with this condition. On occasion, however, certain virulent bacteria that are left over after an antibiotic has killed much of the helpful flora produce toxins that trigger bleeding, discomfort, intense diarrhea, and sometimes life-threatening disorders.

If you experience significant diarrhea and/or bleeding when taking antibiotics, speak with your physician immediately. Chances are a change or discontinuation of antibiotics will be in order.

MYTH 4: THERE IS NO LONGER A THREAT OF COMING DOWN WITH TRAVELER'S DIARRHEA ONCE YOU RETURN HOME FROM A TRIP TO A FOREIGN COUNTRY

Traveler's diarrhea—the diarrhea you contract in a foreign, often exotic, country—can plague you for several days, weeks, or even months after you return home. The timetable depends on the incubation period of the bug that causes the diarrhea. And do not underestimate the seriousness of these bacteria. In some cases, traveler's diarrhea is implicated in chronic problems of irritable bowel syndrome, as well as inflammatory bowel disease, parasitic infection, and worse.

The point is, when returning from exotic climes, do not consider yourself out of the woods until you are home for at least a week, and better, two. If you begin to develop serious diarrhea or related symptoms during this period, consider the possibility that you have an infection, and consult with your physician.

MYTH 5: IF YOU DRINK WHISKEY WITH ICE IN A COUNTRY WHERE THE WATER IS CONTAMINATED, THE WHISKEY WILL KILL ALL BACTERIA LURKING IN THE ICE

Don't believe it. Even undiluted or high-proof liquor/whiskey is not strong enough to kill certain disease-causing bacteria that lodge in ice.

What about carbonated beverages (without ice) or beer and wine? These tend to be harmless, and do not usually cause traveler's diarrhea.

On a similar note, just because the sauce you are eating is the hottest in town does not mean that bacteria cannot survive in it. Often they can. Dr. Adachi and colleagues from Houston studied the popular table sauces served in restaurants in Guadalajara, Mexico, and Houston, Texas. Writing in the journal *Annals of Internal Medicine* (2002), the authors report that these sauces were frequently contaminated with pathogenic bacteria (though more so in Guadalajara).

Myth 6: Cooking Food Always Kills All Infectious Bacteria

The adage goes: "While in a foreign country, if you cannot boil it, cook it, or peel it—forget it." True. But don't forget, if cooked food, even well-cooked food, is exposed for even a few minutes to germs, flies, or dirty hands, this food quickly becomes contaminated. Be especially vigilant of food purchased from street vendors, both at home and more so in countries where hygiene is questionable. Home-cooked food, on the other hand, is usually—not always, of course, but usually—a safe bet.

Myth 7: Intestinal Gas Is a Harmful and Unnatural Phenomenon

Intestinal gas erupting at inappropriate times can certainly make us the laughing stock of the party. This we all know. But, medically speaking, gas is an integral and inevitable by-product of our digestive processes, and a thoroughly normal one as well. Every living human being has gas, usually all the time. Nothing to worry about here; it's perfectly normal. See Chapter 13 for an in-depth look at the subject of gas and digestive health.

MYTH 8: FLATULENCE (GAS) IS PRODUCED BY SWALLOWING AIR WHEN DRINKING OR EATING

Sounds logical. You may have had this dictum repeated to you many times, usually as a warning when you slurp your drink. But don't worry; it is only a tiny bit true at best.

Most of the air we breathe during the day by whatever means is absorbed across the bowel wall into our bloodstream. Some of it is belched out, but very little—if any at all—reaches the rectum and is expelled as flatus (gas). Ninety-nine percent (or thereabouts) of colonic gas is produced by the fermentation of unabsorbed carbohydrates broken down by bacteria in the colon. We discuss the question of gas and gastrointestinal health in Chapter 13.

MYTH 9: REPORTS OF GAS EXPLODING INSIDE A PERSON ARE PATENTLY FALSE

No, they are actually true. Not that such a dire event is going to happen to you. With the high level of medical and surgical precaution taken in hospitals today, chances of an intestinal blowup are infinitesimally small. Just for the record, though, you might be interested to know that during surgery in times past, explosions of the bowels in patients undergoing electrocautery are known to have occurred.

How could such a thing be? When stool is present in the colon, unabsorbed carbohydrates ferment, causing a buildup of gas. Many of these gases are explosive, especially when acted on by an electric current. During surgery, great care must thus be taken not to electrify these gases. Today, while performing a colonoscopy, doctors diligently avoid using electrocautery unless a patient's colon is first purged with cathartics and enemas.

Myth 10: Older People Are More Likely to Have Gas Than Younger People

Well, technically no, we do not produce more gas in our golden years than we do when we are young. But in practice, yes, seniors do tend to be more flatulent.

Here's how it works. As we age, our bowel wall becomes increasingly sensitive to smaller and smaller amounts of gas, and, at the same time, we become correspondingly less capable of controlling these swelling reserves. Thus, while the volume of gas in our gut remains essentially the same through the years, our gastrointestinal equipment becomes less and less capable of holding it in. Hence, the reputation some seniors have for flatulence.

Myth 11: It Is Harmful and Unhealthy to Hold in Gas

Holding in gas is a harmless practice, even for long periods of time. At the same time, though, the prolonged holding of intestinal gas can be an oppressive and sometimes painful ordeal. For some people, holding gas becomes a habit, and over time, it gives rise to chronic feelings of bloating and discomfort. Nothing injurious here, but plenty that's uncomfortable.

In short, while there is no harm in holding gas, there is even less harm in letting it out—at least when social circumstances allow.

Myth 12: When Your Stools Float, It Is an Indication That You Suffer from Indigestion and Malabsorption of Nutrients

The notion that floating stools are a sign of improperly digested food and especially fats is a misconception that was taught in medical schools even up to a few years ago. This theory holds that stools float because of excess fat deposits, which in turn are due to fat malabsorption during the process of digestion. This concept is entirely untrue. Although excess fat does cause stools to float, most floating stools are not related to fatty stools or fat malabsorption.

The reason stools float in the toilet is that air gets trapped inside them, giving the wastes buoyancy, and causing them to rise in the water rather than sink. Large amounts of fiber in the stool can also play a part.

MYTH 13: BLAND DIETS HEAL ULCERS

The origin of this myth goes back several decades to a time when doctors assumed that ulcers were caused by improper eating habits. We know today that what you eat, be it nutritious or junky, has little to do with this condition. Most ulcers are caused by bacterial infection in the stomach and, in some cases, by the effects of medicinal drugs.

A bland diet, therefore, plays little or no role in healing these painful ulcers. Over time, it may promote improved nutrition and digestive strength, and that's good. Just don't expect diet alone to cure your ulcers. In most cases, acid-suppressive and antibiotic treatment is necessary.

MYTH 14: STRESS TRIGGERS STOMACH ULCERS

Wrong again. As explained above, we now know that ulcer formation has little to do with food and just as little to do with stress, worry, or psychological problems. Ulcers, we also know, are primarily caused by the *Helicobacter pylori* (*H. pylori*) bacteria, and medications such as aspirin and ibuprofen. Therapy used to prevent ulcers from recurring depends entirely on the cause of the ulcer.

There is, however, one exception to this rule: When a person undergoes an extreme physical trauma such as a head injury, severe burns, or intense respiratory problems (usually the kind that requires a breathing machine to sustain life), these stressful conditions occasionally cause an ulcer to develop spontaneously in the stomach, producing pain and severe bleeding.

Other than such worst-case scenarios seen in the intensive-care unit, you do not have to worry that taxes and unruly children will put you on the ulcer ward. They won't.

MYTH 15: ALL PEOPLE WHO HAVE *H. PYLORI* INFECTION IN THEIR STOMACHS WILL EVENTUALLY DEVELOP ULCERS

H. pylori bacteria do indeed lead to the development of ulcers of the stomach and duodenum in some people. This is the bad news. The good news is that millions of people are walking around with this bacteria living in their abdominal regions and are doing fine, just fine, with no sign of ulcers. Indeed, only a small percentage of people who carry this infection ever develop symptoms.

Why some people are adversely affected by *H. pylori* and others are not is a medical mystery; though, as is often the case, the question appears to revolve around the battle between the body's host defenses and the virulence that a given strain of *H. pylori* can produce. Other factors that increase the chances of developing ulcers are taking NSAIDs (nonsteroidal anti-inflammatory drugs) such as aspirin and ibuprofen, and a family history of the disease. But as far as the actual presence of *H. pylori* in the stomach goes, it is by no means a sentence of disease.

MYTH 16: THERE IS NOTHING I CAN DO ON MY OWN TO HELP MY ACID REFLUX CONDITION (ONLY MY DOCTOR CAN HELP)

There is actually a great deal you can do on your own to help acid reflux, some of it natural, some of it based on lifestyle changes, and some of it plain common sense. Most people with acid reflux never see a doctor, and even fewer consult a digestive disease specialist. Many control this problem entirely on their own. We discuss acid reflux at length in Chapter 16.

MYTH 17: ALL ANTACIDS ARE THE SAME

They aren't. The primary function of antacids is to neutralize excess acid present in the stomach. But be warned: There are different types of antacids, each with its own particular action and side effects in the bowels.

For example, antacids containing calcium (such as Tums) and aluminum (AlternaGel) tend to cause constipation. Antacids with magnesium promote a laxative effect, though newer versions of Maalox and Mylanta combine magnesium with calcium or aluminum to counteract this problem. Mylanta AR Acid Reducer and Maalox H2 Acid Controller contain acid-blocking ingredients, but, technically speaking, no antacids at all (though the effect they exert is the same).

Finally, keep in mind that calcium-containing antacids provide a much-needed source of this valuable mineral for people who suffer from a deficiency. To find out if calcium is included in an antacid, check the label.

MYTH 18: HEARTBURN IS CAUSED BY EXCESS ACID IN THE STOMACH

This popular belief is buttressed by the common practice of self-medicating with commercial antacids in order (we think) to neutralize excess acid pooling in our stomachs. This view is further reinforced when doctors prescribe medicines to suppress the production of acid.

The truth is that heartburn has nothing to do with excess stomach acid. In most cases, people with heartburn have the same amount of acid in their stomachs as people without heartburn. The real problem is that the acid is in *the wrong place doing the wrong things*, that is, it is moving up from the stomach into the esophagus and, along the way, is producing ugly burning sensations. This sensation is felt from the heart area in the middle of the chest all the way up to the throat, that is, along the area spanned by the esophagus.

While antacids may help heartburn, chemically speaking they are simply neutralizing the acid, not lowering the amount produced in the stomach. In some cases they may actually cause rebound secretions of acid as well. Chapter 16 tells all about heartburn and its related discomforts.

MYTH 19: MEDICINES THAT SUPPRESS STOMACH ACID SHOULD NOT BE TAKEN WHEN DRINKING ALCOHOL

This fallacy is based on the fact that some acid blockers, such as Tagamet, are known to slow down the detoxification of alcohol. This decrease produces higher levels of blood alcohol in drinkers per the amount of alcohol ingested. However, the increase in alcohol level generated is so small that it has little or no clinical effect on drinkers.

At the same time, though, it is always wise to be prudent when drinking and taking medications, even over-the-counter medications. If you have any questions concerning the compatibility of a certain drug with alcohol, discuss this matter with your physician.

MYTH 20: SURGICAL REMOVAL OF THE GALLBLADDER DOES NOT CAUSE LONG-TERM PROBLEMS

It doesn't always. But sometimes it does.

While most patients who undergo a cholecystectomy (gallbladder removal) become symptom-free, 5 to 15 percent suffer from postoperative digestive symptoms that are more serious than the digestive problems experienced before the operation.

In addition, approximately one-third of patients who undergo this operation continue to suffer from the preexisting discomfort in the gallbladder region *despite the fact* that the organ has been removed.

In general, postsurgical gallbladder problems occur more frequently in women than in men, and, oddly, in persons who show little or no significant abnormality in their gallbladders before or during surgery. A few postoperative patients also develop chronic and sometimes debilitating cases of diarrhea. These and other medical aftereffects can occur shortly after the operation, or they may appear years later. There is no telling. This means, in turn, that even if you feel a good deal better following your cholecystectomy, you are not necessarily out of the danger zone. A few years must pass before you can consider yourself thoroughly cured. And, even then, there is a rare possibility of a stone in the bile duct causing problems years or even decades later.

MYTH 21: REMOVAL OF THE GALLBLADDER CAN SOMETIMES CAUSE CANCER

Attempts to link surgical removal of the gallbladder (cholecystectomy) to the development of cancer have consistently failed. There is absolutely no sound clinical evidence to show a relationship between the two. If you are going to undergo a cholecystectomy, give yourself a break and don't add this worrisome myth to your list of concerns.

MYTH 22: EVERYONE WITH GALLSTONES SHOULD HAVE THEIR GALLBLADDERS REMOVED

Gallstones are a common condition and usually do not cause serious problems. You may even have gallstones this very moment and not know it. Or, if you do know it, the management of asymptomatic stones often involves conservative treatment, or just simple observation. It is only when gallstones start to cause pain or other symptoms that dramatic measures become necessary.

At one time, it was also believed that all diabetics who suffered from gallstones should automatically undergo prophylactic cholecystectomy. Thinking on this matter has changed today. Unless the stones are actively bothering diabetic persons and causing pain, it is considered better medicine to keep the condition under watch, and leave things be.

Does the risk of cancer increase if gallstones are left untreated, as some medical professionals claim? Possibly. But if there is a risk, it is so small, statistically speaking, that the dangers of surgery far outweigh the benefits of removal in asymptomatic subjects. Exceptions to this rule are (1) when a person's gallbladder becomes calcified, (2) when a gallbladder polyp grows larger than 1 cm, and (3) special high-risk cases, such as Native-American females, young sickle-cell patients, and patients awaiting organ transplantation.

MYTH 23: THE OLDER PEOPLE GET, THE MORE LIKELY THEY ARE TO SUFFER FROM CONSTIPATION

The older people get, the more likely they are to be constipated. This is true. But—it is *not* true that constipation is a natural consequence of aging. What we mean by this ambiguity is that the digestive tract is built to last a lifetime, and that getting older itself does not cause constipation. In most cases of non-disease-based constipation, this ailment is caused simply by poor lifestyle habits.

It therefore follows that if people exercise regularly; are properly nourished; stay away from rich, binding foods; drink plenty of water; get enough rest; avoid stress; and live a wholesome lifestyle, there is no biological reason why they should become constipated at *any* stage of life. In Chapter 14, we talk about ways to avoid constipation, and what to do when it strikes.

MYTH 24: IF I DO NOT HAVE A BOWEL MOVEMENT EVERY DAY, I AM CONSTIPATED

Only 10 percent of the population has a bowel movement every day, which means that it is perfectly normal, or at least statistically the norm, to have a bowel movement every other day.

More specifically, the range of bowel movements reported in outpatient surveys varies from four movements a day to three movements a week. All these schedules are within the realm of normalcy. Anything less than three movements per week is officially termed "constipation." However, any recent change in bowel habit, even if within the normal range, may be a danger signal. Consult your doctor immediately.

It should be added that many health-care providers insist that the longer toxic wastes remain inside the digestive system, the greater the chance there is of developing disease. The faster these wastes are moved through the gut, they insist, and the more bowel movements we have per week, the better it is for our health. In the chapters to follow, we discuss natural ways in which sluggish digestion and slow-moving bowels can be tuned up and improved.

MYTH 25: IN MOST CASES, A DOCTOR CAN PINPOINT THE CAUSE OF CONSTIPATION

Nine times out of ten, constipation is a symptom, not a primary condition. It may be caused by a spectrum of ailments ranging from poor nutrition to medications to cancer to scores of other possibilities in between.

So don't expect your physician to make an instant diagnosis. Though doctors are skilled at investigating and identifying known causes of constipation, a general diagnosis is the best that can be expected in many cases. This is not, by the way, to say that the constipation cannot be cured—it almost always can—only that in some instances its precise etiology remains unknown.

MYTH 26: A COLONOSCOPY IS PAINFUL

It's not. Where this myth comes from I do not know. In fact, statistics show that approximately 90 percent of patients who undergo colonoscopies report that the laxative purge they receive before the colonoscopy causes more discomfort than the procedure itself. And since most men and women take an intravenous sedative before undergoing a colonoscopy (not a general anesthetic, as some people think), a sizable percentage of patients has no recollection of the procedure whatsoever.

If you have a digestive ailment, and if you have not been able to cure it with conventional or alternative methods, a colonoscopy may be just what the doctor ordered to pinpoint the problem. Do not overlook this valuable and sometimes indispensable health tool.

MYTH 27: CHANGING A MEDICATION FROM PILL OR CAPSULE FORM TO SOLUTION FORM HAS NO EFFECT ON THE DIGESTIVE TRACT

This is a common misconception, even among many health-care providers. The fact is that, though the active chemical in the drug may remain intact when changing from pill or capsule to solution, the inactive ingredients frequently change, sometimes causing gastrointestinal distress.

For example, while pill and capsule forms of most medications are housed in inert delivery systems, many liquid solutions or suspensions come in sweeteners such as sorbitol. Sorbitol is a poorly absorbed sugar, and in some people it acts as a laxative, causing diarrhea and gas. In addition, the rate of absorption and blood levels may be altered by this change and, with it, the therapeutic effectiveness and toxicity of the drug.

Before switching from a pill or capsule to solution form, *always* discuss the matter with your doctor.

MYTH 28: OCCASIONAL BLOOD IN THE STOOL IS NO CAUSE FOR ALARM AND DOES NOT REQUIRE MEDICAL ATTENTION

A statement I commonly hear in my examining room is "Oh, doctor, I only had blood in my stool *one time*." But once is once too often. Occasional blood in the stool can, of course, be due to a number of causes, many of them, such as hemorrhoids, benign. But since polyps and cancer can also bleed intermittently, even occasional blood may signal real disease.

Similarly, the *amount* of blood seen in the stool should not be a deciding factor. Blood is blood. "But doctor," patients insist, "I only saw a tiny drop!" No matter. In this case, a little is a lot. Medical attention should be sought immediately.

The same rule applies when using a stool card kit at home to check for occult blood. If just one out of the three samples tests positive for blood, this is cause for concern. See your physician immediately.

MYTH 29: LIGHT-COLORED STOOL MEANS I DO NOT HAVE BLEEDING FROM THE DIGESTIVE TRACT

The amount of oozing blood in the bowel can sometimes be so incremental that it produces no noticeable changes in stool color. This means that a person can continue to lose blood at a slow but steady rate for weeks and months without realizing it, and without producing dark-colored stools. It is more common for a doctor to detect blood in a patient's stool during a routine screening using stool test cards than it is for patients to see it on their own.

For example, I once examined a sixty-year-old man whose complexion was unnaturally pale. It turned out this man had been losing small quantities of blood for months without knowing it. His hemoglobin count was now a life-threatening 2 g percent. An ordinary count is greater than 12.5 g percent.

The moral here is do not rely on the visual examination of stool alone. Take advantage of home occult blood tests as well, and get regular checkups.

MYTH 30: ANGINA IS A DISEASE OF THE HEART AND DOES NOT INVOLVE THE GUT

The restriction of blood flow in the intestines results in exactly the same condition that it does in the heart—angina pain.

To be more specific, angina of the heart is called *angina pectoris* and is associated with chest pain. Angina of the bowels is called *intestinal angina* and causes belly discomfort. In intestinal angina, pain typically comes immediately after eating, eventually with fear of eating and consequent weight loss. Like angina of the heart, intestinal angina is more likely to strike the elderly than the young. And, like heart angina, the severity of intestinal angina is dependent on the degree and advancement of its underlying cause, which is almost always arteriosclerosis.

MYTH 31: BOWEL POLYPS ARE ALMOST ALWAYS BENIGN AND ARE ALMOST NEVER ANYTHING TO WORRY ABOUT

A polyp is merely a protuberance on the lining of the bowel wall. Whether it is benign or cancerous can only be determined by examining its structure under a microscope.

True, the majority of polyps are harmless. But be aware that some types of polyps can be diagnosed as benign and still have a high cellular predilection toward malignancy at some time in the future. These troublesome growths are labeled as *premalignant* and must be carefully watched.

In general, a bowel polyp is nothing to make light of. If you or members of your family have been diagnosed with colon polyps, discuss what to do next with your doctor immediately.

MYTH 32: ALL POLYPS EVENTUALLY BECOME CANCEROUS

The myth that every polyp is a cancer waiting to happen is the reverse of Myth 31, that polyps are never dangerous. The fact is, some are dangerous, many aren't.

If a polyp is benign, the risk that it will become cancerous varies according to its cellular structure. The *hyperplastic* type of polyp, though very common, does not appear to increase the risk of colon cancer in any way. The *adenoma* type of bowel polyp is, on the other hand, potentially malignant. Most cancers of the colon arise from preexisting polyps.

There is a general safety rule to observe as far as polyps go: A colon that is predisposed to developing adenomas is also predisposed to developing cancer of the colon. Your family history plays an important role here. If any of your close relations have developed this ailment, be especially vigilant.

Though only a fraction of adenoma polyps turn malignant (the risk depends on the size of the polyp and the type of adenoma it happens to be), if you are diagnosed as having an adenoma, schedule regular follow-up colonoscopic exams as directed by your physician. Persons with hyperplastic polyps, on the other hand, usually do not have to be so concerned, and often do not require regular surveillance exams.

MYTH 33: ISCHEMIC COLITIS USUALLY REQUIRES SURGERY

Medically speaking, "ischemia" refers to a reduced blood flow to a particular organ in the body. Ischemic colitis is thus an inflammation caused by an insufficient movement of blood to segments of the colon, a kind of "heart attack" of the bowels.

In most cases, ischemic colitis is a mild disorder and can be resolved with drugs and conservative treatment. In a few patients, however, the inflammation becomes life threatening, and surgery is required.

MYTH 34: ONCE ISCHEMIC COLITIS STRIKES, IT KEEPS RETURNING

In most cases, attacks of ischemic colitis do not recur. Period.

MYTH 35: APPENDICITIS IS STRICTLY A DISEASE OF THE YOUNG

Approximately two-thirds of appendicitis cases occur during the early decades of life. This means that one-third of appendicitis cases occur during midlife and later.

One-third doesn't sound like much, perhaps. But consider this: According to a recent count, there are approximately 250 million people in this country, 6 percent of whom have suffered from appendicitis. Given the fact that 6 percent of 250 million is approximately 15 million, and that one-third of 15 million is 5 million, you can see that appendicitis is no respecter of age, and that it can strike at any point in the life cycle.

The myth that older people do not get appendicitis is also dangerous as well as incorrect. Why? Because when symptoms occur in elderly people, they tend to be mild and frequently nonspecific. Many senior citizens thus ignore the warnings, thinking themselves immune from appendix problems, and believing the pain to be nothing more serious than a stomachache. Statistics show that as many as one out of four older patients stricken with appendicitis delay getting medical help for up to seventy-two hours. The result is an increased chance of a ruptured appendix, with the consequent development of peritonitis and infection, plus more pain, more complications, longer hospital stays, and a higher death rate.

If you think you have appendicitis, seek medical help immediately, no matter what your age. Symptoms include a progressively sharp pain in the lower right side of the abdomen, plus one or more of the following: fever, loss of appetite, nausea, vomiting, and constipation (or occasionally diarrhea).

Myth 36: All Body Fat Is, Metabolically Speaking, the Same

The fat that is deposited in your abdomen and that helps swell your waist-line is chemically different from the fatty tissue located below your gut, in your hips and thighs. Abdominal fat also poses more medical problems than lower-body (hip) fat.

Abdominal fat, however, is metabolically more active than lower-body fat, and is the first form of adipose tissue to dissolve when you lose weight. Lower-body fat is built to store nutrients for the long term and is more difficult to shed.

Myth 37: Most Overweight Adults Were Overweight as Children

Most children who are overweight, it is true, grow up to be overweight adults. It is also true, however, that a majority of obese adults did not suffer from weight problems when they were young.

Myth 38: Exercise Alone Is Sufficient to Lose Weight and Keep It Off

I frequently hear my patients complain: "I work out a lot, I go to the gym, I do my exercises. But I still can't lose weight!" Why not? they want to know.

Because, I tell them, exercise unaccompanied by an appropriate and healthy weight-loss diet plan, while a great boon to mental and physical health, is by no means an effective way to shed pounds.

Remember, I remind them, it takes a grown man, walking four miles per hour, approximately thirty to forty minutes to use about 200 calories. And how long does it take to add 200 calories to your waistline? As long as it takes to eat a cookie or a container of low-fat yogurt with berries. That is, not very long. A beer with a pretzel after an hour's worth of exercise makes the exercise worthless from a weight-loss standpoint.

Further, the more time you spend exercising, the stronger your appetite becomes, and the stronger your urge to eat becomes, a vicious circle for exercisers who want to lose weight.

So what's the best way to shed pounds?

Watch your calorie intake, follow a reasonable weight-loss diet, and control snacking and junk-food cravings. And, of course, exercise. It's a wonderful supplement to dieting and acts as a catalyst to any dietary regimen. Exercise is also an excellent method for toning up your body and maintaining a particular weight once your target weight has been reached.

Myth 39: Today, Surgery Is a Highly Viable Treatment for Obesity

Why don't I just have a liposuction, strapling, or bypass than put up with these impossible diets? Implied in this question is the dangerous myth that surgery is simply one of many safe and effective ways to lose weight. Such a casual attitude toward such a serious undertaking is not, in my opinion, an appropriate way to negotiate weight control.

First, an operation, *any* operation, carries risks: risk of failure, risk of complications, even risk, slight as it may be, of death. What's more, the long-term success of a surgical operation for obesity is highly dependent on a patient's motivation, and on his or her willingness to make—and then stick with—appropriate postoperative lifestyle and dietary changes. In my own practice, I have seen more than one person undergo this operation, suffer through the discomforts that surgery brings, only to eat back most of the weight removed during the operation within a short period of time.

Obesity surgery, in other words, is best looked on as a last-ditch measure to be taken only after all dietary, therapeutic, and lifestyle methods fail.

If you are thinking about undergoing this surgery, it is suggested that you learn as much as you can about the procedure, both the pros and cons, then discuss the matter thoroughly with your family, with medical experts, and with others who have gone this route before. And remember, most insurance companies do not pay for weight-loss surgery except under exceptional circumstances.

MYTH 40: DIVERTICULITIS AND DIVERTICULOSIS ARE THE SAME DISEASE

Diverticulosis is a disease caused by the presence of diverticula—sacs or pockets in the wall of the bowel, usually the colon. Diverticulosis can also occur in other parts of the digestive tract, though with far less frequency than in the colon.

A single sac is called a diverticulum. Multiple sacs are known as diverticula. Approximately 10 percent of men and women in the West develop diverticulosis by age forty. Almost 50 percent have it by sixty, then 70 to 80 percent by age eighty and above. Diverticulosis is an ailment of modern civilization and is practically unknown in rural parts of Asia and Africa. Though its causes are not entirely understood, lack of adequate fiber and roughage in the diet certainly plays a major role in its development.

Diverticulitis, on the other hand, is a disorder that strikes when a diverticulum and the surrounding area become inflamed and infected due to leakage in the diverticulum. It starts as an impaction of solid concentrations of stool in the bowel. Sometimes, the wall of the diverticulum is too weak to withstand pressure and gives way entirely, producing a small perforation or hole that leaks fecal material through the bowel wall. As a result, patients develop abdominal pain, fever, tenderness, and other signs of abdominal infection.

Antibiotics, soft diet, and bedrest usually resolve episodes of diverticulitis, though if symptoms are especially severe, liquid diets, intravenous feeding, and even surgery may be necessary. A follow-up colonoscopy is usually undertaken about four to eight weeks after surgery to exclude the possibility of cancer masquerading as diverticulitis. Chapter 16 deals in depth with this disagreeable ailment, along with a number of other common digestive disorders.

chapter four

The Importance of Sleep
to Digestion
(and Vice Versa)

A complex network of different organs powers the human body. From the outside, these organs appear to operate independently of one another, sometimes almost in a vacuum. With careful observation, we discover that the work these organs perform is not separate at all; they are all working marvelously in sync, all part of a single integrated and interconnected machine.

Indeed, in certain schools of Chinese medicine, our organs are considered to be "divine officials," each striving to operate in harmony with the others to keep the "kingdom" of the human body working productively and well. The flows, secretions, and metabolic processes that take place inside us every day, which on casual glance appear to be unrelated, are, from this standpoint, all components of a single unified biological ecosystem.

Take, for example, the two seemingly unconnected functions of sleep and digestion. The digestive system processes food and eliminates wastes. These are its exclusive purposes. Sleep, on the other hand, is a quiescent state of the body and mind when vital functions such as breathing, heartbeat, body temperature, and blood pressure decrease, and brain activity grows largely dormant. It is a time of physical rest and repair, a product of brain chemistry and of the neurological workings of the unconscious mind.

These two functions appear to have little to do with each other. But just as the electrical system and the fuel system of an automobile perform separate but interrelated tasks, so digestion and sleep work together to promote overall body health—or, when out of sync, to generate a number of physical problems that trouble both of these functions.

What kind of problems? Take heartburn, for example. Though heartburn begins in the stomach, its waves of burning acid cause us to lose hours of sleep at night. Or indigestion. It starts in the gut, yes, but ends up waking us from our beauty rest. Or an overload of carbohydrates taken in at lunch can make us somnambulant for the rest of the afternoon.

Gas, stomach cramps, burping, the bloated feeling that comes from stuffing down too much dinner, all contribute to uneven sleep patterns and, some experts maintain, disturbing dreams. (The Japanese refer to nightmares triggered by overeating as "fish and dumpling dreams.") And, of course, we know that ingesting too much caffeine during the day keeps many of us wide-eyed at night.

The affiliation between these two physiological functions is thus a powerful and inescapable one; this is a good thing, as there is a positive side to it as well.

Chamomile tea, for example, calms both the stomach and the dreaming mind, as do other herbal potions. (More on these later in the chapter.) A glass of warm milk with honey in it, or maybe a dish of yogurt before bed, helps millions of people fall asleep every night. And how often do we note the way in which that delicious Sunday lunch rolls around comfortably in our stomachs, making us mellow and ready for an afternoon snooze? It works the other way too: a deep, restful sleep can help promote digestion.

In short, the biorythmic relationship between sleep and digestion is a subtle but substantial one. It is evident from the fact that sleep pattern is often disturbed in digestive disorders like irritable bowel syndrome and functional dyspepsia. A good restful sleep allows the body's vital energies to focus on the digestion, absorption, and assimilation of the nutrients. It is also a relationship that we ignore at our peril. Remember, sleep is one of the three pillars of life, the other two being food and sex. Our bodies' natural rhythms demand that we work during the day but that we sleep at night. This rule of nature must be obeyed for optimal health and longevity.

MANY ROADS TO A GOOD NIGHT'S SLEEP

Fifteen percent of Americans suffer from chronic insomnia, and a far greater number—according to the Mayo Clinic, 60 million Americans—suffer from some variety of sleep disorder. What's more, this is just the tip of the sleep-deprived iceberg.

According to a survey carried out by the National Sleep Foundation in Washington, D.C., two-thirds of Americans experience difficulty falling asleep at night, along with severe restlessness once in a state of slumber. As many as one-third of severe heartburn sufferers must sleep in a recliner.

Also common are early awakenings, "the up-at-four-A.M.-and-not-able-to-get-back-to-sleep" agony so many of us know so well. Twenty percent of subjects interviewed by the National Sleep Foundation claimed they were so tired and muddleheaded from early risings that their productivity at work was substantially reduced.

In some cases, sleeplessness triggers accidents on the job. In other instances, accidents occur while traveling to and from work as a result of sleep deprivation. The National Highway Traffic Safety Administration estimates that drivers who doze off at the wheel cause 56,000 automobile accidents every year.

UNDERSTANDING YOUR INSOMNIA—
AND DOING SOMETHING ABOUT IT

Insomnia takes two forms. The first form prevents us from falling asleep when we first get into bed. The second interferes with the quality and depth of rest once we fall asleep, and causes us to wake—and remain awake—at odd times of the night, usually between the hours of 2:00 A.M. and 5:00 A.M.

Some people suffer from the first form of insomnia but not the second. Many experience both kinds. In either scenario, insomnia is clearly a burden, keeping us up, making us tense and irritable, and provoking dullness of mind, depression, and lethargy the next day.

How much sleep is enough sleep? The "average" man and woman, medical research tells us, requires approximately seven to eight hours of quality slumber every night. This figure is ballpark at best, and, in reality, the amount of sleep needed varies considerably from person to person.

Clearly there are people who sleep no more than five or six hours a night, wake up refreshed, and go about their day's business with purpose and zest. Such people are well within the range of normalcy. Others find that unless they get eight or nine hours of dozing time, they are tired and gloomy the next day and their on-the-job performance sags accordingly. These people are also normal. Still, others sleep for many hours every night, but wake up feeling unrested. Some people in this category consider themselves insomniacs, not because they don't sleep, but because their quality of sleep seems like no sleep at all.

A famous experiment carried out in different forms at sleep laboratories across the country demonstrates how tricky the question of measuring one's own sleep patterns can be. In this experiment, people who suffered from various forms of insomnia were bedded down for the night in comfortable quarters and were asked to press a button every time they heard a buzzing sound.

The results of the experiment showed that when the buzzer went off at different hours throughout the night, most subjects made no response at all. Why? Because the subjects were asleep, sometimes deeply so, and they had the brain-wave mappings and tape-recorded outbursts of snoring to prove it. Yet, when quizzed the next morning, a majority of these subjects insisted that they had not slept a wink the entire night. This phenomenon is called *sleep state misperception*.

For many people a good night's sleep is thus an elusive goal, and one that is made even more challenging by the fact that so many external and internal pressures affect it.

Occasionally, for example, insomnia is caused by a serious disorder such as chronic depression or neurological disease, in which case a physician's assistance is necessary. More commonly, stress is the culprit; not far behind stress come poor nutrition and digestive problems. Finally, there are environmental stimulations such as noise, light, room temperature, an uncomfortable mattress, and bodily irritations such as indigestion, cramped positions, and labored breathing, all of which profoundly reduce the quality of sleep.

What factors most affect and disturb your own sleep patterns? Consider the following questions:

- Is your mattress too hard? Is it too soft? Is your pillow comfortable? Do your blankets scratch or tickle? Do not overlook such items as mattress firmness or bed coverings as potential sleep irritants.
- Do you sleep under enough blankets at night, or maybe under too many? (Being too cold or too hot are common sleep disrupters.) If you feel cold when you crawl into bed at night, try wearing socks and gloves. Studies show that people who go to bed with warm hands and feet tend to fall asleep quickly. Conversely, if your room is too hot and humid in the summer, consider installing an air conditioner or using a fan. Both measures improve sleep quality.
- What is the light level in your room at night? Many people discover that simply turning off a lamp or using curtains to block a neighbor's porch light improves their rest. Placing curtains or blinds over windows stops morning light from filtering in and waking us up too early. The darker the room, the better it is for sleeping.

- What is the noise level in your sleeping quarters? Is there a busy road close to your bedroom window? A high volume of city noise right outside? Are there crying children in the vicinity? Barking dogs or yowling cats? A favorite way around the noise dilemma is to sleep with earplugs. Another is to move your bed to a quieter place in the home. The less noise there is, the better one sleeps.

- How much liquid do you drink during and after dinner each evening? A full bladder can wake you up once, twice, three times, or more. If you find yourself continually plodding to the john in the middle of the night, avoid all liquids for, say, three to four hours before bed. After five or six o'clock in the evening, avoid fluids that have a diuretic effect like coffee and alcohol. Empty your bladder just before retiring.

- Do you sleep with a partner who snores? If so, do not underestimate this inescapable irritant as a cause of sleeplessness. If your partner snores excessively, and if you feel unrested each morning, the noise may be seriously cutting into your quality of sleep. To remedy the snoring situation, consider 1) sleeping with ear plugs, 2) talking to your partner about entering a snore-reduction program, 3) using a snore-reduction medication or device, or 4) sleeping in a separate room. Another trick is to wake sleepers up each time they snore and tell them to roll on to their side. Since most snoring is done while lying on the back, many people who snore can be "trained" to sleep on their sides.

- During the day, do you use your bedroom for work or entertaining? Does it serve as an office? A play space for children? A family room? Studies show that people sleep better in bedrooms that are used exclusively for sleeping rather than for multiple daytime activities.

- Do you frequently wake up in the middle of the night feeling thirsty, with a dry, parched throat? If so, consider placing a cool-air humidifier in your bedroom. Also, consider keeping a thermos of fresh water and/or a portable urinal near your bed to render the dreary midnight walk to the bathroom unnecessary. Often, it's the walk that wakes us up.

- Do you sleep on your stomach? Many stomach sleepers are light sleepers. Though there is much discussion on the subject of sleep posture, a number of sleep experts believe that sleeping on one's back and side are the best ways to fall asleep and stay asleep. Patients with chronic heartburn should always sleep on their left side.

- Do you burn the candle at both ends? Many people have noticed how dramatically sleep cycles are disturbed after staying up into the wee hours one or more nights in a row. Studies show that people who rise early every weekday, then sleep late during the weekends, often suffer from sleep difficulties. As far as sleep goes, routine is all-important. Go to bed at the same hour every night, and get up at the same hour each morning. Stick to this routine as closely as possible. It helps.

- Do you attempt to get as much sunlight as you can immediately after waking up each morning? Studies show that exposure to sunlight or, if sunlight is not available, to bright artificial light after rising helps the body set its internal biological clock. Many health-care professionals recommend that persons suffering from sleep disorders receive at least one-hour exposure to sunlight every morning. When traveling, immediate exposure to several hours of daylight at one's new location also helps prevent jet lag.

- Are you a frequent daytime napper? If so, repent. Sleeping during the day is a major cause of nocturnal wakefulness, especially if you are already prone to sleep problems and insomnia. When that tired feeling steals over you at four in the afternoon, try taking a walk or doing some exercise. These activities wake you up, help you sleep at night, and keep you from the dangerous deed of daytime napping.

- Are you a couch potato? Do you get enough exercise? Studies show that a half hour's worth of exercise every day keeps insomnia away. If you exercise already, avoid exertions immediately before going to bed. The goal is to lower your heartbeat, pulse, and circulation, not speed them up. Optimally, exercise performed in the morning, or at least three to four hours before bed at night, is most effective against sleep problems.

An Effect, Not a Cause

Through the years, a number of remedies have been put forth to ease the anxieties of sleepless nights. Some of these remedies are psychological and some are medicinal. Best known, perhaps, are prescription sedatives, especially sedatives in the *benzodiazepine* family (such as Halcion and Valium). These drugs provide a potent and usually foolproof counter to many forms of insomnia. Take the medicine and you fall asleep. End of story.

The problem with sedatives, though, as many people have discovered, is that they produce an unpleasant array of side effects, including headache, irritability, dizziness, upset stomach, dry mouth, and next-day drowsiness. Unpleasant too is the fact that over time prescription sedatives and, to a lesser degree, nonprescription sedatives (such as Nytol and Sominex) become tolerated; that is, they lose their effectiveness with repeated daily use. Moreover, with long-term use, benzodiazepines often interfere with natural patterns of sleep, *causing* sleep abnormalities rather than curing them.

While conventional sedatives certainly have their place in medical practice, and while sedatives are a powerful first line of help for insomniacs, people who are interested in achieving stable slumber over the long run are advised to think of sleep difficulties as an indication of overall physical imbalance, the origins of which are located in different parts of the body, especially in the gut.

What do we mean by "imbalance"?

When important biochemical processes such as digestion or elimination are not functioning at full capacity, the entire organism is thrown off kilter, with poor-quality sleep (among other symptoms) resulting.

What's more, poor sleep results in poor digestion, and vice versa, and soon a vicious cycle ensues. In such instances, disturbed sleep may be your body's way of telling you that things are not operating as efficiently as they should in your gut. The sleeplessness is telling you to pay attention. Changes need to be made.

Sleep disorders, in other words, are often an effect rather than a cause, a secondary reaction that traces its origins back to careless living habits or to metabolic imbalances caused by improper nutrition, poor elimination, and impaired digestion. Although it is difficult to quote exact statistics, my own experience as a physician tells me that a number of the sleeping difficulties I see in patients are not caused by nervous ailments or serious disease, but by some disturbance of the nutrition-digestion-sleep biorhythm.

The following sections on sleep improvement are thus designed to address the forms of insomnia whose origins lie in the digestive tract. Once certain gastrointestinal issues are cleared up, I have frequently observed, not only does sound sleep return, but improved health results as well. At the very least, by following the suggestions offered in the sections below, you will gradually come to feel more awake, more alive, cleaner inside, and better able to sleep at night.

NUTRITIONAL AND DIGESTIVE DO'S AND DON'TS FOR A BETTER NIGHT'S REST

Each of the sections below should be looked on as a separate cog in the wheel of a good night's sleep. You do not have to apply every suggestion provided in these sections or follow every bit of advice. However, by putting as many of these methods to work for you as possible, you attack sleeplessness at its roots and increase your chances of success.

Be aware that the information offered in these sections emphasizes natural approaches to sleep. These methods are all inexpensive, accessible, easy to apply, side-effect-free, and, for many people, quite effective.

At the same time, remember that what works for one person does not necessarily work for another. For some sleepless patients, the herb valerian is the perfect natural sedative. For others, it barely works. Natural remedies are gentle healers working on the body's subtle energy structure. Many of them take time to heal. Occasionally, they do not work at all, and others must be taken in their stead. With persistence, however, you will almost always find one that suits your needs.

It is suggested, therefore, that you give these methods a bit of time to do their work. Many people see results in a few days, but others must be more patient and let nature take its course. Chances are if you stick to this regimen and remain consistent, you will not be disappointed.

Foods That Help Us Sleep

Foods High in L-Tryptophan

Why is it that after a heavy lunch we often feel drowsy? Why does a cup of warm milk before bed do the same? Why does a dinner rich in carbohydrates make us drop off in our easy chair or nod off in front of the TV? The reason is simple: certain foods act as natural soporifics, calming the mind, slowing heart rate, quieting the nerves, and producing a state of body and mind that is receptive to sleep. The food substance that is perhaps most effective in this way is the essential amino acid *L-tryptophan*.

For many years, L-tryptophan supplements could be purchased at any vitamin shop or health-food store. Insomniacs far and wide knew it to be a quick, side-effect-free means of improving sleep. Due to a contaminated batch of L-tryptophan from Japan that reached this country in 1989, which triggered a rare and serious disorder called eosinophilia-myalgia syndrome (see P. K. Hertzman's article in the *New England Journal of Medicine,* 1990, for the whole story), commercial L-tryptophan products were seriously discredited. A kind of hysteria followed this event in which the finger of guilt was pointed at L-tryptophan itself rather than at the company that had botched its production. In response, the FDA yanked all L-tryptophan supplements from the shelves across America, and so for years this helpful substance was largely inaccessible. Today, it is making something of a commercial comeback in an indirect way, though caution is still the word. Also see the section on 5-HTP, a good alternative to tryptophan.

Fortunately for the sleep deprived, L-tryptophan occurs naturally in many common foods including grains, meat, and dairy products. Once eaten and digested, it is then converted by the brain into *serotonin,* a powerful neurotransmitter that plays a key role in controlling mood, pain levels, and our ability to fall asleep.

Interestingly, adults who suffer from insomnia are often found to have low levels of serotonin in their blood. Elderly people are notoriously deficient in this substance and tend to suffer from insomnia more frequently than younger people. Depression, which often accompanies chronic insomnia, can also be caused by an imbalance of serotonin levels in the brain.

For people who suffer from sleep problems, therefore, a dietary increase in foods containing this critical amino acid is recommended. Especially strong in L-tryptophan are the following:

Turkey, beef, and veal   Whole-grain breads and cereals
Tuna fish   Dates
Yogurt   Milk
Cottage cheese   Rice
Peanut butter

Carbohydrate-Heavy Meals

Many insomniacs find that eating meals heavy on carbohydrates makes them drowsy. This occurs because a high-carb diet results in a quick rise in blood glucose level and associated hormonal changes leading to sleepiness. On the other hand, the same high-carb meal in other individuals may lead to sleep disturbance because of the inappropriate and ill-timed secretion of insulin, causing blood glucose levels to drop. A diet replete with vegetables, whole grains, fruits, nuts, and seeds—and light on the meat—works for many poor sleepers.

More Protein

Go heavy on protein for your evening meals. Protein produces fewer (and less dramatic) rises and drops in insulin secretion than carbohydrates, and its digestion is less troubling to sleep. Pack your proteins into the dinnertime meal for a week or two and see if this helps.

Avoid Foods and Drinks That Interfere with Your Sleep

The following foods and drinks have all at one time been implicated in problems of sleeplessness and insomnia.

Sugar

All signs indicate that sugar places a burden on digestion. Certainly Shakespeare thought so, as this quote from *Richard II* shows: "Things sweet to taste prove in digestion sour." It is a metaphor for living, perhaps, but also a solid piece of physiological observation.

The prime nutritional bad guy in the1970s and 1980s, sugar has recently taken a backseat as dietary demon to even more objectionable substances like fats, alcohol, and tobacco. Still, the sweet stuff continues to have its perils and its deleterious effects have become a household name thanks to Dr. Atkin's weight-loss program. Over the years, many scientific journals, including the conservative *Journal of the American Medical Association,* have featured articles describing the ways in which sugar contributes to indigestion, gallbladder disease, diverticulosis, cancer of the colon, and, yes, in some cases, insomnia. Although clinical proof is not absolute, and although the controversy swirls, there is enough evidence to suggest that persons bothered by poor sleep are well advised to cut down on their daily intake of this delicious substance.

In physiological terms, when sugar eaters first ingest a sweet, they are rewarded with a sudden shot of energy, the famous "sugar rush." In some people, this rush then triggers hypoglycemia, a blood-sugar drop, causing the person to experience a sudden dip in energy accompanied, in many cases, by a sense of lethargy, malaise, and even restless depression.

Response to sugar varies from person to person, of course, depending on tolerance and metabolism, and not everyone reacts in this way. But some do, and sometimes in extreme ways. For people who suspect that sugar is keeping them up nights via nocturnal hypoglycemia, here are some steps that can be taken:

Test yourself. If you are not diabetic but suspect that sugar is affecting your slumber, try this experiment. Eat a liberal amount of sugar every day for a week. During this period observe your sleep patterns. The following week abstain from all sweets, and see what the night hours bring.

If your sleep is poor during the first week while eating sweets, then dramatically improved during the second week of abstinence, you have made an important discovery. Consider continuing on a low-sugar or sweet-free diet to reduce sugar's harmful effects on your rest.

Avoid certain foods. Cut back on your daily intake of candy, ice cream, cake, soft drinks, and other foods that contain inordinately large stores of sugar. If you eat a balanced diet, your body will receive the sugar it needs from fresh fruit, vegetables, and grains. Avoiding sugar will not endanger your nutritional health in any way.

Be aware of hidden sugar in your food. Be on the alert for foods that contain hidden stores of sugar. Included in this category are the following:

Most commercial breakfast cereals	Pasta
Salad dressings	Pickles (especially sweet pickles)
Processed meats and sausage	Cigarettes (yes, cigarettes)
Canned fruits and vegetables	Almost all canned soups
Mustard	Mayonnaise
Vitamin pills (check the label)	Nondairy creamer
Some smoked foods	Most bread
Peanut butter (natural peanut butter is a better choice)	Some cheeses
	Beer, wine, and liquor
	Ketchup

Caffeine

You have already heard all the arguments for caffeine, pro and con, and no doubt you have come to your own conclusions whether or not to include caffeine drinks on your menu. Still, be careful. Over time, the familiar and, for many of us, reassuring presence of coffee, tea, and cola drinks at breakfast, lunch, and dinner makes us take these stimulating refreshments for granted, and in the process we forget the real dangers they pose.

Caffeine, for example, besides having diuretic properties and being mildly addictive, continues to affect us long after its wake-up benefits have come and gone, sometimes for as long as eight to twenty hours. This time lag between cause and effect can disguise the role that caffeine plays in triggering insomnia. "What the heck," people say to themselves, tossing and turning in bed at 2:00 A.M. "I had my last cup of coffee more than twelve hours ago. That couldn't be what's keeping me up."

But perhaps it is. It all depends on your tolerance. Some people, for example, are relatively immune to caffeine's sleep-disturbing effects. They process it quickly and excrete it before it does them any harm. Others, however, are affected by even the small amount of caffeine found in chocolate, green tea, cocoa, medications (both over-the-counter and prescription), and soft drinks. For people with low caffeine tolerance, the challenge is to discover just how sensitive they really are, and to act accordingly.

What is the best way to determine one's caffeine sensitivity? If you are a regular caffeine user, try the following technique. On morning one, drink a cup of coffee or tea at eight o'clock. Then refrain from taking any caffeine for the rest of the day. Observe how well you sleep that night. If your sleep is sound, push the coffee-or-tea hour up a notch next morning, to nine o'clock.

Still sleeping well? Next day, push the hour up to ten o'clock, then to eleven the next day, then twelve, and so on, until you reach an hour when you begin to feel that the caffeine is affecting your sleep.

Now calculate. Let us say the coffee or tea begins to impair your sleep at around four in the afternoon. Do you normally go to bed at, say, eleven? Good. Then subtract four (as in four o'clock in the afternoon) from eleven (as in eleven o'clock at night), giving you seven. You now know your caffeine limit—seven hours. That is, it is best to take your last cup of coffee or tea at least seven hours before going to bed.

This hour gauge is not written in stone, of course. There are daily varia-tions depending on your mood, the strength of the drink, and body chemistry. Nonetheless, this method provides a good approximate measuring gauge.

Finally, there's one more caffeine-foiling trick that is better than all the others: give up caffeine entirely. Abstinence is the one foolproof way to avoid the caffeine jitters and to maintain maximum health. Consider it.

Tobacco

Inveterate smokers often require a regular intake of nicotine during the night as well as during the day. This need launches them into a continual state of mini nicotine withdrawal, forcing them to wake up several times during the night for a smoke.

In Vienna, Dr. Reider and colleagues have recently described a new symptom they call "nocturnal sleep-disturbing nicotine craving," or simply NSDNC. As reported in *Acta Medica Austria* (2001), this disorder forces smokers to wake up several times during the night and to smoke a ciga-rette before being able to fall back to sleep. The restless sensations asso-ciated with NSDNC are due to declining nicotine concentrations in the blood, the doctors report, and manifest as an intense, almost irresistible craving.

More subtly, some inveterate smokers fall asleep promptly at bedtime, then wake up a number of times during the night in response to their nico-tine needs. Though they do not necessarily remember these awakenings, their bodies remember them quite well. The next day, these people feel strangely tired, listless, and sleep-deprived. "But I slept eight hours last night," the smoker exclaims. "I can't figure out why I'm so tired."

Beside these obvious disadvantages, there is some evidence to show that smoking interferes with the brain's actual sleep mechanism, causing sleepers to spend less time in the deep stage IV and REM states so nec-essary for a sound night's rest.

Dr. D. J. Davila and colleagues from the Mayo Clinic, as reported in the *American Journal of Respiratory Critical Care Medicine* (1994), studied the effects of nicotine on healthy nonsmokers. He found that nicotine decreases total sleep time, sleep efficiency, and precious REM sleep.

Dr. B. A. Phillips and Dr. F. J. Danner, as reported in *Archives of Internal Medicine* (1995), compared the sleep patterns of 484 subjects, half of whom were smokers. The smokers, it turned out, had more difficulty falling asleep than the nonsmokers. They also experienced high rates of daytime sleepiness, breathing difficulties, minor accidents, depression, and increased caffeine intake. Yet again, more reasons to stop smoking.

Alcohol

Though alcoholic beverages help many people relax and unwind, innumerable studies show that heavy intake of alcohol interferes with basic sleep patterns in a number of ways.

First, excessive alcohol intake reduces the number of hours we sleep at night and tends to make us restless and fitful. It lessens the amount of time we spend in non-REM and REM states of sleep. It likewise discourages regular body movements and posture changes so necessary for a good rest.

Heavy drinking also taxes the bladder, causing drinkers to wake up repeatedly throughout the night to urinate. It releases adrenaline into the bloodstream, producing anxious sleep. It interferes with the transport of L-tryptophan to the brain, reducing the serotonin supplies needed for a good night's rest. Finally, it is believed by some that the long-term REM sleep deprivation experienced by alcoholics contributes both to aberrant behavior and to delirium tremens when the heavy drinker is trying to withdraw or detox.

The moral here is to drink in moderation, especially at night and especially if you are already sleep sensitive.

Supplements That Help Us Fall Asleep

With the recent upsurge of interest in natural cures, a profusion of herbal sedatives and tranquilizers both familiar and exotic are appearing on the vitamin store shelf. Unlike conventional prescription and over-the-counter medications, these potions are believed to produce few side effects when taken appropriately. They are rarely toxic, and are mostly easy on digestion. Though the price of some of these products is becoming inflated, and though these mixtures do not necessarily work for everyone, herbal sedatives still appear to be, as the advertising copy tells us, "true gifts from nature."

As with any medicine, of course, it is wise to make haste slowly. Use common sense. Before you use an herbal sedative, consider the following suggestions:

- Be sure to follow all dosage guidelines presented on the package. Though herbal sedatives are safe, their harmlessness is not an invitation to overuse. Too much of anything can cause problems.
- Use one sedative herb at a time. Try it out for a few weeks. If it does the job, fine. Stick with it. If not, try another. Avoid the scattershot method, taking several herbal medications at once. Even if this method works, you will never know which herb is really doing the trick. One sleep remedy at a time is best.
- If your insomnia persists, or if you find that you cannot fall asleep at night without using some form of medicinal remedy, it may be time to delve more deeply into the cause of the problem. Check the dietary sections of this chapter for hints and suggestions. Talk to your doctor and to specialists. Read up on the subject. Most important, make a frank evaluation of your own lifestyle. Most sleeplessness is provoked by stress, digestive problems, and poor habits of living.

Also, deficiencies of several vitamins are known to encourage sleep disorders. Fortify yourself with adequate supplies of these nutrients and your chances of a good night's sleep increase accordingly.

Kava Kava

Perhaps the most popular and best known herbal sedative today, kava kava has long been used in Polynesia as the centerpiece for sacred communal ceremonies. Producing a tranquilizing effect and, it is believed in the South Pacific, a mystical sense of harmony with the environment, kava kava is a specific against stress, anxiety, and, most of all, poor sleep.

A study of twenty-nine patients reported in the journal *Phytomed*

(1996) focused on patients diagnosed with anxiety disorders. Given 100 mg of kava kava extract three times a day for four weeks, subjects were evaluated according to several standard psychological profiles. At the end of the study, most subjects found that their sleep was measurably improved, and that physical and mental side effects were minimal.

Dr. J. S. Cauffield, writing in the journal *Lippincott's Primary Care Practice* (1999), states that kava kava is superior to placebo in the treatment of anxiety and is roughly equivalent in its sedative effects to the drugs oxazepam and bromazepam.

Many other studies, especially those carried out in Europe where funding for alternative sedative remedies is readily available, testify to kava kava's powerful calming effects. Kava kava can currently be purchased at most pharmacies and health-product stores in the United States. The liquid extract is the most potent, but it has a harsh, bitter taste. Capsules are easier on the taste buds, but slightly less effective in helping promote sleep. Both forms do the trick.

A note on possible problems: Though kava kava causes no short-term side effects, this herb has recently come under suspicion by conventional medical authorities who claim that prolonged use generates liver damage and is harmful to persons suffering from Parkinson's disease. Although these studies are inconclusive, and although the definitive decision is not yet in concerning how serious the side effects really are, it cannot hurt to err on the side of caution. Let your doctor know you are taking kava kava, and avoid using this herb for more than two weeks at a time. Do not take with alcohol or any other sedatives. It should not be used by pregnant or breast-feeding women or by patients with kidney or blood disorders.

Valerian Root

A safe, powerful, and increasingly popular nervous system depressant, valerian root has been used in Russia, China, and Europe for centuries as a specific against tension, depression, anxiety, insomnia, and hysterical conditions. Its effects are both sedative and tranquilizing.

According to a study published in *Pharmacology, Biochemistry, and Behavior* (1982), valerian root produces a decrease in sleep latency and improves the quality of sleep. This effect is most prominently seen in poor or irregular sleepers.

Similar beneficial effects are mentioned in studies by Dr. P. D. Leathwood and Dr. F. Chauffard in *Planta Medica* (1985). Another study by Leathwood and Chauffard, reported in *Psychiatric Research* (1982), shows that valerian decreases sleep awakenings and improves sleep latency and overall quality of sleep. These findings were objectively confirmed during tests by EEG evaluation. In one Swedish double-blind, placebo-controlled study, Dr. O. Lindahl and Dr. L. Lindwall, as reported in *Pharmacological Biochemical Behavior* (1989), demonstrated that valerian led to deep, uninterrupted sleep in 44 percent of subjects, while 89 percent of subjects reported good or improved quality of sleep.

Note that for a small percent of people, valerian acts as a stimulant rather than as a sedative. If you plan to use this herb, start off with a low dose. If you feel calmer, as most people do, and if the herb helps you sleep, take it for several more weeks. Then stop usage, wait two weeks, and begin again. Continue following this cycle. The recommended dose for valerian is 1 to 3 g of the dried root taken once or twice a day.

Chamomile

Not quite as powerful a sedative as valerian root or kava kava, the lovely little chamomile bud still deserves an honored place on the list of sleep inducers. Not only are its relaxing effects quickly felt, but it is also useful for taming nausea, colic in children, indigestion, and the symptoms of colds and flu. Most important, the L-tryptophan and calcium found in chamomile make it useful as both a sedative and stomach relaxant, helping users unwind before bedtime and enjoy a peaceful night's repose.

In one German double-blind study, as reported in *Arzneimittelforschung* (1997), Dr. de la Motte and colleagues showed that children suffering from diarrhea recover faster when given a pectin/chamomile substance than do children given a placebo. Other studies in *Planta* (1979) indicate that, in some cases, chamomile helps prevent the development of ulcers.

Chamomile can be ingested hot or cold as a beverage. Or it can be taken in capsule form. It is often used as an ingredient in commercial herbal sleep mixtures. People who suffer from stress-related sleeplessness may wish to drink two or three cups of chamomile tea throughout the day as a specific against the emotional ups and downs of daily living. The relaxing results of this herb are almost instantaneous. Be careful, though, not to overdo. More than five or six cups a day of chamomile tea can slow down motor reactions and produce feelings of sluggishness.

Other Helpful Herbal Natural Sleep Remedies

There are literally hundreds, perhaps thousands, of herbs that calm the nervous system and promote a sedative effect on the heart and mind. Some of the more potent and readily available of these substances include:

Fennel seed	Lemon balm	Peppermint leaves
Hops	Linden flowers	Siberian ginseng
Lavender flowers	Passionflower	Skullcap

Another helpful sleep remedy is based on Ayurvedic practice. Mix equal amounts of aniseed, chamomile, and dill. Place a half teaspoon of this mixture in boiling water and steep for five minutes. Cool, add a teaspoon of honey, and drink at bedtime. Also try drinking a cup of coconut juice an hour before sleep.

Melatonin

Melatonin is a powerful hormone produced every day in our pineal glands. Studies show that it plays a central role in inducing sound sleep at night and that a deficit of this substance can invite insomnia.

It therefore follows that melatonin supplements are enormously effective for helping people get to sleep—but *only* if users have a lack of melatonin in their brain chemistry to begin with. Persons who suffer from sleep disorders and who maintain adequate melatonin supplies do not profit at all from these supplements. If enough melatonin is already present in the system, more is not going to help. Either way, melatonin is a safe and side effect–free alternative.

Who is deficient in melatonin? Mostly the elderly. In men and women over age sixty, the pineal gland works less vigorously than it once did, and melatonin supplies dwindle. Still, melatonin deficiency is not found exclusively among the elderly. Practically anyone can have it, and many can have it without their knowledge.

How do you find out if you are melatonin deficient? Simply take melatonin for a few days and witness the results. Begin by taking 3 mg several hours before going to sleep. (In many people, melatonin takes at least an hour and sometimes more to kick in.) If the melatonin helps you fall asleep and stay asleep, but if you feel sluggish the next morning, cut down to 2 mg. If you are still tired after this, cut down to 1 mg.

Time-release capsules are usually considered the most effective form of delivery. Melatonin supplements are available at most health-food stores, pharmacies, and some supermarkets. Patients with sleep problems require 75 mg at bedtime. For jet lag, use 5 mg a day, starting three days before travel and continuing three days after the flight.

Caution: Patients with liver disease, stroke, depression, neurological or kidney disease should not take melatonin.

5-HTP

Somewhat of a newcomer to the natural sedative repertoire, 5-HTP is sometimes referred to by its technical name, 5-hydroxytryptophan. A near relative of the amino acid L-tryptophan, 5-HTP is chemically closer to pure serotonin than ordinary L-tryptophan, and is processed more quickly and effectively in the brain. Since it is derived naturally from an African plant (*Griffonia simplicifolia*) rather than synthesized in the lab like L-tryptophan, many health-care professionals believe it is safer and less likely to be tainted than commercially produced L-tryptophan. For many people, 5-HTP serves as a gratifyingly prompt and effective cure for sleeplessness.

Dr. A. Soulairac and Dr. H. Lambinet, in their article, "Clinical Studies of the Effect of the Serotonin Precursor L-5-Hydroxytryptophan on Sleep Disorders," published in *Rundsch Med Prax* (1988), report that 5-HTP substantially improves the quality and depth of REM sleep without increasing actual sleep time, especially during the critical sleep stage 3 and stage 4. Similarly, in the medical journal *Lancet* (1981), Dr. Webb and

Dr. Kirker report a case of severe post-traumatic insomnia effectively treated with L-5-hydroxytryptophan. 5-HTP has been shown to help overcome sleep fragmentation in alcoholics during alcohol withdrawal, as reported by Dr. Zarcone in the *American Journal of Psychiatry* (1975).

When using 5-HTP, start with 250 mg, then reduce or increase the dose as needed. Some nutritionists suggest eating a piece of fruit or drinking a glass of fruit juice with the supplement to boost its effectiveness. In doses over 300 mg, nausea is possible, and can be controlled by using enteric-coated capsules that dissolve in the intestines rather than in the more sensitive areas of the stomach. It is also suggested that, when taking 5-HTP, users increase their daily intake of B vitamins. Interestingly, 5-HTP is being used today with increasing success to treat depression, migraine headaches, overweight, and fibromyalgia along with insomnia.

B Vitamins

An adequate intake of water-soluble B vitamins calms the nerves and relaxes the muscles. Foods containing B vitamins include walnuts, wheat germ, whole-grain bread and cereals, sunflower seeds, legumes, potatoes, leafy green vegetables, brewer's yeast, and blackstrap molasses (interestingly, a teaspoon of blackstrap molasses every evening is a standard early American folk remedy for insomnia). Note that smoking, drinking, and stress significantly reduce the body's supply of B vitamins. If you fall into any of these categories, be sure to take extra-large supplies of supplemental vitamin B.

Pyridoxine

Pyridoxine (vitamin B_6), in particular, plays an important part in calming the nerves. Without supplies of this vitamin in our daily diet, we tend to become crabby, listless, anxious, chronically tired, and sleep deprived. Deficiencies can also cause inhibition of *tryptophan hydroxylase,* an enzyme that plays a part in the conversion of tryptophan to serotonin. Preliminary data from Dr. Ebben in New York suggests that adequate pyridoxine in the diet increases dream vividness and our ability to recall dreams.

For an adequate intake of pyridoxine, take vitamin B supplements and eat more foods that contain this substance such as wheat germ, bananas, and walnuts.

Vitamin D

If you take calcium (see "Calcium" below), you will also need adequate supplies of vitamin D to help your body process and absorb this nutrient. A dosage of 400 IU of vitamin D a day is recommended.

Calcium

Calcium is an inexpensive natural relaxant that is often all that's needed to improve troubled sleep. Foods that contain calcium include green beans, most leafy vegetables (especially broccoli, watercress, and cauliflower), nuts, seeds, tofu, dairy products, and whole grains. Commercial supplements are also useful. For many poor sleepers, 350 to 500 mg of calcium a day does the trick.

Magnesium

Like calcium, magnesium calms the nerves and improves the quality of rest. Take it with calcium for extra sleep protection. Magnesium is found in whole grains, legumes, and dark-green leafy vegetables. A dosage of 250 to 350 mg of magnesium a day is recommended.

Zinc

Both people with insomnia and people with depression are often found to be zinc deficient. Take 50 mg of zinc a day along with the vitamin and mineral supplements discussed above.

Japanese Stomach Massage for Deep Body Relaxation

The following technique, borrowed from the Japanese art of Shiatsu (a close relative of Chinese acupressure), is easy to practice, safe, and, if done properly, amazingly effective for inducing relaxation and sleep. Try it on a friend, a partner, a child, or even yourself.

Start by having the person lie on his or her back with the abdominal area bared. Imagine that the person's navel is the center of a six-inch circle. On the circumference of this circle, imagine that the numbers of a clock are arranged in conventional order from one to twelve, with the number twelve on top nearest the solar plexus. You will use these numbers as location points when applying massage.

Hold your five fingers together, forming them into a kind of beak, and press the spot that corresponds to twelve o'clock on the imaginary clock. Apply pressure for approximately fifteen to twenty seconds, being careful not to press too hard. If the person complains of pain, modify the pressure until the proper comfort level is established.

Now move around the circle clockwise (that is, right to left, following the movement of food in the intestines), applying the same pressure to the point at one o'clock. As before, be careful not to press too hard.

Now move to the point at two o'clock, push and hold; then to three o'clock, four o'clock, five o'clock, and so forth, proceeding all the way around the circle until you return to twelve. Hold the pressure at each point for approximately fifteen to twenty seconds.

Apply four or five rotations of this massage. After going through several cycles, many massage therapists find that their clients are so deeply relaxed that they fall asleep in the middle of the treatment.

You can also stimulate these same pressure points on your own abdominal area and achieve similar results, though this technique is generally more restful and effective when applied by another person.

More Commonsense Advice for a Better Sleep

Finally, here are some tips on digestion and a good night's sleep.

- For a good night's sleep, avoid overeating. Digestion is a complicated process that keeps many organs busy at once and that continues for long periods of time, using many of the body's energies and resources. Reduce the time your body spends at this taxing chore by eating moderately, especially at dinner.

- If you do nap during the day, keep your naps short—no more than forty-five minutes at most.
- When eating, make sure to chew your food thoroughly before swallowing. The more processing that food receives from digestive enzymes in the mouth, the less digestion must take place in the gut, and the sounder you sleep. Yoga practitioners often chew each bite of food twenty-five to fifty times, a time-consuming but worthy goal.
- In my own practice, before a colonoscopy (a scope of the colon) it is standard procedure to clean out the colon with various purging techniques. After the colonoscopy is completed, interestingly, patients' symptoms occasionally resolve themselves without need for further treatment. This sudden healing, I believe, may be due to the fact that the colon-cleaning procedures improve the health of the entire body, including a patient's ability to relax and sleep. Consult Chapter 9 for details on internal cleaning and detoxification.
- Many people have difficulty falling asleep on a full stomach. If you are among them, eat your large meal at least five or six hours before bedtime, and be sure to avoid nighttime snacks.
- If you must snack: Snack no less than two hours before going to bed, and snack on foods rich in tryptophan, such as grains, meat, and dairy products (see "Foods High in L-Tryptophan" on page 74), or on easily digestible foods such as fruit and vegetables. Avoid all junk foods and spicy foods.
- Note that by refraining from food at night before bed, you are rewarded with a welcome side benefit: weight loss. Food eaten in the late hours digests slowly and turns more easily to fat. Avoid the late-night eating habit and you avoid putting on extra pounds as well.
- If you suffer from chronic constipation, there is some clinical evidence to show that the low-level discomfort this disorder brings can interfere with a good night's sleep. Consult Chapter 14 for advice and suggestions on overcoming constipation.
- Avoid foods that are loaded with chemical preservatives. Although the relationship between food additives and sleep disorders is a controversial one, and although the final word concerning the relation-

ship between the two has not yet been spoken, we do know for sure that when certain chemical preservatives are removed from the diet of hyperactive children these children calm down and sleep more soundly. All things considered, it is probably best to avoid highly processed and preserved foods whenever you can, especially if your sleep patterns are easily disturbed.

• Ayurvedic methods for promoting sound sleep include the following. Although some of these remedies seem a bit folksy, the Indian people have been using them for centuries, apparently with impressive success.

- Sleep on your left side whenever possible. This practice is also encouraged by modern medicine, since sleeping on the left side is beneficial for digestion and for controlling acid reflux. Sleeping on the stomach is considered the worst of all sleep positions. When sleeping, always keep your head slightly higher than your feet.
- Before bed, massage your forehead with oil of jasmine, mustard oil, or clarified butter. You can also massage your feet with milk.
- Ayurvedic proponents claim that sleeping with the head facing east promotes a deep meditative sleep, while facing south promotes a physically restful sleep. Sleeping with the head pointing toward the west is said to generate bad dreams. Always avoid sleeping with the head pointing due north; it generates headaches and irritability.
- According to Ayurvedic tradition, the optimal way to sleep is to go to bed three hours after dusk and to awaken one or two hours before dawn. Sleep during this period promotes vigor, vitality, strength, clarity of mind, and longevity.
- Wear as few clothes as possible when sleeping. Be sure all clothes fit loosely and well. Never cover your face when sleeping, even with a pillow.

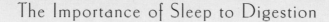

- Never go to bed when angry or upset. If you have had an argument with a friend, spouse, or relative, make up first.
- According to the Ayurvedic tradition, lack or poor-quality sleep at night increases vata and suppresses kapha, causing irritability, anxiety, restlessness, headache, depression, and insecurity. Eat according to your dosha.

chapter five

The Effects of Stress
on Digestion

During the first week of June 1983, when buyers of *Time* magazine
reached for their favorite weekly news magazine, they were
greeted with an unusual cover illustration. Instead of the usual
portraits of politicians and world shakers, the image that greeted them
that day showed an agonized head breaking through a block of stone and
screaming the name of the week's title story: "Stress! Seeking Cures
for Modern Anxieties." The article went on to target stress as the "epi-
demic of the eighties," and to refer to it as the country's number-one medical problem.

Since this edition of *Time* came on the stands two decades ago, little
has changed in the stress level of the average American. If anything, the
anxiety quotient of the common citizen has escalated, some would say by
quantum leaps. In 1983, *Prevention* magazine asked survey subjects if
they experience "great stress" at least one day a week. Fifty-five percent
said yes. Thirteen years later, the same survey was given. This time, 75 percent of respondents answered in the affirmative. Health-care experts esti-

mate that 75 to 90 percent of all visits to a primary care physician are due to stress-related problems.

Today, many health-care professionals have come to agree that the thinking and feeling parts of a human being play a pivotal role in the homeostasis of their bodies, and that any therapy based on a presumed separation between mind and body is less likely to generate healing effects than one that addresses both parts with equal intensity and respect.

MEASURING THE EFFECTS OF STRESS

Due to incomplete information and perhaps to vivid images such as the one that appeared on the cover of *Time*, there is a notion common to professionals and laypersons alike that stress stems exclusively from reactions to loss and adversity. While it is certainly true that troublesome events cause strife, technically speaking, stress is not invariably connected to loss or catastrophe. In some cases, it can also be the result of positive encounters. The Holmes-Rahe Scale, developed to measure stress levels experienced in different life situations, and published for the first time in 1967 in the *Journal of Psychosomatic Research,* is quite clear on this matter.

When you look at the Holmes-Rahe Scale, for instance, the first thing you notice, as might be expected, is that tragedy and loss are the most powerful producers of stress. Number one on the list is the death of a spouse. Number two is divorce, number three marital separation, number four prison, and number five the death of a close relative.

So far no surprises. But read on. Just below these first-rank negative stressors are events that we normally think of as enriching and festive, events such as "marriage" (stressor number seven on the list), "marital or relationship reconciliation" (stressor number nine), "pregnancy" (stressor number twelve), and "birth of a new family member" (stressor number fourteen).

Relatively positive, or at least neutral, events are also on the scale. Examples include "starting a new job," "retirement," "moving one's residence," "vacations," and celebrating big yearly holidays like Christmas.

Most surprising of all, perhaps, is the fact that somewhere in the middle of the scale, just below "in-law problems" and "foreclosure of a mort-gage or loan," is a stressor titled "outstanding personal achievement." Fail-ure, in other words, is not the only cause of stress. Success can provoke it too.

What Is Stress?

If stress is not exclusively defined as a negative reaction to upsetting in-fluences, what exactly is it? In a nutshell, stress is a *physical-emotional re-action resulting from some form of change in a person's life.* "Change" is the operative word here, and under its large umbrella is included any dramatic alteration, be it pleasurable or painful, joyous or tragic, that disrupts a per-son's daily habits of living.

We need to understand that stress results less from events themselves (it is, after all, theoretically possible to undergo the most agonizing trials and tribulations and remain serene) and more from the physical, emo-tional, and mental changes that these events trigger. Once we grasp this important point, it is easy to understand why so many happenings in life that are supposed to bring us enjoyment end up providing nothing better than a pain in the gut.

We understand, for instance, why some lottery winners, instead of jumping for joy when told they are rich, report feeling dazed, disoriented, anxious, even nauseous. We understand why the birth of a child, statisti-cally speaking, is more likely to raise the chances of divorce rather than promote domestic harmony.

Knowing about the relationship between change and physical reaction also helps us understand why in Chinese medicine one of the main causes of disease that physicians look for when examining a patient is a recent experience of intense happiness or joy. The theory behind this diagnostic tactic is that energy balance is the most important element in human well-ness. Any emotional event that disrupts this balance, be it positive or neg-ative, disturbs the flow of a person's inner energies and, with it, his or her health.

THE CAUSES AND SYMPTOMS OF STRESS

Whatever influence causes our specific form of stress, be it (1) bodily stress from sickness or injury, (2) social stress from unpleasant events in life and disagreeable interactions with other people, (3) psychological stress from depression, worry, low self-esteem, or (4) lifestyle stress engendered by alcohol abuse, workaholism, drugs, and plain hard living, this phenomenon almost invariably expresses itself in some form of physical and/or mental symptoms.

What actually causes these symptoms? The answer is an interesting one and is linked to the biological history of all humankind. At one time in the remote past, we know, our ancestors were continually under threat of sudden physical harm. At any moment, a lion or tiger might leap on them from behind a tree. Or members of a neighboring village might launch a surprise attack. Or a violent rainstorm, a hurricane, or a blizzard might suddenly erupt, endangering the life and limb of people who lived largely unprotected from the elements.

As a result of this continual exposure to dangerous situations, the human organism evolved over time in such a way that whenever a threat to life and limb presented itself, a sudden surge of energy prepared the endangered person to either run away as quickly as possible or to stand and do battle. Today we refer to this response as the "fight or flight" mechanism.

The moment this mechanism clicks in, physiologically speaking, the hypothalamus in the brain tells the pituitary gland to release the hormone ACTH. This substance triggers the adrenals, a small but extremely potent set of glands located just above the kidneys. The adrenals pump powerful hormones such as adrenaline into the bloodstream to provide instant stamina and mental alertness. The effects of these secretions send instant rushes of energy coursing throughout the systems. Everything comes alive and awake.

As a result of such sudden and somewhat violent changes in body chemistry, many physical symptoms follow. Breath rate increases in order to bring more oxygen to the blood. Blood pressure rises, and metabolism speeds up. The palms sweat, the heart beats more quickly, pupils in the eyes dilate, the salivary glands go dry, muscles tighten and tense, the sexual drive diminishes, and digestion shuts down as blood from the gut is diverted to the muscles. The body, in short, is preparing—or *thinks* it is preparing—to flee or defend itself.

In our modern world, tigers in the bush or raids by neighboring tribes are unusual, to say the least. Yet, at the same time, analogous if not exactly equivalent dangers lurk, both in our business life and at home where we often find ourselves under attack—not physical attack per se, but the *psychological and emotional* kind.

In which ways? In arguments with a spouse, for example, or in feelings of panic when there is not enough money to pay the bills. When working on a tight deadline at the office. When contemplating a trip to the dentist's office or an audit from the IRS. While driving in rush-hour traffic. When late for a critical appointment. When being yelled at by our boss. When watching our investments sink with the DOW. When warned that the downsizing list has our name on it. . . . The whole collection of harsh pressures that modern life so lavishly pours upon us.

Because of the way we have evolved over the eons, and also by sheer dint of habit, our bodies are unable to differentiate between the actual physical threat of a tiger in the jungle and the emotional threat of an angry neighbor in the next yard.

As a result, at the slightest sign of trouble, real or perceived, physical or mental, our internal stress responses automatically swing into high gear, going into fight-or-flight mode, opening the energy sluices, and overtaxing our bodies with constant and needless metabolic exertions that invariably turn out to be false alarms. Over time, as we habitually erupt into these tempests in teapots hour after hour, day after day, year after year, the inevitable finally happens—stress burnout, with a group of pathological symptoms to show for it.

Mentally, for example, chronic stress clouds memory capacity. It impairs concentration and encourages depression, sleep disturbances, slow judgment, disorganization, restlessness, and mental fatigue. In some cases, it can even trip off a psychosis such as paranoia.

On an emotional level, too much stress spawns apathy, sadness, irritability, crying jags, and despair. In some people, bouts of anxiety develop. Other people experience hopelessness, social withdrawal, or panic attacks.

On a purely physical level, possible reactions to stress include fatigue, headache, insomnia, chest pains, tremors, muscle pains, nervous tics, changes in the menstrual cycle, shortness of breath, asthma, high blood pressure, frequent colds, loss of sex drive, and palpitations.

Finally, in terms of digestive equilibrium, stress can wreak havoc on every part of the gut, causing or exacerbating heartburn, diarrhea, constipation, indigestion, stomach pains, fluttering stomach, colitis, ulcers, and more. In fact, stress tends to aggravate and make worse practically every digestive disease we know—from heartburn to constipation to stomach cancer.

Many studies collaborate the relationship between stress and intestinal disease. For example, Dr. Dumitrascu and Dr. Granescu from Romania studied the correlation between stress and irritable bowel syndrome (IBS). Reporting in the *Romanian Journal of Internal Medicine* (1996), the authors state that 63 percent of persons with IBS experience abnormally high levels of stress in their daily existence, as based on the life events scale designed by Holmes and Rahe. Similarly, at the annual Digestive Disease Week conference in 2002, Dr. H. Mertz and colleagues presented data showing that stress dramatically increases the sensitivity to rectal distension in irritable bowel syndrome patients, but not in healthy control subjects. (Digestive Disease Week is the largest yearly gathering of digestive diseases specialists and scientists in the world.)

Often the stress that causes a particular digestive pain or disease has its origins in the distant past. Many people who were physically and sexually abused during childhood, for example, develop trauma-related stomach and intestinal aliments years later. A group of investigators lead by Dr. Yehuda Ringel recently presented data in *Digestive Disease Week* (2002) showing that in MRI brain scans, painful bowel distention triggers patterns of brain activation in women who were sexually abused. Significantly, these patterns differ substantially from the patterns registered by women who were never abused. Apparently, the memory of this painful event is long kept suppressed, resulting in exaggerated perceptions of bowel pain later on, plus a range of generalized digestive ailments.

THE BRAIN-GUT AXIS

By now it should be clear that the way in which the mind processes high-pressure events is a far more important determinant of health than the actual events themselves. It is also clear that, in many cases, the digestive problems that patients complain of in a physician's office are due not just to a specific physical disorder, but to the weakening of the entire physical system through chronic worry and fret.

An important point to note here is that on a physical level the central nervous system (CNS) and the digestive system are connected in measurable ways, and are continually exchanging electrochemical messages on a variety of different subjects. This relationship is so busy and so interactive that doctors now refer to it as the "brain-gut axis."

We know, for instance, that the central nervous system produces chemicals that trigger peristalsis in the intestines. The CNS also mandates the release of chemicals such as acetylcholine and adrenaline that cue the stomach, telling it when to begin digestion, when to end it, when to secrete more acid, and when to cease and desist.

On its own end, the digestive system constantly sends back messages to the CNS, telling the brain when it is satisfied, when it is hungry, when it hurts, and when it is sick, anxious, or full.

Interestingly, the human gastrointestinal tract boasts approximately the same number of nerve cells as our spinal cord. This fact has caused some medical researchers to posit the theory that the gastrointestinal tract is structurally and neurochemically a kind of second brain unto itself that is medically referred to as the "enteric nervous system" (ENS).

Simply put, the gut has a mind of its own, a thinking and feeling capacity that to some degree is autonomous from the central nervous system, and that constantly interacts with the big brain in the head, just as a state governor confers on important issues with the president.

It is known, for example, that of the thirty chemicals of different classes that transmit messages within the central nervous system, almost all of these are present and active in the ENS. "The ENS," in the words of Dr. Michael Gershon of Columbia University, a pioneer in this field, "is no simple collection of relay ganglia but rather a complete integrative brain in its own right" (*Gastroenterology*, 1981).

There are even similarities in the way that the ENS and the central nervous system react to neurological disease. "The ENS," writes Gershon, "is also vulnerable to what are generally thought of as brain lesions: Both the Lewy bodies associated with Parkinson's disease and the amyloid plaques and neurofibrillary tangles identified with Alzheimer's disease have been found in the bowels of patients with these conditions. It is conceivable that Alzheimer's disease, so difficult to diagnose in the absence of autopsy data, may some day be routinely identified by rectal biopsy" (*Hospital Practice*, 1999).

From a body-mind standpoint, this deep interaction between brain and gut stirs up a great deal of mental and physiological activity, both of a positive and negative kind.

The effect, for instance, of negative thoughts and mental messages on the gut is known to slow down peristalsis and evacuation. It can cause cramping, negative changes in bowel habits, and, some medical researchers believe, encourage the overgrowth of unfriendly intestinal bacteria.

People who are about to perform onstage, give a speech, deliver a group presentation, or go into battle clearly know the rigors of nausea, vomiting, and the bouts of diarrhea that can accompany such frightening encounters. Other persons, pressured by chronic problems at home or at the office, complain of chronic digestive bugbears such as stomachaches, heartburn, nausea, indigestion, and constipation. Clearly, the brain and the stomach are linked.

A very elegant study of the effects of stress on the gut was done several years ago on a group of healthy medical students. The students' colonic movements were assessed during a colonoscopy. As the colonoscopy was in progress, the students all registered normal colonic movements. Then, out of the blue, one of the investigators suddenly shouted the single alarming word "Cancer!" In a moment, the colonic motility of the entire group sped up dramatically, and stayed there until the hoax was explained. The purpose was to see how quickly gut can react to an effect on the brain, and the effect was instantaneous. The hoax was a stressor that caused the colon to get excited; it calmed down once the stress was relieved by explanation of the hoax.

Studies in this area likewise show that the intense stresses generated by life-changing experiences such as divorce, lawsuit, or loss of a job can worsen symptoms in irritable bowel syndrome (IBS) symptoms. People suffering from Crohn's disease or ulcerative colitis experience a similar worsening of symptoms during times of mental and emotional distress. A recent study of college students found that among students who were experiencing diarrhea and constipation, almost two-thirds were currently under severe stress.

Moreover, it is common wisdom among doctors that many of the functional gastrointestinal problems complained of in the examining room are due to or associated with emotional distress rather than to digestive disease. It is known, for instance, that patients who visit physicians for functional gut ailments are *three times* more likely to suffer from anxiety or depression than patients who complain of other symptoms.

To treat such complications, some doctors prescribe psychotropic medications such as antidepressants, not just to lower patients' stress but to act on their gut brain or ENS as well. Other practitioners employ mental techniques such as relaxation exercises and hypnosis. Numerous published studies report the positive therapeutic effects of hypnosis on nausea and vomiting, especially in people undergoing chemotherapy or surgery and in pregnant women.

In one study published in the journal *Alimentary Pharmacology and Therapeutics* (1988), Dr. Whorwell shows that, in addition to relieving the symptoms of IBS, hypnotherapy markedly improves a patient's quality of life and helps reduce his or her absenteeism from work. The positive effects of hypnosis also extend to other digestive disorders such as peptic ulcers. Dr. Whorwell's group conducted a controlled trial using hypnotherapy in relapse prevention of duodenal ulceration, and reported the results in the prestigious journal *Lancet* (1988). After healing the ulcers with ranitidine (a popular ulcer drug), patients were given either hypnotherapy or placebo for ten weeks. Yearlong follow-up studies showed that while all the patients in the placebo group had relapsed, only 53 percent of those given hypnotherapy experienced a recurrence of ulcers.

Finally, when looking at the brain-gut axis on a less technical level, consider the implications involved when we speak of having a "gut feeling," when we undergo a "gut reaction," when we quip that "the way to a man's heart is through his stomach." Some people even invent their own graphic terms that unconsciously show just how linked the gut and emotions really are. Over the years I have heard patients describe maladies with telling phrases such as "stressed-out stomach," "garbage gut," "heartbreak heartburn," and "timid tummy."

In Japan, a man or woman of accomplishment is known as a "person who acts from the belly." In show business, actors in training are taught to "speak from the gut." Martial artists tell us that a majority of power and combat wisdom emanates from their abdomens. In Hinduism, the stomach is marked as one of the seven *chakras*, or energy centers, and is described in Hindu writings as the center of power and will. Zen monks still practice a form of meditation involving the *hara*, or lower abdomen, in which they place awareness two inches below their navel. Sitting silently and passively, the monks are trained to allow the intelligence embodied in this region to awaken their higher spiritual capacities.

Looked at from this purely intuitive perspective, the Laughing Buddhas, the Taoist Ho Tais, the Hindu god and goddess statues, and all the other large-bellied figures from Eastern religions appear to have a meaning that is more than just whimsical or aesthetic.

Clearly, our stomach and bowels do more than process food and excrete wastes. In their own way, they "think" and "feel" as well. If we are to become fully health conscious, we are advised to heed this fact, and to give our gastrointestinal tract the attention, respect, and respite from stress that it needs and deserves.

TREATING STRESS IN YOUR OWN LIFE

Once we understand that many of the vague and undiagnosed digestive symptoms we suffer from are due to the stress of everyday living rather than to infection or disease, we can turn our attention toward various "soft," nonchemical methods of healing these problems.

Many people visiting the physician's office are relieved to learn that there is nothing clinically wrong with their stomachs or bowels, that their problem lies in the more controllable realms of the heart and mind. Doctors who are friendly to alternative methods respond to these situations by putting patients on a regimen of natural cures and relaxation techniques. These methods are often all that is needed to get the digestive and elimination systems back on track.

Simple things are easy to do. Remember what mom said: "Calm down before you eat." Even this piece of homespun advice appears to have a scientific basis. Dr. Barbara Parker and colleagues from Australia studied the factors responsible for food intake. Presenting at the annual Digestive Disease Week in 2002, they stated that not only pre-meal hunger but also pre-meal calmness are independent predictors of how much food we will eat at a sitting.

The natural modalities discussed in the sections to follow are widely in use today to reduce tension and to establish a better and friendlier balance between gut and mind.

Exercise

Many people consider exercise the number-one antidote for stress, and with good reason. The number of physical and psychological benefits that result from regular exercise is amazing. These benefits include the following:

- Increased muscle strength, endurance, coordination, and balance
- Heightened stamina, vigor, and daily energy level

- Improved immune-system functioning, with a corresponding lack of colds and flus each year
- Improved circulation and blood supply to muscles and heightened ability to utilize oxygen. The risk of heart disease or stroke is also reduced
- Lowered systolic and diastolic blood pressure
- Lowered total cholesterol, including lowered counts of LDL ("harmful") cholesterol and heightened counts of HDL ("helpful") cholesterol
- Weight loss and healthy weight maintenance
- Improved bone-mineral density to avoid osteoporosis. Increased joint flexibility and increased range of motion
- Reduced rate of colon cancer, breast cancer, and perhaps other forms of cancer
- Reduced risk of developing diabetes
- Improved quality of sleep and help relieving insomnia
- For pregnant women, a reduction in the chance of developing complications during and after childbirth
- Reduced risk of ulcers, irritable bowel syndrome, indigestion, constipation, and other gastrointestinal ailments
- Reduced chances of premature death plus a possible increase in overall longevity

The psycho-emotional benefits of exercise, induced by raised endorphin levels and rebalancing of the same neurotransmitters addressed by chemical antidepressants, are likewise impressive. Included are reduction in anxiety, mood enhancement, improved physical appearance, increased states of relaxation, heightened self-esteem and confidence, greater concentration and clarity of thought, and an overall improvement in general outlook and quality of life.

All of these benefits, needless to say, go a long way toward reducing stress levels in our lives and improving digestive health. It is estimated that every half hour of vigorous exercise we perform pays us back with approximately two hours of increased relaxation and relief from tension.

As always, it is a good idea to check with your doctor before beginning any type of rigorous exercise, especially if you have been largely inactive up until now. Once you receive the green light, look for a fitness system that best suits your physical goals. Most people prefer workouts that increase endurance, strength, flexibility, and balance; raise heart rate and blood circulation; and that make exercisers feel relaxed and energized. Most of all, training should be fun. The "make it burn" credo so popular a few decades ago has been replaced by the concept of comfortable fitness—finding the degree of exercise that best suits your needs and sticking with it.

What are your choices? Start by considering a sport such as tennis, martial arts, basketball, racquetball, skiing, volleyball, cycling, or swimming, all of which offer social fun along with aerobic stimulation and physical training. Endurance and fitness exercises are also good. These include fast walking, jogging, stair climbing, walking on treadmills, and using rowing machines. Think also of the more formal and choreographed exercise programs such as dancing, gymnastics, calisthenics, and aerobic exercise classes. Weight training, though less of a stress reliever than aerobic exercise, also helps people relax and unwind. Finally, there are the "soft," low-impact exercise systems such as yoga, chi gung (qi gong), and tai chi that are especially well geared for seniors and for people who wish to combine a meditative practice with their exercise plan.

The list of exercise options these days is endless. Check your local gym to see what it has to offer. You might also want to buy a book or two on general exercise guidelines.

Mood-Enhancing Herbs

In Chapter 4, we profiled a selection of herbs and supplements that help promote a sound night's sleep. Several of these same herbal potions are beneficial for fighting stress and for inducing a calm stomach.

Kava Kava

An extract taken from the kava kava plant, a native of the South Pacific, is a mood enhancer and antianxiety herb that has been much in the spotlight these days. A 1996 report in the journal *Phytomed* focused on twenty-nine patients diagnosed with a variety of anxiety problems including restlessness, free-floating anxiety, and panic disorder. Subjects were given 100 mg of kava kava extract three times a day for four weeks. A majority of the subjects claimed their symptoms were measurably improved, with no ill side effects.

In laboratory tests, kava kava has consistently proved itself to be superior to placebo in the treatment of anxiety. Its antistress effects, as reported by Cauffield and H. J. Forbes in the 1999 journal *Lippincott's Primary Practical Care,* are estimated to be roughly equivalent to those produced by conventional sedative drugs such as oxazepam and bromazepam.

Based on studies reviewed by Dr. Pittler and Dr. Ernst in *Cochrane Database Systematic Review* (2002), the side effects of kava kava are mild, transient, and infrequent. It is not considered addictive and, unlike Valium, Xanax, or alcohol, does not appear to promote hangover or depression.

A note on kava kava: Since this herb tends to enhance the sedative effects of conventional barbiturates and sedatives such as Valium, it is suggested that the two types of medication not be taken together or mixed. Several studies report that in prolonged use, kava kava produces liver damage, and that it may be harmful to persons suffering from Parkinson's disease. Though these claims remain unsubstantiated in randomized, controlled trials, some physicians feel that patients who use kava kava for long periods should visit a physician after three to six months use to check for possible liver damage. Better yet, until the verdict is in on the long-term safety of kava kava, take it only on an as-needed basis, and limit its use to a week or two at most.

Valerian Root

A safe and powerful central nervous system depressant, valerian root has been used for centuries in countries throughout the world as an antidote to anxiety, depression, sleeplessness, restlessness, hysteria, and nervous conditions of all kinds. Its effects are both sedative and tranquilizing.

Dr. Houghton in the *Journal of Pharmacy and Pharmacology* (1999) writes that valerian, in addition to containing GABA (which causes sedation), inhibits the breakdown of GABA in the brain, prolonging its sedative effect. An added bonus of valerian is that unlike conventional tranquilizers and sedatives, and unlike recreational relaxants like alcohol and marijuana, it may not have any negative impact on coordination. Dosages of valerian call for 150 to 300 mg in capsule form taken during times of stress.

Caution: Valerian should not be taken with alcohol or other sedatives or by patients with liver disease. Do not drive or operate machinery while taking any sedative. Many products contain alcohol. Do not take during pregnancy or while breast-feeding.

Kava Kava and Valerian Combination

Kava kava and valerian taken together produce a combined effect that appears to be stronger than the effect generated by each individual herb. Dr. Cropley and colleagues, as reported in *Phytotherapy Research* (2002), studied the effect of kava kava and valerian on response to stress in fifty-four healthy individuals. At the end of the trial, lowered blood pressure readings were reported among a majority of subjects, along with improved heart rate and relief from feelings of stress and pressure. The authors of the study conclude that the kava kava/valerian combination improves health by reducing physiological activity during stress and by generating the same calming influences that promote healthy sleep.

Caution: Although helpful as an antispasmodic during stomach distress, it can occasionally cause stomach upset and is believed to induce abortion.

Dr. Wheatley from the Psychopharmacology Research Group in London also studied the role of kava kava and valerian on subjects with stress-induced insomnia. As reported in *Phytotherapy Research* (2001), the authors claim that these herbs used in combination not only reduce the severity of stress among patients, but help subjects get a better night's sleep. For more information on valerian and kava kava, see Chapter 4.

Chamomile

Chamomile is mentioned many times throughout this book, primarily as an aid to digestive health. It is also a first-class relaxant. Though perhaps not as powerful as kava kava or valerian, chamomile exerts a subtle, quieting effect on body and mind, and clearly deserves a place in every overstressed person's medicine cabinet. Chamomile also helps relax spastic intestinal muscles and calms queasy stomachs. It acts as a mild sedative to sooth the nerves and focus the mind. It is nonaddictive, and, though relaxing, does not impair motor function.

St. John's Wort

St. John's wort is another recent star in the herbal antistress tool chest. In more than thirty double-blind studies conducted worldwide, St. John's wort has been shown to engender significant antidepressant effects in mild to moderate cases of chronic depression. It works by exerting a substantial serotonin-boosting effect on the central nervous system, reducing depression for many patients as successfully as commercial prescription antidepressants such as Paxil or Prozac. Even for people who are not clinically depressed, St. John's wort appears to exert a mood-enhancing effect.

Note that, like prescription antidepressants, this herb requires several weeks to build up a sufficient blood level, which means that time and patience are required until the positive effects click in. The optimal safe and effective dose, as determined in clinical tests, is 300 mg of the extract taken three times daily.

Some vendors of St. John's wort, especially those who market cheaper products, simply crush and process the herb, selling it in a less powerful, non-extracted form. The term "0.3 percent hypericin" on the label tells you that the useful chemicals in the herb have all been extracted and potentized.

Caution: St. John's wort occasionally interacts poorly with conventional antidepressants, especially SSRIs such as Prozac or Paxil. If you are taking medications, especially a prescription antidepressant, be sure to discuss St. John's wort use with your doctor before putting it to the test.

Siberian Ginseng

Botanically speaking, Siberian ginseng (*Eleutherococcu senticosus*) is not ginseng at all, although it exerts many of the same healing effects as its namesake. Its primary use is as an "adaptogen," that is, an herb that protects the body from a host of perils including adverse weather conditions, environmental hazards, and the general effects of stress, sorrow, and overwork.

Physiologically, Siberian ginseng bolsters adrenal function and strengthens immune response. It is often prescribed for persons suffering from chronic fatigue syndrome. In one double-blind trial, as reported by Drs. Bohn, Nebe, and Birr in *Arzneimittelforschung* (1987), a group of healthy volunteers were given 10 ml of fluid extract of Siberian ginseng, while another group was given a placebo. Subjects taking the extract showed strong health benefits, including a dramatic increase in T-helper cells, which power the immune system to fight off infection. The placebo group showed no improvement.

The recommended dose of Siberian ginseng is between 100 and 200 mg taken once or twice a day. After two months, it is recommended that its use be discontinued for two weeks, then resumed for another two-month course.

Other Useful Herbs for Overcoming Stress

Other herbs known to reduce stress levels and elevate mood include the following:

- Hops
- Lavender flowers
- Lemon balm
- Peppermint leaves
- Passionflower
- Linden flowers

Rest and Relaxation

It is easy to overlook the part played by rest and relaxation in the battle against stress. But when you think about it, leisure, wholesome recreation, and time away from the daily grind are some of your strongest allies in this area.

This statement may seem obvious. Yet, as a doctor, I am amazed to find some of my most highly pressured patients complaining about a host of stress-related gut problems and then seeking relaxation through sedatives, alcohol, drugs, pick-me-ups, and antistress medications. These overburdened men and women ignore the most obvious fact: the best way to unwind is simply to slow down and take it easy.

Following are discussions of high-quality rest-inducers, many of which may seem obvious, but are often overlooked and clearly worth heeding.

Get a Good Night's Sleep on a Regular Basis

Sound sleep is one of the strongest bulwarks we have against stress. At least seven or eight hours of sleep each night is ideal. Conversely, lack of sleep causes stress—often a great deal more stress than we suppose.

Eat Better

Do certain foods cause tension and stress? Absolutely. How about that extra cup of coffee? Or tea? Both are loaded with caffeine, as are many cola drinks. Don't underestimate their overstimulating effects on the nervous system. For some people, hot, spicy foods are disturbing to mental equilibrium, which is why Chinese and Ayurvedic physicians often discourage them. Junk foods, too many sweets, skipping meals, eating when exhausted or upset—such careless habits weaken the system, and a weakened system is a tense system.

In general, eating properly is one of the least talked about yet most important methods of fighting stress. Consult Chapters 1 and 2 for information on the relationship between eating well and good digestive health.

Allow Yourself More Breaks During the Day

Many of us become so hypnotized by the work in front of us, so driven by deadlines and must-dos, that we forget a crucial fact of life: at a certain point in the day, non-stop exertion generates tension and fatigue, which in turn causes a decline in the quality of work. It's a case of diminishing returns.

Happily, the fix is an easy one. Get up from your desk for a few minutes every hour or so. Walk around. Stretch. Breathe deeply. Drink a glass of water or a cup of herbal tea. Talk to a friend or coworker. Look out the window. Go outside for a few minutes. Get in the habit of taking small rests a number of times a day. The therapeutic benefits add up.

Workaholism is a disease of our time, and many people do not allow themselves the luxury of slacking off—*ever*. This attitude is not only counterproductive to health but also to the quality of the work produced. Time away from the responsibilities of life recharges our batteries and allows us to do a better job when we return. Afford yourself the luxury.

Take a Vacation

Even a weekend getaway is invigorating, defusing the tensions of the week, the month, the year. Take a trip to that historical monument you've wanted to see. Go on a cruise. Visit that friend in Ohio or California. Attend that ballgame. Have a whirlwind weekend in Las Vegas. Make a short retreat. Or simply take an occasional day off from the office, store, and household chores. Leave the kids with the grandparents. Park the dog at a friend's house. Go for it. No doubt you've more than earned the time off. Breaks from the routine work wonders on composure and self-esteem. Just do it.

Cultivate Outside Interests

Studies find that dedicated involvement in a personal interest is an important element in maintaining health and longevity. The moral is to fill your leisure time with pleasant and diverting activities such as gardening, photography, cooking, quilting, reading, sketching and painting, raising tropical fish, computer programming, breeding dogs, hiking in nature, woodworking, needlepoint, bicycling, fixing up old cars, collecting collectibles, maintaining your own Web site, learning a language, playing a sport, editing home videos, or volunteering at a local school, animal shelter, hospital, or fire department—you name it. The trick is to find a pastime that involves you emotionally and mentally, and give yourself to it fully. The rewards can be tremendous.

Strive to Stay Positive

It's been said a thousand times, but it is always true: It is better to see the glass half full than half empty. Good things are on the way. Life is reasonably happy, and sometimes really great. Bad things come along, sure, but so do good things. Studies show that people who cultivate an upbeat attitude toward their work, their friends, their love lives, and their families live longer, stay healthier, recover from disease more quickly, and enjoy life to a greater extent than those who dwell on the negatives.

A hundred years ago, the French pharmacist Emil Coue introduced a simple exercise that swept Europe and America. Subjects were told to stand in front of a mirror every morning and repeat the following statement twenty times: "Every day in every way I am getting better and better."

Participants did not have to ponder these words or even think about them while reciting. The words themselves did the job. "Every thought that completely fills our mind becomes true for us, and has a tendency to transform itself into action," wrote Coue in his essay "Instructions for Practitioners of the Method."

Though laughed at by turn-of-the-century experts, today we know that Coue's deceptively simple method is a well-structured exercise in positive autosuggestion. At the time, thousands of men and women claimed that their lives were dramatically improved by repeating this phrase, and a number of people still recite Coue's happy mantra to their mirrors every day.

Pessimists among us will counter by saying that life may not, in fact, be getting better and better. This is true. On the other hand, it may. Who knows? Who can predict? And, anyway, why practice what Fritz Perls, founder of Gestalt therapy, once called "catastrophic expectation"? Why assume the worst? Why not assume the best? It's just as easy to do, just as likely to happen, doing it feels a whole lot better than dwelling on the negative, and in the long run it brings better results.

The essential point to remember is that, the more you repeat positive affirmations to yourself, the deeper they penetrate into your subconscious, and the more likely they are to become self-fulfilling prophecies. Ultimately, we are what we think we are.

Deep Breathing

Deep breathing is one of the fastest and most efficient methods we know of to achieve body-mind relaxation and to still the diverting thoughts that continually flow through our brains. Spiritual practitioners both East and West have long been privy to this secret, that deep breathing quiets the mind as well as the body. For this reason, they often begin their meditations with a round of deep inhalations and exhalations, both to steady their concentration and to create a sense of well-being that directly encourages tranquillity.

A set of therapeutic breathing exercises is featured in Chapter 6; see "Practicing Breathing and Breath Control Exercises" on page 132. I suggest that you incorporate the powerful breathing techniques described there into your antistress regimen.

Biofeedback

Many of the body's physiological functions work on their own without our knowledge or participation. Circulation, skin temperature, respiration, heartbeat, and digestion are all autonomous functions that require little or no attention from our conscious minds. We are, in fact, the passive recipients of these functions, if not their total prisoners.

Still, recent developments in medical electronics have made it clear that the mind can exert greater command over these functions than we previously supposed and that, if certain unconscious functions like blood pressure or involuntary muscle movements are monitored electronically, the mind can learn to modify these processes to some extent and even control them.

One device ideally suited to this task is the biofeedback machine, both the sophisticated models used in professional clinics and the scaled-down commercial appliances designed for home use.

Clinical biofeedback machines monitor tension changes in the subject's muscular system. These changes are registered by a series of high-pitched sounds (or sometimes flashes, beeps, and the like) that rise and fall in sync with a person's shifting tensions. As relaxation increases, the machine emits correlative sounds or flashes. While monitoring this feedback, the patient and the biofeedback therapist often work together to interpret responses or to perform visualization and relaxation exercises.

Biofeedback, in other words, is a kind of benevolent Pavlovian interface between human and machine. Eventually, by participation in regular biofeedback sessions, patients learn to relax many of the physiological functions they once thought were involuntary and to gain control of the way these functions respond to stress. The final goal is to become free of the machine entirely and to relax one's internal functions by the power of the mind alone.

Many overstressed persons have found a substantial measure of relaxation and relief from disease pain and stress by using biofeedback, both on their own and assisted by biofeedback experts. Dr. Heymann and colleagues from Germany, as reported in the *American Journal of Gastroenterology* (2000), found that patients suffering from irritable bowel syndrome (IBS) showed faster recovery and greater improvement using biofeedback than patients treated with conventional methods alone. The authors conclude that the combination of medical treatment along with multicomponent behavioral treatment such as biofeedback is a superior method to medical treatment alone. Dr. Emmanuel and Dr. Kamm from the United Kingdom, as reported in the journal *Gut* (2001), likewise report that biofeedback not only positively affects the pelvic areas but also improves the activity of direct brain signaling to the gut, hastening the movement of feces through the bowels and speeding up elimination. The beneficial effects of biofeedback in fecal incontinence and constipation have also been documented in several studies.

Self-Suggestion Exercises and Meditation

Over the past few decades, medical researchers have come to realize that the practices of self-suggestion and in-depth meditation can, when properly applied, produce significant long-term benefits in health and in a person's ability to improve performance on the job.

Both of these methods, self-suggestion and meditation, relax the muscles, lower blood pressure, decrease pulse rate, sharpen concentration, elevate mood, improve the quality of sleep, and refresh the mental and physical faculties, enabling a person to deal more effectively with the stresses of daily living.

At the present time, there is abundant amount of clinical information supporting the positive role that meditation and relaxation exercises play in personal health. According to Dr. G. D. Jacobs of the Harvard Medical School, studies presented in several hundred peer-reviewed articles demonstrate conclusively that relaxation exercises and mind-body interventions are useful in the treatment of a variety of diseases caused by or made worse by stress. Recent data suggest that these techniques are useful in relieving insomnia, helping chronic headaches, strengthening immune response, and improving the prognosis of heart disease. Dr. Jacobs cautions, however, that mind-body therapies are not panaceas and that they often work best when used in conjunction with standard medical care.

In one study, as reported in the *American Journal of Health Promotion* (2000), Dr. Herron and Dr. Hillis evaluated the collective impact of transcendental meditation (TM) on the government health-care system. Their findings showed that long-term practice of TM can help lower national health-care costs considerably. Over a six-year period, regular TM meditators spent 5 to 13 percent less annually for medical expenses than members of the control group.

Dr. Mason and associates, as reported in the journal *Sleep* (1997), compared the sleep patterns of people practicing TM with the sleep of control subjects. Investigators found that people who practiced TM slept better than those in the control group.

There is, of course, an enormous amount of instructive material on relaxation and meditation currently available. If the subject interests you, a short sampling of books and tapes on the topic is featured in the Appendix. Meanwhile, discussed below are two effective, get-you-started exercises—one a mind-body relaxation via self-suggestion and the other a beginner's meditation. Both will give you a taste of how these techniques work and how they reduce stress both on a physical level and on a mental level.

Body Mind Relaxation Exercise

Lie down on a comfortable surface, stretch out, and take several deep breaths. Keep your hands at your sides and your legs comfortably spread about a foot apart. Start by concentrating on your scalp. Tense this area as tightly as possible, holding the pressure for five seconds. You can maintain tension longer if you wish, but never less than five seconds. Now release, feeling the looseness in the scalp area that results. Tense your forehead for the same amount of time, or longer if you wish. Hold. Relax. Breathe deeply. Now tense your eyes. Nose. Mouth. Tongue. Ears. The back of your head. Tighten each of these areas for a minimum of five seconds, then release and let go. Feel the pleasant sense of ease and lightness that follows.

From the head continue down your body, section by section. Tighten your neck, release, and relax. Then tighten your upper back. Do the same with your shoulders, chest, upper arms, lower arms, wrists, and hands. Tighten and release your rib cage, stomach, abdomen, and your lower back. Tighten and release the hips, buttocks, groin, thighs and knees, calves, ankles, feet, and toes.

By now, you should be experiencing a kind of dreamy, comfortable vacuum throughout your entire body. Enjoy the many pleasant sensations that are flowing through you. Pent-up stress in your muscles is being released like the tension from a spring. Your blood is circulating faster. Your lymph glands are being toned. Savor the feeling.

While tightening and releasing, keep your mind as blank as possible. Quiet. Empty. If you find this task difficult, dwell instead on pleasant thoughts, on beautiful landscapes you have enjoyed in the past, on happy memories. Disturbing images or arousing images should be dismissed. They cause tension and tightness.

After you have moved down your entire body in this way, tensing and relaxing all its parts, take several more deep breaths. Your body is now deeply relaxed, and your mind is more receptive than usual to suggestion. Continue as follows.

Imagine that your body is filled with water from head to toe. Make a mental picture of it—you are a container full of water.

Imagine that you are about to slowly drain this water down and out of your body. Tell yourself that when you finish the draining process, you will feel delightfully buoyant and empty. A sense of release and relaxation will surely follow.

Start at your head. Imagine that the water is slowly flowing downward, level by level, from the top of your head to the soles of your feet. Picture the volumes of water moving down from your head to your neck, then to your chest and stomach. Picture the water running down your arms and out your fingers.

Continue bringing the water level down through your abdomen and groin, through your thighs and calves, into your feet, and finally out a hole in the middle of each foot. In Chinese acupuncture, this point in the center of the foot is known as the "bubbling spring" and is used in many exercises to rid the body of negative energy or what acupuncturists refer to as "evil chi."

Repeat this mental draining exercise two or three times. At the end of the second or third session, shift your point of concentration to the "holes" on the bottom of your feet. Imagine that the water is continuing to run out through these holes. Imagine that jets of water are shooting out of the holes like the spray from a fountain, emptying your entire body. Maintain this image for five to ten minutes, or longer if you like.

The water, of course, represents the tension in your body, and the draining is a visualization technique that, with the help of your own mental self-suggestions and a trick of the mind, helps eliminate the stress that has been storing itself up inside you for days, weeks, months, or years. At the end of the session, you will experience a delightful sensation of refreshment and invigoration. Some people feel as if they have taken a nap or are just getting up in the morning.

When you have finished the exercise, take a few deep breaths, stretch a bit, get up, and get on with your new day.

A Simple Exercise in Meditation

Sit in a comfortable chair, keeping your back as straight as possible. An erect spine is a prerequisite to any form of meditation. It allows the energy to circulate freely through your nervous system and keeps you focused and awake.

Take several deep breaths. At this point, you may wish to practice one or two of the breathing exercises featured in Chapter 6.

Now close your eyes and start to count from one to ten, picturing each number in your mind's eye as you count. One. Two. Three. Four. Five . . . A useful trick is to imagine that the numbers are being written on a blackboard in front of you, or on a piece of white paper in black ink.

At first, this exercise seems simple. The numbers flow easily. Then, soon enough, vagrant thoughts start to enter your thinking space and the mind wanders, carrying you off in a river of daydreams and images. Concentration is lost.

When attention wanders this way, simply bring your awareness back to the counting process and continue. Over and over and over. The meditating mind has two compartments, the visual compartment and the verbal compartment. Both must be kept fully involved if the mediation is to work properly. In this exercise, the verbal part of the mind is kept fixed on a single point of concentration by counting the numbers. The visual part is occupied by picturing the numbers. In this way, ideally, no part of the cognitive faculty is left over to dwell on idle thoughts.

Keep on counting. When you reach the number ten, start counting backward—ten, nine, eight, seven . . . After counting back to the number one, begin counting upward again from one to ten, and so on, continuing the cycle.

As you go, try to keep distracting thoughts to a minimum. It doesn't matter if these distracting thoughts are happy or sad, creative or useless. You can think them all at a later time. Right now, your goal is to fix your attention solely on the numbers.

When your attention does wander, as it inevitably will, simply bring it back to the numbers and keep counting. For reasons not entirely understood, the simple act of harnessing the mind and keeping it riveted to a single image (or prayer, invocation, mantra, or whatever) slows down brain waves and allows vital functions such as heartbeat, respiration, circulation, and digestion to rest, heal, and restore themselves—the mind-body connection at its best. This is where meditation really earns its stripes. When your mind does stray from time to time, as it must, avoid feeling irritated or self-critical. These feelings are distractions too and will quickly carry you away.

To achieve a successful meditation practice, one should sit every day for ten to fifteen minutes, once in the morning and once in the evening. Try not to skip a day. Some people meditate right before going to bed. This is a good idea, as meditation is known to enhance sleep as well as relaxation.

Over time, as you improve, you may wish to extend your sitting time and also to seek formal meditation instruction. There are many books and tapes on the subject (see Appendix), as well as a number of spiritually and psychologically oriented organizations that teach these techniques.

Meanwhile, the exercise presented here is simple enough for any beginner to master, challenging enough to awaken a taste for the inner stillness and peace of mind that result from this ancient technique. If you are a first-time meditator, consider yourself in for an adventure. Good luck.

In a nutshell, your big brain is connected to—and interacts with—the little brain in your gut. While the gut has a mind of its own, stress in this area can be alleviated by reducing stress on the big brain and thus keeping your digestive system running like a well-oiled machine.

chapter six

Improving Digestive Function and Eliminating Stomach Distress with Yoga

In the West, when stomach distress strikes, we reach for the medicine bottle. In India, where the art of yoga has been practiced for centuries, physical stretches and breathing techniques are the first line of defense for millions of men, women, and children.

How can this be? How can simple (and sometimes not so simple) body postures and breathing gymnastics offset the pains of indigestion, diarrhea, constipation, and other common gut problems? In several ways. First, followers of yoga know that, by assuming prescribed physical positions and by bolstering these efforts with breath control, a number of physiological changes result in body metabolism.

Increased blood circulation is one of these changes. Muscle relaxation and relief of tension in stressed areas is another. Certain yoga postures activate the production of enzymes or the stimulation of hormones. Others promote lymph circulation. Still others accelerate oxygen assimilation during respiration and activate electrical nerve impulses that run up and down the spine.

119

These effects, in turn, boost our immunological lines of defense. They balance metabolism and strengthen the muscular and skeletal systems. They make the joints, tendons, and spine more supple; encourage the release of helpful hormones into the blood; and increase the effectiveness of the body's natural healing powers.

Since each yoga exercise is designed to stimulate a different set of organs and a different set of muscles, a major part of the science of yoga is matching the right postures—called *asanas*—to the right physical problem. Some asanas benefit the heart. Some improve joint flexibility or heighten mental clarity. And some are designed specifically to improve the health of the gut.

Yoga postures may, for instance, massage the organs of digestion and stimulate digestive juices. Others increase stomach acid, tone abdominal viscera, rid the colon of toxins, speed up elimination, and increase circulation throughout the entire digestive system. That's for starters.

As modern medicine now knows, so-called "simple stress" is the hidden trigger behind an amazingly large number of physical problems. When stress strikes, the tendons tighten and stomach muscles become knotted. The heart races and the blood pressure elevates, sometimes to a dangerous degree. Breathing turns choppy and uneven, and a general sense of anxiety and dis-ease follows. For people with vulnerable stomachs, the aftermath of these tense moments is often centered directly in the gut area where tension triggers a number of physical symptoms, including diarrhea, constipation, heartburn, stomach cramps, and indigestion.

Enter the ancient art of yoga. Perhaps the one benefit that everyone reports from practicing this exercise system is release from tension. After an hour's session of stretching, bending, twisting, and deep breathing, agreement is unanimous that stress levels decrease dramatically, that a sense of centeredness and gravity prevails, and that an overall feeling of well-being pervades the entire body. The negative side effects of stress wane and, with them go stress-related stomach and intestinal problems.

Finally, on a more mystical level, yoga exercises, as well as other Eastern exercise systems, are designed not only to boost physiological response, but also to improve the flow of subtle body energies. Known to followers of yoga as *prana* and to practitioners of Chinese exercise systems as *chi,* this subtle energy, it is believed, is compromised by the insults visited on our bodies during the course of everyday living. Poor diet, overweight, smoking, alcohol abuse, insufficient sleep, lack of physical activity, workaholism, environmental stressors such as pollution and noise, and even negative emotions such as anger and depression, all contribute to the weakening of the prana, and thus to a decline in physical health. Again, yoga to the rescue.

Like all parts of the body, the stomach, bowels, and related digestive organs depend on a steady flow of prana for their well-being. When this flow is disturbed, discomfort follows, and ultimately illness takes hold. According to Eastern medical theory, the root cause of most diseases is not bacteria or viruses—these are secondary invaders that thrive only when the body's lines of defense are weakened. Sickness originates when the flow of prana is weakened.

Remedy? Yoga. By practicing a regimen of yoga exercises for a few minutes every day, yoga practitioners firmly believe that we can offset the prana-destroying effects that modern lifestyle brings. These exercises neutralize the toxins that enter our bodies and minds. They keep the flow of subtle energies properly moving inside us. They bring psychological wellness and physical fitness. As a famous yoga text puts it, practice yoga faithfully every day and good health follows "as surely as the plow follows the ox."

DEGREES OF COMMITMENT

There is no need to become a dedicated, full-time practitioner of yoga to profit from its postures and exercises, however. Benefits can be gained by practicing these techniques for as little as ten to fifteen minutes a day. Full-time commitment is by no means required. A little yoga goes a long way.

At the same time, as you put the following stretches and breathing exercises to work for you on a regular basis, you may gradually find that the calmness, well-being, and confidence that yoga engenders become addictive. Yoga asanas not only improve digestive function, but also enhance physical, mental, and emotional function, thereby improving mood, heightening sensitivity, curing old aches and pains, increasing energy, and making the world a brighter, nicer place to live in.

Many followers of the yogic arts begin the practice of yoga simply to improve their health and end up becoming full-time devotees.

Finally, while performing yoga, some people like to play soothing music, while others prefer silence. Exercisers can suit themselves in this regard, though traditionally yoga is practiced in a tranquil, meditative environment.

MORE THAN AN EXERCISE PROGRAM

In the pages that follow, you will be introduced to a series of basic yet powerful yoga postures, all of which have earned their stripes for centuries as a way to prevent gut problems before they occur and as a way to heal them when they appear. Before beginning this unique and sometimes exotic method of healing, there are several important things you should know.

The first point to note is that, contrary to popular notion, yoga is not simply an exercise system. It is an ethical philosophy and a spiritual path as well. In India, yoga is recognized as one of the six schools of orthodox Hinduism, a practical refinement of ideas originally presented in ancient Hindu texts such as the Bhagavad Gita, the Vedas, and the Upanishads. Using an array of contemplative tools such as chanting, music, dance, mantra repetition, meditation, prayer, and personal interaction with a guru, yogis (yoga practitioners) strive to induce states of higher consciousness and to gain control over both body and mind. The study of yoga, as a yoga teacher once told me, involves the taming of the body, the study of the mind, and the enlightenment of the soul.

The strange and wonderful physical exercises now so popular in the West are thus only a part of yoga. For its literally millions of practitioners around the world, yoga is a method for keeping fit and trim, yes. But it is also a road to spiritual development.

IDENTIFYING YOUR INVISIBLE ENERGY CENTERS

The map of the human body used by yogis differs dramatically from the anatomical charts you are likely to see on the walls of a Western physician's office.

While yoga exercises are engineered to work directly with physical organs such as the heart, stomach, and lungs, yoga practitioners also believe that the body consists of separate energy centers that cannot be seen with the eye but that exert a profound influence on every person's physical and spiritual destiny. These centers are known in yoga as chakras.

Most schools of yoga recognize seven basic chakras, or centers. These seven centers, they believe, are situated on a vertical axis starting in the pelvic area and moving upward along the spine to the top of the head.

The first chakra is located at the base of the spine where it contains raw, instinctive energy. The second chakra is in the genital area, the center of sex. The third chakra resides in the stomach, the seat of power. The fourth chakra is in the heart, the source of emotions and love. The fifth chakra is in the throat where it corresponds to the intellect. The sixth chakra is located directly between the eyes, ruling intuition and second sight (for which reason it is known as the "third eye"). And the seventh, or "crown chakra," is located at the top of the head. Once opened by practice and meditation, it is believed to bring spiritual enlightenment and cosmic vision.

Each of these centers also corresponds roughly to (although it should not be mistaken for) one of the body's endocrine glands and/or one of its principal nerve/energy centers.

There is no need for most readers to concern themselves too deeply with this esoteric anatomy, and most of us will wish to concentrate on the healing aspect of the exercises alone.

Nonetheless, it is a good idea to keep the theory of the chakras in mind when doing yoga, as practitioners report that when performing these exercises one or more of their vital centers is stimulated, with strange and sometimes profound sensations resulting. For this reason, serious practitioners are urged to work with an instructor who is familiar with the physical and mental reactions that sometimes occur during yoga sessions.

Some yogis, for example, note that after a brisk workout they experience a tingling or sense of warmth at the base of the spine. In yogic terms, this means that their first or lowest chakra has been aroused. Others describe unusually strong emotions of compassion after a yoga session, an indication that the heart chakra has been touched.

THE EXERCISES

You should consult a good comprehensive book on yoga, such as *Yoga: the Path to Holistic Health* by B. K. S. Iyengar; *How to Use Yoga: A Step-By-Step Guide to the Iyengar Method of Yoga, for Relaxation, Health and Well-Being* by Mira Mehta and Eláine Collins; and *I Can't Believe It's Yoga!: The Ultimate Beginner's Workout for Men and Women* by Lisa Trivell and Peter Field Peck, in order to learn the basics before engaging in these exercises. Once you're ready, the following sequence of yoga exercises should take twenty to thirty minutes to complete. Make it a point to perform these asanas (postures) in the same sequence at every session.

Uddiyana Bandha Asana (The Stomach Lift)

Abdominal benefits: Uddiyana Bandha is a superb exercise for energizing the entire abdominal area, as well as for exercising the lungs, heart, and diaphragm. It kneads the gastrointestinal region, toning and massaging the rarely exercised internal organs of the lower trunk. While performing this posture, the organs of digestion are stimulated, especially the liver and pancreas, and the lower parts of the intestines are drained of residual digestive juices. Relief of constipation follows, and over time abdominal fat is reduced. The central nervous system is relaxed, and there is substantial improvement in the assimilation, processing, and digestion of food substances.

Time: Several minutes.

Performing: From a comfortable standing position, bend forward and place your hands on your knees. As you bend forward, exhale briskly, forcing the air out of your lungs and stomach. Empty as much air as you can from the lungs—all of it, if possible. After you exhale intensely for several seconds, you may think the job is done. But there's still more air left to expel. Don't believe it? Try humming or making an "ahhhhh" sound as you continue to exhale. You'll be surprised to discover how much air is still left in your stomach and lungs.

After pressing out as much air as possible, tighten the muscles of your stomach and rectum, and pull your abdomen in toward your spine, raising your diaphragm as you do. This movement produces a kind of concave hollow across the abdominal region. Now push your stomach out, pull it in again, back and forth, in and out. This undulating motion produces a ripple or wave effect that deeply massages the internal organs. Continue the in-out movements as long as you can hold your out-breath, then relax and breathe in deeply. Rest for a minute, relax, and repeat. Uddiyana bandha should be performed at least four times in a row. People who are constipated can help the effectiveness of this exercise by drinking several glasses of water before they begin. The combination of water and stomach undulations has a positive and sometimes immediate effect on the bowels.

Caution: This exercise—and in fact all yoga exercises—is meant to improve your health, not to challenge your endurance. Don't hold your exhalation to the point of pain. When you feel a comfortable need to inhale, do so, then relax and enjoy the benefits the exercise brings. Pushing beyond one's limits always produces negative results.

Uttanasana Asana (Forward Bend from a Standing Position)

Abdominal benefits: Compressing the lower abdominal areas expels gas, activates digestive juices, and brings healing supplies of blood to the digestive organs. Since stress tends to manifest itself in the form of stomach tension for many people, a deep sense of relaxation is often noticed after performing this exercise. As a side benefit, blood is brought to the face and brain, helping focus mental attention and improving the complexion.

Time: Approximately three minutes.

Performing: From a standing position, raise your arms over your head. Exhale slowly and bend as far forward as you can. If you are limber, you may wish to touch the floor with your hands. If not, dangle your arms as close to the floor as they will comfortably go. Remain in this position for approximately a minute, breathing slowly and evenly. Then, very slowly, straighten up. As you come up, imagine that each vertebra of your spine is aligning itself with the one below it, click, click, click, like a row of blocks. Keep this image in mind as you slowly come up. When you reach the standing position, picture all of the vertebrae aligned in a straight row and perfectly in place. Stand quietly for a minute or two. Experience the stretch and increased movements of energy along your spine. Repeat one more time.

Caution: If you suffer from chronic lower back problems, consult with your doctor or physical therapist before adding this exercise to your routine.

Eka Pada Pavanamuktasana Asana (One Leg to Chest Gas-Reducing Posture)

Abdominal benefits: Eka Pada Pavanamuktasana is a wonderful exercise for expelling gas from the abdomen and for toning the gut. It is helpful if you frequently experience bloating after a meal. It also is an effective digestive for people who overeat.

Time: A set of five leg lifts done with each leg takes from three to four minutes. No rush.

Performing: Lie on your back with your legs out straight. Relax. Take several deep breaths. Clear your mind.

Inhale deeply. Bend your right leg at the knee. Clasp your hands around the knee and pull it to your chest. Remaining in this posture, and maintaining the in-breath, lift your head and slowly move it as close as possible to your raised knee. Hold this stretch for a few seconds, release, exhale, and return to the lying position. Do not force the movement by overstretching. Perform the same movement with the left leg. Alternate between the right leg and the left leg lifts, five knee hugs each side.

Yoga Mudra Asana (Sitting Position)

Abdominal benefits: Yoga Mudra is a classic posture for aiding problems of digestive distress such as indigestion, stomachache, loose bowels, constipation, and bloating. It is also used to reduce burping and to relieve intestinal gas.

Time: Five to ten seconds each repetition.

Performing: Sit on the floor in a cross-legged position, keeping your spine as straight as possible. Sit quietly for a moment or two. Breathe deeply. Relax. Now place your hands behind your back. Slowly bend forward as if to touch your head to the floor, exhaling as you go. Extend as far forward as you can, breathing normally. Hold for five to ten seconds, then straighten up.

Repeat this movement five or six times in a row, pausing to relax for a moment or two between each forward lean. As your limberness increases, attempt to hold this position for progressively longer periods of time. Two to three minutes per forward lean is a reasonable goal.

Caution: Do not push this one, especially in the beginning. Easy does it.

Sarvangasana Asana (Shoulder Stand)

Abdominal benefits: Known as "the whole body pose," this classic yoga stance increases circulation throughout the head and torso, stimulates digestive juices, helps the liver process wastes, brings blood to the brain, and tones the nervous system. It is often used as a specific against constipation and liver problems. Moreover, by assuming an upside-down posture, the normal pull of gravity is reversed, making Sarvangasana a corrective against prolapse, stomach paunch, and sagging abdominal muscles. This exercise is an excellent asana for people who cannot (or do not wish) to try a full headstand.

Time: Beginners should hold this position for approximately a minute. As time goes on, work to build up to several minutes.

Performing: Lie on your back for several minutes. Relax as deeply as you can. Keeping your legs together, raise your body slowly into a shoulder stand. Help the movement out by pushing the small of your back upward with your hands.

In the final position, your torso is almost vertical to the floor, your hands are locked into your lower back as support, and your chin is pressed tightly against your chest. The more perpendicular you keep your body, the better the results will be. Feel the blood rushing into your stomach, filling your body with warmth and well-being. This is one of the best of all yoga asanas for stomach problems, and also for general flexibility, circulation, and health.

Sitting Twist

Abdominal benefits: The slow, twisting motions performed in this exercise deeply massage the gut, ridding the gastrointestinal system of toxins, stimulating circulation, speeding up metabolism, loosening the spine, and generally strengthening the organs and muscles of the abdomen. With constant practice, digestion improves, regularity is maintained, and chronic gas subsides (including both the abdominal and burping varieties).

Time: Several minutes.

Performing: Sit comfortably on a chair or stool with your hands in your lap and your legs planted firmly on the floor. Place your feet about a foot apart. Take several deep breaths, then slowly twist your upper torso to the left, keeping your hands in your lap and your legs in place as you go. Take about thirty seconds to complete the full twist. Avoid straining or placing undue pressure on your spine. Most important, do not rush it. The slowness and steadiness of this movement are key ingredients to its effectiveness.

When you have reached your comfort zone, remain there for ten to twenty seconds, then slowly return to the starting position, again taking approximately thirty seconds to complete the movement. Repeat the same twisting motion to the right side.

In the beginning, perform one set of twists to each side. Over time, you can build up to two or three twists to each side. Breathe evenly and deeply as you perform this motion. When finished, sit for a few minutes, experiencing the subtle but very real sensations of energy flow that follow. These feelings are no illusion—they are the results of heightened blood circulation, muscle release, and increased circulation of the prana throughout the trunk and spinal areas.

Caution: As mentioned, do not twist beyond your comfort zone, especially if you have back problems. If you feel any pain at all, stop and consult with a doctor or physical therapist before continuing.

Paschimottanasana Asana (Forward Bend)

Abdominal benefits: Every organ in the abdomen, including the stomach, intestines, pancreas, kidneys, and liver, is nourished by this classic yoga posture. As a side benefit for men, the prostate gland profits from the extra blood that is moved into the lower trunk areas, and the sexual system is toned. Peristaltic action in the colon is likewise stimulated, and persistent cases of constipation and heartburn are known to clear up within a few weeks time by daily performance of this asana.

Time: Approximately three to four minutes.

Performing: Lie on your back with legs straight out and your arms straight over your head. Slowly raise your torso into a sitting position, keeping the legs straight. Place your hands on your knees. From this position, reach forward, grab your ankles, and pull your torso forward and downward. Be careful not to bounce. Simply let the forward and downward movement expand on its own. Increased flexibility in yoga does not come from forcing a stretch but from relaxing into it and letting the natural weight of the body do the work. Over time, you will notice that your flexibility improves and that your skill at particular exercises increases.

While the goal of this posture is to touch your head to your knees and hold it there, this is a difficult movement for many people, and it is suggested that in the beginning you simply bend as far forward as you can, find your comfort zone, and hold it there for approximately ten to fifteen seconds. Then slowly return to the lying position and relax. Repeat two more times. Breathe evenly and deeply as you stretch, but do not hold your breath at any point. Do not push your limits.

Hasta Pada Asana (Forward Bend Holding the Ankles)

Abdominal benefits: Each time you perform Hasta Pada, waste matter is forced to move more quickly through the intestines, cleansing the colon and preventing waste buildup in the gastrointestinal tract. Flabbiness and stomach bloating are reduced, and gas is eliminated. As a side benefit, this exercise is useful for stopping headaches, bringing blood to the head and face (and hence, for improving the complexion and clearing the mind), and for warming up cold hands and feet.

Time: One to two minutes.

Performing: From a standing position, exhale and bend your trunk forward at the waist, slowly sliding your hands down your legs until they grip your ankles. Once in this position, press your head as close as possible to your knees. Do not strain or overextend. Simply stretch as far forward and down as you can. Hold for five seconds, then slowly return to the standing position, inhaling as you rise. Repeat two to three times.

Caution: As usual, do not force this stretch or bounce as you bend forward. Let the weight of gravity do the stretching for you. The ability to move your head closer and closer to your knees will increase over time. The goal is not to achieve a perfect posture but to get the best stretch possible.

Utkatasana (Sitting in an Imaginary Chair Pose)

Abdominal benefits: This asana is usually referred to as the "chair pose." In Sanskrit, however, the term "Utkatasana" means "the power position." Besides strengthening the legs and hips, and helping straighten and align the spine, this asana brings blood to the stomach, strengthens the organs of digestion and elimination, and combats constipation and sluggish peristalsis.

Time: Approximately one minute to do three repetitions.

Performing: Stand with your feet shoulder-width apart and firmly planted on the floor. Exhale. Raise your hands over your head, inhale, and squat down halfway, as if you were sitting in a chair. You will immediately feel pressure on your thighs and a kind of burning warmth at the base of your spine.

Hold this position and your breath for ten seconds, then exhale and return to a standing position. As time goes on, try to increase your "sitting" time in the imaginary chair to thirty seconds. Perform three repetitions each session, resting a few moments in between each set.

Caution: Do not hold this position to the point of pain. If your legs shake, this is a danger signal from the knees. They are telling you to stand up immediately.

Padmasana (Lotus Posture), Siddhasana, and Vajrasana

Abdominal benefits: The three sitting postures featured in this entry are closely related in form and function, and are all used for exercise and during meditation. Designed to balance the body and center the awareness, all three postures calm the nervous system and increase intestinal relaxation.

Time: Five minutes or more, at the sitter's discretion.

Performing: First, the simple Padmasana: Sit on the floor in a cross-legged position. Keep your spine as straight as possible. Gaze straight ahead, focusing on a point in the air approximately three feet in front of you. Relax your stomach and expand your chest. Breathe deeply and evenly. Simply sitting in this position a few minutes every day brings therapeutic results. It is also a classic posture for meditation.

The advanced form of the Padmasana calls for sitting in the same position, but this time place your right foot on top of your left thigh, and your left foot on top of your right thigh. This stretch takes a bit of doing, and usually requires a few months' work before it can be mastered. Don't push it.

Next, the Siddhasana, a modified form of the Padmasana. Sit cross-legged as above, but this time place your right foot on top of your right calf. This posture produces a wonderful stretch to the hamstrings and calves of both legs. Many yogis prefer it for meditation.

Finally, the Vajrasana: Assume a full kneeling position, placing one hand on either knee. Look straight ahead and keep your spine erect. Try sitting in this posture for a few minutes. It helps speed up digestion and relieve stomach pain. The Vajrasana is also used as a meditation posture, both by yogis and Zen practitioners.

PRACTICING BREATHING AND BREATH CONTROL EXERCISES

Breathing exercises, or *pranayama* as they are called by yogis, are used in yoga to relax and to amplify the healing force generated by the physical postures. Both disciplines should be performed at the same session—first exercise, then breath control.

Find a quiet, well-ventilated space. In the beginning, ten minutes of breathing exercises is adequate. Over time, you may wish to increase the time and add further breathing exercises to your regimen.

Advanced practitioners of breathing exercises prefer sitting in the lotus posture or Padmasana (see page 132). Most beginners find the normal cross-legged "tailor" posture conducive to keeping the spine straight, a prerequisite when performing pranayama. If the cross-legged position is inconvenient, sit in a straight-back chair, keeping your neck and back as straight as possible. A zafu or meditation cushion, available from suppliers of yoga equipment (see Appendix), also makes an excellent seat. Some yoga teachers recommend sitting on silk or fur while performing breathing exercises and facing north or east. Both practices are said to improve the flow of prana.

The following three breathing exercises provide a taste of the serenity and centeredness that result from yogic breath control. The benefits of this discipline are many and are usually experienced right away, even during the first session. Besides bringing deep relaxation and relief from tension, deep breathing stimulates the lungs, the stomach, and the internal organs, and helps clean and oxygenate the entire system. The effectiveness of the immune system is accordingly enhanced.

Although deep breathing is not absolutely required, it is a wonderful complement to the physical exercises and is highly recommended. The regenerative powers of deep breathing help fortify and heal the gut almost as effectively as the postures themselves.

Breathing Exercise One:
The Three-Stage Cleansing Breath

Most people are chest breathers. That is, most people breathe only from the upper part of their lungs, while the lower lungs and stomach remain largely inactive. You can verify this statement by observing your own breathing patterns during the day.

Note how shallow your breath is when you are seated at a desk or walking down the street. Notice how little your stomach and lower rib cage are involved in the rhythms of breathing. Even when performing vigorous aerobic exercise, the tendency is to breathe—"pant" might be a better word—from the upper rib cage. The lower areas of the thorax go largely unexercised and unused.

When performing pranayama, however, the muscular movements of the abdomen, lower lungs, and upper lungs all work as a unit and are all integrated into a single long, deep breath. The depth and pumping action this method produces multiply oxygen intake many times. Soon you find yourself breathing in a new way.

Here's how three-stage breathing works:

1. Inhale. For the first third of the inhalation, bring the air directly into your abdomen, expanding your stomach into a pot belly.
2. For the second part of the breath, bring the inhalation up from the abdomen into the chest and the mid region of your lungs.
3. For the third part of the inhalation, inhale into the upper regions of the chest and lungs. Raise your shoulders and upper torso slightly as you perform this maneuver. Then exhale in one steady breath.

These three motions, breathing into the abdomen, into the mid lungs, then into the upper lungs, are done in one long, continuous inhalation. Do not pause at any point. The entire process takes five to ten seconds, depending on a person's experience and lung capacity. When you perform this exercise properly, the movement of air from the lower trunk to the middle and upper trunk flows naturally and produces a feeling of total inflation.

Next, we apply this three-part breathing to what yogis call the Cleansing Breath. Start by inhaling, keeping your eyes open and spine as straight as possible. Fill your lungs to capacity using the three-stage method described above. Hold the inhalation for three to five seconds, then slowly exhale. Perform ten inhalations and ten exhalations in this way. When breathing in, keep your back straight. When breathing out, bend slightly forward.

Many people like to further enhance the benefits of breath control with a visualization. For example, as you perform the Cleansing Breath, picture yourself walking in a beautiful mountain landscape or flower-filled meadow feeling joyous and free. Or imagine that you are visiting a loved one, talking happily, laughing, embracing. Some people picture themselves at work, coping beautifully with the day's tasks, or dealing with daily problems in a clear and mindful way. The type of visualization you choose is at your discretion. Be sure the pictures you form are friendly, positive, and healing.

After performing one round of the Three-Stage Cleansing Breath, rest for a minute or two and savor its effects. People who practice the Three-Stage Cleansing Breath for the first time are often amazed at the degree of relaxation and well-being it brings. Deep breathing is nature's own tranquilizer. No side effects to worry about, no hangover, no addiction. If you wish, you can repeat this exercise one more time.

Breathing Exercise Two: The Rhythmic Breath

A bit more advanced than the Three-Stage Cleansing Breath, the Rhythmic Breath is done, as its name describes, by breathing in and out to a prescribed number of beats. While advanced rhythmic yoga breathing exercises require complicated counting procedures, this exercise is simple and straightforward yet extremely powerful.

Let's begin. With your spine, neck, and head straight, inhale evenly to a count of eight, using the three-stage technique described above. Count slowly to yourself as you inhale—one, two, three, four . . . Each beat should be approximately a second in length.

When fully inflated, hold your breath to a count of four. Then exhale to a count of eight. Repeat the cycle again, inhaling to count, holding your breath to count, breathing out to count. Do not stop in between breaths. Do ten complete breaths.

Savor the feelings of emptiness and repose the breathing brings. You may wish to complement this exercise with visualizations, as described for the Cleansing Breath above. As with the Three-Stage Cleansing Breath, it is important to empty your mind of unpleasant thoughts as you breathe.

Breathing Exercise Three:
Alternating Nostril Breath

A still more advanced breathing exercise is the Alternating Nostril Breath. Although this exercise sounds complicated when described, with a little practice it can be quickly mastered. It provides excellent relief from stress and from stage fright when facing a new and difficult situation. It helps focus the mind and is useful before sitting down to any challenging mental task. People with common digestive problems such as heartburn and stomach cramps often find this exercise helps lesson their symptoms. At the least, Alternating Nostril Breath promotes deep feelings of relaxation and builds powers of concentration. Buddhist monks and yogis often practice it as a prelude to meditation.

Sit in a comfortable position with your spine, neck, and back straight. With your index finger, tightly close your right nostril. Using the three-stage breathing technique described above, inhale into your left nostril slowly and evenly to a count of eight.

When you have inhaled to capacity, hold your breath for a count of four. Then cover the left nostril, and exhale evenly through the right nostril to a count of eight. Hold to a count of two when all the air is exhaled.

On the next breath, continue to keep your left nostril covered and inhale again through your right nostril, again to a count of eight. Hold your breath to a count of four. Then close the right nostril and exhale through the left to a count of eight. Continue to alternate nostrils in this way, performing ten repetitions. One inhalation and one exhalation equals one full breath.

When beginning this exercise, you may feel a bit light-headed. If you experience dizziness after the first few breaths, stop the exercise, breathe normally, and wait for the symptoms to subside. Then continue. After practicing this breathing exercise for a few days, these sensations will pass.

When beginning your practice of yoga breathing, ten repetitions at a time is adequate. As the Alternating Breath becomes more familiar and easier to do, you may wish to extend the number of breaths. Try to practice every day.

OTHER YOGA PRACTICES FOR THE HEALTH OF THE GUT

By now, it should be apparent that yoga is a true holistic form of healing, a total body-mind system designed to treat the entire person. If you work with these exercises on a regular basis, you may thus want to take advantage of other yoga techniques that complement these practices and that enhance their effectiveness. Some of the more accessible of these techniques are described below.

Reduce the Amounts of Mucus in Your System

Yogis believe that too much mucus building up in the chest, head, and intestines is "impure." In medical terms, this means that mucus traps wastes and bacteria along its sticky surfaces, holds toxins in the body, and triggers colds, flu, and more serious diseases.

To eliminate mucus, yogis avoid phlegm-producing foods such as hot, spicy foods. Long-time practitioners also use a method known as *neti*. Neti is done by taking a length of rope and immersing it in salt water. The rope is threaded through one nostril and out the mouth, then pulled back and forth several times to clean and scour the nasal areas. Do not try this technique without guidance from an expert practitioner.

Some yogis simply sniff warm water directly into the nostrils and spit it out. You can also use salt water for this purpose if you prefer. For people prone to allergies, taking water into the nose can curtail sneezing fits. It also exerts a healing effect on stomach problems such as indigestion that are frequently exacerbated by mucus drip. Special neti cups are available from yoga supply stores. See the Appendix.

Breathe Deeply Whenever Possible

During the day, remember to breathe more with your entire abdominal and thorax areas and to increase the depth of each breath. If you live in a

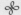
polluted area, keep an air filter in your home or apartment. Clean air purifies the digestive system and increases mental acuity.

Clean Your Tongue Regularly

Many yogis clean their tongues at least twice a day with a scraper, twig, or spoon. The process is known as *dhauti*. In the West, a toothbrush does the job just tolerably well. Use it to brush the top and bottom surfaces of the tongue for thirty seconds, or until the tongue feels clean and scoured. Keeping the tongue clean removes toxins and bacteria from the saliva. Since we also know that many cases of halitosis are produced by tongue bacteria, bad breath is also minimized by tongue brushing. Many drugstores sell plastic tongue cleaners.

Cleaning the tongue stimulates the taste buds and increases the flow of saliva. Since many important digestive enzymes are found in saliva, including ptyalin, a substance that breaks down the starches that cause indigestion and constipation, tongue cleaning aids digestion as well as increases personal hygiene.

Swallow Your Saliva Frequently

Saliva contains many digestive enzymes, and the intentional pooling of saliva and swallowing it throughout the day is a boon to digestive health. In Chinese medicine, saliva is known as the "Golden Elixir." There are many exercises in this system designed to increase saliva production. Swallowing copious amounts of saliva is believed by Chinese doctors to improve digestive function and to promote better health.

Chew All Food Thoroughly

Thorough mastication of food is stressed for yoga practitioners. Some yogis go so far as to chew each bite of food fifty times or more, though this is not a practical method for everyone. Simply chew your food as carefully and thoroughly as you can at each meal—twenty-five times each bite is a reasonable goal—and avoid swallowing large chunks of unmasticated food. Make an effort to keep the food in your mouth for as long a time as possible, allowing it to disintegrate and dissolve on its own. Thoroughly chewed food digests well and makes bowel movements larger and smoother.

Eat Slowly and Never to Excess

Leave the table feeling three-quarters full—that's the rule of thumb. Within twenty minutes, after the food has reached your stomach, you will then feel completely satisfied but not stuffed. Yogis and many practitioners of other natural health systems believe that chronic overeating is a prime cause of stomach distress and of ill health.

Drink Plenty of Pure Water During the Day

Everyone agrees: Drink at least eight glasses of pure water a day. Water cleanses the gastrointestinal tract and helps swell the size of the feces in the gut, stimulating elimination and fighting constipation.

Avoid Tight-Fitting Clothes

The body is built to breathe fully and easily, and to move in an unencumbered way. Tight bras, elastic stockings, binding shirts, and form-fitting pants, all cut off blood circulation and choke the natural flow of energy through the body. Whenever possible, wear loose-fitting, comfortable clothes, especially around the stomach area. In Chinese medicine, the stomach is considered the center of the life force as well as the processor of digestion. Strapping the stomach up with tight belts and elastic bands is, in this sense, a violation of a person's source of fundamental energy. There are cases of people who have become free of chronic gut distress simply by loosening their belts or by avoiding a belt entirely.

Meditate

In-depth meditation is the last and final stage of yoga, and is ordinarily taught to yoga pupils by a qualified teacher.

Although meditation practice is not a prerequisite to better health, it tends to enhance the healing effects of yoga postures and, at the same time, promotes a delicious sense of relaxation that is a soothing balm to the soul as well as to the digestive system. Why not give it a try?

chapter seven

Curds Are the Way:
The Many Healing Powers
of Yogurt

Some time ago, a number of professional health-care specialists were asked to name the three foods they considered to be the most contributive to human nutrition and good health in order of preference. Can you guess which ones made the final cut? Here's the result:

1. Yogurt
2. Salmon
3. Honey

Yogurt leads the pack, as it often does in such surveys. Perhaps this is one reason why a national survey of more than 500 primary-care general practitioners, carried out by Monroe Mendelsohn Research Company in July 2001, revealed that when physicians do, in fact, take the time to discuss nutrition with their patients, two out of three recommend that yogurt be added to the daily menu.

Health-care specialists and nutritionists all have their personal choice of favorite foods, of course, and there is always the expert who pops up and points out that honey is, after all, not an ideal food for diabetics, or that really, *some* people suffer allergic reactions to dairy products. Granted. Whatever the exceptions happen to be, however, generally speaking there is no doubt that yogurt is high on the universal good-for-you list of eatables, and for good reason.

Long a popular food in countries throughout the world, yogurt was already a staple when the Babylonians and the Assyrians were marching across the Middle East. A medical tract from seventh-century Syria, *The Great Explanation of the Power of the Element and Medicine,* states quite emphatically that yogurt aids digestion, regulates the intestinal tract, and is an excellent specific for "strengthening the stomach." According to Persian folklore, Abraham regularly ate yogurt in the belief that it contributed to his enhanced productivity and longevity. Perhaps it is coincidental, perhaps not, that the geographic areas of the planet where longevity rates have always been impressively high—the Caucasus, Bulgaria, southern Russia, Hunza in northern Pakistan—are also places where the population, young and old, eats yogurt several times a day. Interestingly, in one ancient Middle Eastern language, the word for yogurt is derived from the same linguistic root as the word for "life."

One yogurt legend, probably apocryphal, has it that yogurt first appeared in the Western world at the French court of Francis I. The ailing potentate was supposedly restored to health by a "secret formula" administered to him in a secret ritual by a mysterious Turk from Istanbul. The court physicians were so amazed by the healing properties of this marvelous elixir that they paid the Turk a king's ransom for his formula—which turned out to be none other than goat's milk yogurt.

According to Drs. Water, Keene, and Gershwin, in their article published in the *Journal of Nutrition* (1999), the beneficial effects of yogurt were first brought to the attention of Western medicine by a Dr. Metchnikoff in the early twentieth century. At the time, Dr. Metchnikoff attributed his own health and longevity to yogurt, going on to claim that "when people have learnt how to cultivate a suitable flora in the intestines of children as soon as they are weaned from the breast, the normal life may ex tend to twice my 70 years" (quoted in O. Metchnikoff, *The Life of Elie Metchnikoff.* Boston: Houghton Mifflin, 1921).

Following World War II, yogurt began to appear regularly on the Western supermarket shelf. For some time it languished there, a prisoner of its reputation as a sour-tasting sibling of buttermilk. By the 1960s, its star was on the rise, although now it was identified mainly with crunchy granola-eating hippies and "health-food" cranks.

Today, of course, all this has changed. According to the United States Department of Agriculture, the average American now eats between four and six pounds of yogurt a year. The market for this creamy treat has recently topped the $2.2 billion market in the United States and is expected to grow at a rate of 3 percent per annum.

We could go on extolling yogurt's popularity for some time, as well as the virtues of its derivatives, acidophilus milk and kefir (both soured milk, yogurtlike products in liquid form). Indeed, the sections below focus specifically on yogurt's digestive benefits, explaining how this wonder food remedies such common gastrointestinal tract problems as diarrhea, constipation, lactose intolerance, reactions to antibiotics, and more.

First, however, we must ask these basic questions: What are the ingredients and nutrients in yogurt that make it so healthy? How does it work inside the gut to deliver so many powerful benefits? And what does it really do to help our bodies and our minds?

INSIDE THE GUT: BACTERIA FRIENDLY AND UNFRIENDLY

Composed of countless numbers of living bio-organisms (one cup of cultured yogurt contains literally *billions* of helpful bacilli), once ingested these cultures make their way into the gastrointestinal tract. Here, they join other varieties of intestinal microflora, some of them neutral, some friendly, most transient, where they perform a variety of useful services for the body. These services include the following:

- Breaking down food and helping digest it
- Maintaining a healthy level of bile salts in the digestive system (bile salts fight toxic flora in the gut)
- Slowing the growth of health-threatening pathogens
- Reducing cholesterol
- Suppressing tumor growth. There is some indication that friendly microflora in the gut actually inhibits carcinogenesis and thus delays or prevents cancer formation. Some evidence suggests that certain bacteria helps shrink tumors, including the cancerous types
- Discouraging the proliferation and colonization of harmful microorganisms inside the wall of the gastrointestinal tract
- Stimulating the production of interferon, a group of proteins that increases the strength and activity of killer cells that form the core of the human immune system and are one of the body's first-line defenses against cancer
- Generating a natural antibiotic affect that destroys unfriendly putrefactive bacteria living in the bowel. These bacteria clog the digestive system, produce toxic wastes, and, in many cases, initiate disease.

The larger the number of friendly bacteria that live in our bowels, the more healthy our gastrointestinal systems become. Conversely, when friendly bacteria are destroyed in the gastrointestinal tract—that is, when they are, for example, washed away by laxatives, wiped out by antibiotics, starved by poor-quality food, or withered by high levels of stress—the biological ecology of our bowels is thrown out of kilter. The unfriendly organisms then multiply unchecked and quickly gain the upper hand. Possible results include constipation, diarrhea, stomachache, bloating, indigestion, and, in some cases, the development of serious internal disease.

One remedy for friendly microflora depletion is yogurt.

THE PREVENTIVE AND CURATIVE POWERS OF YOGURT

Which ailments in particular does yogurt protect us against? Which disorders does it actually cure? Before we discuss yogurt as healer, understand that at the present time many physicians remain somewhat skeptical concerning certain medicinal claims made for soured-milk products in general, and yogurt in particular. The mighty FDA refuses to allow food manufacturers to list medical claims on their soured-milk product labels, and perhaps this is a good thing, as claim-makers in the natural food business have been known to overstep their bounds.

At the same time, health-care professionals who are friendly toward natural remedies swear by yogurt as a specific against a number of digestive and other physical conditions, and certainly there are endless anecdotal tales, many of them heard in my own office, concerning the surprising and sometimes remarkable healing effects of yogurt.

As with many natural remedies, the way to discover whether yogurt is a boon to your digestive problems is simply to try it. Yogurt is cheap, easy to find, delicious, healthy, and nutritious. Try it.

Meanwhile, let's have a look at some of the common ailments yogurt is reputed to help.

Helping Diarrhea

Acute diarrhea with its many possible vexations—dehydration, high frequency of defecation, increased fluidity of stools, and large watery volumes passed—is ordinarily considered the symptom of an underlying disorder rather than a disease per se. At the same time, diarrhea is clearly triggered by commonplace rigors of daily living such as colds, flu, alcohol, travel, infected food, and stress. Happily, transient bouts of this unpleasant condition respond gratifyingly well to the healing virtues of yogurt.

According to popular wisdom, dairy products tend to make diarrhea worse, not better, and therefore diarrhea sufferers should avoid these products entirely. Doctors will even tell you that dairy foods actually *cause* diarrhea, not cure it, especially in persons with allergies or lactose intolerance. All this is true *except* in the case of yogurt and its soured-milk by-products. Why? Because when diarrhea strikes, it kills a high percentage of *Saccharomyces boulardii* and a number of other bacteria that live in the gut. Both of these bacteria are necessary for regularity and smooth digestion. As it turns out, active yogurt cultures, as well as other forms of *Lactobacillus* in liquid or powder form, are loaded with digestive flora. Introducing these products to the diet helps replace the friendly bacteria wiped out by the diarrhea, and is often all that is needed to reestablish normal bowel function.

In the case of antibiotic-caused diarrhea, yogurt and its derivatives are an even more appropriate form of medicine. Once antibiotics enter the digestive system, their killing powers become indiscriminate. Willy-nilly, they purge friendly microflora along with unfriendly, allowing the harmful microorganisms that instigate diarrhea (such as *Clostridium difficile*) to proliferate unchecked. Once in the gut, antibiotics can also trigger the growth of the bacteria *Candida albicans,* which, in turn, may produce virulent yeast infections.

In all these scenarios, yogurt and its derivatives are a possible antidote, returning large stores of helpful bacteria to the gastrointestinal tract, and crowding out and killing the harmful infectious bacteria.

Try eating yogurt the next time you are stricken with loose bowels. And, by the way, for children who suffer from frequent diarrhea, yogurt is known to be a gentle and tasty restorative. Dr. Boudraa and colleagues, as reported in the *Journal of Pediatric Gastroenterology and Nutrition* (2001), studied the effect of yogurt on children with diarrhea aged three months to twenty-four months. A portion of stricken children was given an infant formula fermented with yogurt culture bacteria. At the end of the study, the duration of the diarrhea and the number of stools measured were substantially less among the yogurt group than among the control group. In fact, forty-eight hours after the study began, fewer than 20 percent of the yogurt-fed babies still had diarrhea, while 75 percent in the control group continued to suffer from it.

Helping Constipation

If you suffer from occasional constipation caused by diet, stress, medications, or whatever, try adding a cup of live-culture yogurt to your daily menu. Eat it preferably for breakfast every morning when peristalsis is most active.

Yogurt and other soured-milk derivatives help the body manufacture vitamins in the intestines, which are crucial for building friendly flora, and thus for fighting slow-moving bowels and constipation. See Chapter 14 for the specifics of treating constipation naturally.

Strengthening the Immune System

Recent studies at the University of California at Davis demonstrate that people who eat generous supplies of live-culture yogurt show increased rates of interferon production. As mentioned earlier, interferon is a protein that promotes immune response by potentiating both immune cells and antibodies required to fight infections and cancer. As a pharmaceutical, interferon is used to combat leukemia and a variety of cancers, as well as hepatitis B and C, and to help fight infectious diseases in people who suffer from immunodeficiency disorders.

Besides increasing interferon production, yogurt stimulates the production of interleukin, a chemical that plays a critical role in reducing allergic response. Yogurt also provides the body with a host of essential nutrients, including protein (one eight-ounce serving of yogurt a day delivers almost a quarter of the daily recommended quota), vitamins, potassium, magnesium, and calcium. These nutrients strengthen the immune system and keep the body energized and in good repair.

Dr. Meydani and Dr. Ha from Tufts University, as reported in the *American Journal of Clinical Nutrition* (2000), conclude that evidence for yogurt's immunological-boosting qualities is compelling and strong. They recommend that people with compromised immune systems, especially the elderly, consume yogurt on a regular basis to increase resistance to disease.

Remedying Calcium Deficiency

Yogurt's strongest claim in the nutrient department is, like all milk products, its lavish stores of calcium. Calcium is *the* key player in helping maintain a strong and enduring skeletal system. Nearly 99 percent of the calcium in the body is located in the bones and teeth. Indeed, deposits in the bones make up around 1.5 to 2 percent of the body's total weight.

Besides strengthening the skeletal structure and preventing bone diseases (such as osteoporosis), calcium plays a role in maintaining blood clotting, muscle contraction, heartbeat, blood pressure, and a smoothly functioning nervous system. Lack of calcium manifests itself in muscle cramps, nervous disorders, softening of the bone, irregular bowel movements, and colon cancer.

Of all the ways of satisfying one's daily requirement of calcium, eating yogurt is no doubt the easiest and most pleasant. Six ounces of yogurt contain around 250 to 400 mg of calcium (cottage cheese has only 120 to 140 mg per cup). This count is higher in some brands of yogurt, lower in others, depending on the quality of the milk and the way in which the yogurt is processed (or not processed). Studying the label on a nutritious brand of commercial yogurt, we learn that a single cup of yogurt provides approximately 40 percent of an adult's daily calcium requirement. Another brand boasts 45 percent. Adjust your daily intake accordingly.

Other important nutrients found in yogurt include protein, potassium, vitamin A, vitamin C, and several other important vitamins. All come in different percent and measure, depending on the brand.

Bypassing Lactose Intolerance

Many people, including a large number of infants, are incapable of processing the milk sugar lactose because of a lack of the digestive enzyme lactase. This peculiarity of the digestive system is known as lactose intolerance. Reactions to this disorder include bloating, stomach pain, and intense diarrhea. Symptoms can last for a few minutes or for as long as a day.

While fewer than 15 percent of the population of northern Europe (or

Americans of northern European descent) suffer from lactose intolerance, it is estimated that nine out of ten Asians, Native Americans, and African-Americans have few enzymes to digest lactose. This same condition is present, though to a lesser extent, among people with a Mediterranean heritage.

Since dairy products such as milk, cream, cheese, and sour cream contain large amounts of lactose, individuals who suffer from lactose intolerance are cautioned to avoid dairy foods, or to eat commercial lactose-reduced and/or lactose-free milk products. With one exception: Due to a relatively simple chemical process that takes place during fermentation, people who cannot tolerate other types of dairy products can ordinarily eat yogurt and related sour-milk products with impunity.

Why? Because when milk is fermenting and being transformed into yogurt, its live bacterial cultures manufacture stores of the enzyme lactase. Once ingested, lactase helps break down the lactose that might otherwise result in lactose intolerance. The result is that people with lactose intolerance can usually eat yogurt products to their hearts' content, with no fear of intestinal discomfort.

Note, by the way, that freezing destroys much of the lactase in dairy products. For this reason, people who suffer from lactose intolerance are advised to avoid frozen yogurt and its derivatives.

Healing Yeast Infections

First, let it be said that not every health-care professional believes that eating yogurt cures yeast infections. Many researchers believe that studies are inconclusive, and that most stories of miracle yeast cures are anecdotal. Perhaps. Still, the evidence is compelling.

In one controlled trial, women who ate eight ounces of unpasteurized, live-culture *Lactobacillus acidophilus* every day showed a substantial decrease in frequency of *Candida* colonization in their vaginal areas. In another trial, women suffering from stubborn cases of yeast infection ate five ounces of unpasteurized, live-culture yogurt every day and, at the end of the test, showed more than a 50 percent reduction in recurrence (women who ate the pasteurized varieties showed little or no reduction). Dr. Hilton and colleagues from Long Island Jewish Medical Center in New York studied the effects of live-culture yogurt as a preventive for *Candida* yeast infection. In their study, eight female subjects ate eight ounces of yogurt every day for six months, then stopped eating the yogurt for another six months. Reporting their results in the journal *Annals of Internal Medicine* (1992), researchers reported a decrease in infection among the women while they were eating the yogurt, then an increase once they stopped.

Clinical evidence notwithstanding—and there is a good deal more of it than many researchers realize—the question of yogurt's yeast-killing powers remains a controversial one.

At times, of course, critics go a bit too far. In 1972, two founders of the Federation of Feminist Women's Health Centers in Los Angeles were arrested at their self-help clinic for advising women to self-treat their vaginal yeast infections with yogurt. The trial became known as the "Great Yogurt Conspiracy," and its outcome was as predictable as you might expect: the clinic was found innocent on all charges, and the instigators of the raid turned out to be several local physicians who apparently looked on the clinic as a threat to the health of the female race, and perhaps to their own profits as well.

The origins of yeast infections stem from an acid-base pH imbalance in a woman's vaginal area, and not from actual bacterial infection (technically speaking, there are no causative bacteria present in yeast infections). Poor diet (especially too much sugar), stress, antibiotics, and the effect of birth control pills can all serve as triggers.

The most common form of yeast problem, *Candida* (or *Monilia*), produces high-profile, easily recognizable symptoms including itching in the vaginal area and a lumpy white discharge that is sometimes odorous, and that is often compared in its consistency to cottage cheese. Other possible signs of candida include small superficial fissures in the vaginal region, a burning sensation while urinating, and pain during intercourse.

Once an infection of this kind appears, it tends to be persistent and sometimes maddeningly recurrent. Bacterial vaginosis, a related vaginal infection, has many of the same qualities.

According to information posted on the Web site of the Feminist Women's Health Centers, there are several simultaneous and effective first-line health measures that women can take against yeast infections. These include the following:

- When suffering from a yeast infection, insert unpasteurized, live-culture, unflavored yogurt into the vagina. Perform this maneuver using a spoon, spatula, or vaginal-cream applicator. The Center suggests that you apply the yogurt culture at night, and wear a pad.
- Using unpasteurized, live-culture yogurt mixed with water, apply regular vaginal douches.
- Drink acidophilus milk or eat acidophilus powder until the infection improves. Both forms of culture are available at health-food stores.
- Besides the yogurt treatments described above, the Center suggests that women drink plenty of cranberry juice, eat lots of garlic, and/or paint their vagina, cervix, and vulva with gentian violet, a disinfectant available at most pharmacies. "This usually works," the Center's Web site tells us, "after one treatment."

Other Possible Curative Benefits of Yogurt

Many other claims have been made for the medicinal wonders of yogurt—some marginal, some accepted, and some possible but unproven. Some of these possible benefits include antitumor effects, cholesterol-reducing properties, and healing effects with yeast infections.

From time to time, yogurt has been credited with healing ulcers, remedying nervous fatigue, combating insomnia, and reducing depression. All quite conjectural. But who knows?

In India, many women apply yogurt to their skin, believing it to be a moistening agent, a skin purifier, a hair conditioner, and a preventive for blemishes and skin infection. One popular Indian cosmetic recipe calls for mixing a teaspoon of turmeric into a cup of yogurt. Make a paste of the mixture and apply it to the skin for beautification. Some women claim this mixture also reduces dandruff. Try it and see for yourself.

KNOW YOUR YOGURT

From the standpoint of intestinal health, the type and the quality of the yogurt you eat are almost as important as the fact that you are eating it at all. And remember: not all yogurts are created equal. Know, for example, that many of the commercial brands you purchase at the supermarket are made from only two bacterial cultures, *Lactobacillus bulgaricus* and *Streptococcus thermophilus.*

These cultures are fine as far as cultures go, and are, in fact, the two necessary ingredients to make yogurt yogurt. Brands that are more health-oriented, however, contribute several other strains of friendly bacteria to the mix including *B. bifidus, L. casei,* and *L. reuteri.* These extra organisms add measurably to the intestinal flora supplied by the yogurt and provide first-line medicinal value.

Also keep in mind that, during production, some commercial yogurt makers heat-treat their milk after pasteurization to boost its shelf life. In the process, they kill most of the live cultures, which, as you know, are the substances that give yogurt its digestive and healing clout. Heat treatment neither detracts from the taste or flavor of yogurt nor reduces yogurt's stores of protein, calcium, and other nutrients. But, when intense post-pasteurization heat is applied, it is just about a sure thing that yogurt's friendly microflora will be cooked away. When this happens, all that remains is a tasty dessert.

Thus, a yogurt rule of thumb: If you see a logo on the yogurt container in the shape of an A and C (standing for "Active Cultures"), and/or if the label tells you the product *contains* "active" or "live" cultures, this means the product's microflora are alive and ready to do good things in your gut.

The operative word here is "contains." Some yogurt brands tell you that they are *made* with active cultures. What they do not tell you is that these active cultures are destroyed by processing and heating. And, of course, if the label announces (as it is now required to do by law) that a particular yogurt is "heat-treated after culturing," this is proof positive that the friendly bacteria are mostly dead and gone.

Note that around 85 percent of yogurt sold in the United States is sweetened with fruit, strawberry being the most popular flavor. This is fine if you are eating your yogurt as a refreshment, but not so fine if you are using it to treat symptoms, especially symptoms of yeast, which may be exacerbated by sugar.

Also, if you suffer from yeast infections be wary of frozen yogurt. Frozen yogurt is loaded with sugar, fat (as much as 14 grams per cup), and calories (sometimes as high as 400 per serving). Most frozen yogurt has also had the delicate microflora chilled out of it. At the same time, it should be said that a few frozen yogurt manufacturers go to lengths to preserve the friendly cultures in their product and to keep its nutrient levels reasonably high. Like regular yogurts, not all frozen yogurts are the same. Check the label before purchase.

Make Your Own Yogurt

Why not? It's fast, easy, and the quality of yogurt you make at home is as good and often better than the products you buy at the supermarket. It's also cheaper and fun to make. It's always a great kitchen project to do with children.

Start by procuring a dry yogurt starter culture (see the Appendix for sources). Or simply use any high-quality yogurt you buy at the store. Either will do. If you use the store-bought variety, make sure it contains no fruit.

The following are the ingredients and tools you will need:

- One quart of one-percent milk or skim milk if you want to prepare a low-fat yogurt; or one quart of whole milk if you prefer something richer and more liberal on the butterfat
- Three teaspoons of fresh, active-culture yogurt or an equivalent amount of dry yogurt starter
- Sterilized jars with tops
- Kitchen thermometer

First, sterilize your jars in boiling water and set them aside.

Pour the milk into a saucepan and bring it to a boil. Some people scald the milk rather than boil it, the theory being that more of the nutrients are left alive this way. Perhaps, but many people still prefer boiling. The moment the milk has boiled, remove it from the stove and let it cool to a temperature of 110°F. You can use your thermometer to get a precise reading. Or you can employ the old-fashioned system, allowing the milk to cool down to the point where you can insert your finger and keep it immersed in the milk for ten seconds without burning.

When the milk has reached 110°F or thereabouts, add the fresh yogurt starter or the starter culture, and stir gently. Make sure to remove all lumps as you mix. Then ladle the mixture into your sterilized jars, and cap them tightly.

The goal now is to keep the jars of fermenting milk at around 110°F for three to eight hours. There are two ways to do this:

1. Use a commercial yogurt maker. The instructions are in the box.
2. Use one of a number of homemade methods described below:

    • Place the jars in a saucepan with a few inches of warm water on the bottom, then place the pot on the stove. Set the flame under it to low.
    • If it is winter, cover the bottles with a towel, and place them on a warm radiator.
    • Preheat your oven to 300°F. When it reaches that temperature, turn off the oven, let it cool for twenty minutes, and place the yogurt bottles inside.
    • Place the jars in an electric heating pan filled with several inches of water, keeping the temperature set at low.
    • Place the jars in a crockpot set at low.
    • Some people simply turn on the oven light and place the jars inside (the oven light is all the heat that's required). Others use a

box with a lit light bulb inside. Still others place a heating pad over the jars.

As you can see, incubating yogurt is an approximate science, and you may wish to experiment on your own with these different techniques. Don't worry if the temperature fails to remain at exactly 110°F every moment your yogurt is cooking. These improvised methods seem to get the job done despite the imprecision.

At the same time, it *is* wise to check your temperature readings from time to time, preferably with the kitchen thermometer or, in a pinch, with the ten-count finger test. If the yogurt gets too cold and stays this way for too long, it will not jell. If it is too hot, the friendly bacteria will die and the milk will curdle.

Yogurt made with fresh yogurt culture usually requires three to six hours of cooking time. Yogurt made with dry culture takes eight to twelve hours.

How can you tell when the yogurt is ready? Test it by tipping one of the jars slightly to the side to see if it is solidified. Or insert a knife into the yogurt to test for firmness. The yogurt will firm up even more once it sits in the refrigerator for several hours.

YOGURT RECIPES

Yogurt can be used as a base for salad dressings, as a side dish (especially with hot food), or as a dessert. Here are some recipes from the land of India (mostly for salads and raitas) where yogurt is considered a special treat and is often served at every meal of the day.

❧ Plain Raita ❧

Serve as a side dish with hot, spicy food.

1 cup yogurt (regular,
  homemade, or fat-free)
½ cup water
½ cup shredded
  peeled cucumber

¼ teaspoon salt
½ teaspoon roasted cumin seed
¼ teaspoon pepper
Chili powder to taste

1. Mix the yogurt with the water and blend it to a semi-solid paste.
2. Add the remaining ingredients and mix well. Refrigerate for thirty to sixty minutes before serving. (Waiting is essential; it allows the flavors to blend.)

❧ Mint Raita ❧

1 cup yogurt (regular,
  homemade, or fat-free)
½ cup water
½ teaspoon freshly picked
  shredded mint leaves

½ teaspoon roasted cumin seed
¼ teaspoon pepper
¼ teaspoon salt
Chili powder to taste
¼ teaspoon powdered mint

1. Mix the yogurt with the water and blend into a semi-solid paste.
2. Add the remaining ingredients except the powdered mint and mix well.
3. Sprinkle the mint powder over the top. Refrigerate for thirty to sixty minutes before serving.

Variation: If the weather is hot, consider adding chopped cucumber to the mixture.

❧ Yogurt Vegetable Salad ❧

2 cups yogurt (regular, homemade, or fat-free)
1 cup water
⅓ teaspoon freshly picked, shredded mint leaves
1 small onion, chopped
½ cup chopped fresh spinach
1 tablespoon roasted cumin seed

1 tablespoon vegetable oil
⅓ cup shredded peeled cucumber
1 medium tomato, chopped
1 fresh carrot, shredded
¼ teaspoon salt
Chili powder to taste
¼ teaspoon powdered mint

1. Mix the yogurt and water together and blend into a semi-solid paste.
2. Add the remaining ingredients except the powdered mint and mix well.
3. Sprinkle the mint powder over the top. Refrigerate for thirty to sixty minutes before serving.

❧ Banana Raita ❧

2 cups yogurt (regular, homemade, or fat-free)
1 cup water
1 medium banana, cut into bite-sized pieces

1 tablespoon sugar (or to taste)
⅓ cup raisins
4 to 6 cardamom pods
2 walnuts, crumbled

1. Mix the yogurt with the water and blend into a semi-solid paste.
2. Add the remaining ingredients and mix. Refrigerate for thirty to sixty minutes before serving.

✤ Apple and Banana Raita ✤

2 cups yogurt (regular,
homemade, or fat-free)

1 cup water

1 medium apple, cut into
bite-sized pieces

1 banana, chopped

⅓ cup raisins

1 tablespoon sugar (or to taste)

4 to 6 cardamom pods

2 walnuts, crumbled

1. Mix the yogurt with the water and blend into a semi-solid paste.
2. Add the remaining ingredients and mix. Refrigerate for thirty to
   sixty minutes before serving.

✤ Mixed Fruit Raita ✤

2 cups yogurt (regular,
homemade, or fat-free)

1 cup water

1 cup dairy or non-dairy Cool
Whip or sour cream

½ medium apple, chopped

1 banana, chopped

10-ounce can mandarin orange
slices, drained

⅓ cup raisins

Sugar to taste

4 to 6 cardamom pods

2 walnuts, crumbled

1. Mix the yogurt with the water and blend into a semi-solid paste.
2. Add the remaining ingredients and mix. Refrigerate for thirty to
   sixty minutes before serving.
   Enjoy.

By now, I hope I have convinced you that yogurt provides not just nutritional benefits but also healing and preventive benefits during health and sickness. Use this power food as an essential component of your diet—many doctors do!

chapter eight

Probiotics: The New Digestion Technology

Happily ensconced inside our winding, tunnel-like gastrointestinal tract lives a vast civilization of teeming microorganisms that weighs as much as four pounds in a healthy gut and that includes approximately 400 species.

A small portion of these microorganisms lives in the stomach. Many more thrive in the small intestine, and still more in the large intestine. Basically uncountable—over a twenty-four-hour period, billions of these bacteria are born and die—they number somewhere in the trillions. Around a third of the fecal matter that we void every day is made up of these organisms. In fact, bacterial populations in the wastes number up to *one hundred billion microorganisms per milliliter,* which is about the thickest density of living creatures it is possible to support on earth. By some estimates, there are more microorganisms living in the gut than there are cells in the entire body.

Not all of these bacteria are friendly, as we have seen. Some cause infection. Others secrete harmful wastes, while others are simply squatters, along for the ride, and useless as far as digestion goes. Dr. Eamonn Quigley, editor-in-chief of the prestigious *American Journal of Gastroenterology*, in a recent lecture to digestive disease specialists at the annual Digestive Disease Week in San Francisco in 2002, made this provocative and definitive statement: "The enemy is within the fecal stream."

Moreover, unfriendly and imbalanced bacteria in the gut may not just cause local disease. Consider this example, which shows how digestive problems affect seemingly unrelated parts of the body: Dr. Cordts and colleagues studied the role of gut disorders in chronic venous insufficiency. Reporting their results in the journal *Vascular Surgery* (2001), the researchers observed that, among patients suffering from venous insufficiency, high amounts of yeast were found in seven out of nine of their stool samples, whereas no yeast was detected in the stool of control subjects. The doctors concluded that gut disorders may promote systemic inflammation and white blood cell abnormalities, which, in turn, lead to diseases of the *leg veins!*

In Chapter 7, we learned about the glories that friendly bacteria bring to the digestive tract, especially the varieties that come in soured milk. These products, we know, contain bacterial flora that are remarkably helpful to just about every stage of human digestion.

Yogurt, with its many active bacterial cultures is, of course, the high-profile star here, along with related acidophilus derivatives. There are, however, other products that contain similarly helpful bacterial strains, and that provide users with a veritable cornucopia of beneficial digestive services.

Some of these bacteria-containing foods are natural; some are developed in the laboratory. Some come in yogurt and acidophilus products; others are sold separately in capsule, liquid, or powder form. And, while some of these foods have been familiar to scientists for years, researchers in Europe, Russia, and Japan are continually discovering new ones. Today, although you may not be aware of the fact (few people are), there is a burgeoning industry of these bio-food products. The name of this new industry is probiotics.

❦ Probiotics: The New Digestion Technology ❦

INTRODUCING PROBIOTICS

"Probiotics" is a term used to describe the helpful microorganisms that live inside the gastrointestinal tract. Any food that is labeled "probiotic," such as yogurt, contains these supportive organisms and distributes them throughout the gut. The word "probiotics" itself is derived from the Latin *pro,* meaning "for," and *bio,* meaning "life." Probiotics, in other words, means "for life" or, more poetically phrased, "life enhancing."

The theory behind what advocates now call "the probiotic revolution" is simply this: In our modern world, we are constantly being exposed to an array of pollutants, toxins, and biohazards that 100 years ago were unknown to the average American. The friendly flora that colonizes our gut, and that in more natural conditions thrives, is severely depleted by these environmental contaminants and makes our digestive systems vulnerable to a wide variety of infections and disorders that under more normal conditions would be fought off with ease.

What are these biohazards exactly? How do they harm us?

Throughout other chapters in this book, we have enumerated the various environmental and infectious insults that besiege the modern digestive system, and by now the roll call is a familiar one. The short list of antagonists that attack the friendly flora in our gut includes the following:

- **Antibiotics**—An antibiotic is just what its name implies, a force of anti-life (recall that *bio* means "life"). This feature is a great boon when we are suffering from an infection. But, as most of us know, there is also a downside to this medical miracle: the antibiotic destroys good bacteria along with bad.

    Antibiotics have, moreover, a special predilection for the friendly flora coating the inside of our intestines. After a round or two of a broad-spectrum antibiotic like ampicillin or clarithromycin, these helpful bacteria become seriously depleted, allowing harmful bacteria and fungi such as *Candida* to move in and take their place. In one study of antibiotics and intestinal flora, it was found that 25 percent of patients treated with prolonged courses of tetracycline suffer from yeast infections.

- **Poor diet**—A majority of the foods we eat are grown with synthetic fertilizers and processed with chemical additives that include flavorings, colorings, taste enhancers, rancidity retarders, preservatives, and more. A majority of these substances are unfriendly to intestinal flora, and some are downright poisonous. Still others are known to be carcinogenic (cancer causing). The fact that these chemicals are added to our food in small quantities in no way reduces their toxicity.

    Complicating the contaminant dilemma even more is the fact that many of the cattle husbanded in the West are fed foods containing antibiotics. When these cattle are slaughtered, the antibiotics inside them do not necessarily go away. They often remain embedded in the animals' meat, and are passed on to human eaters every time a beef dinner is served.

    What this means in terms of intestinal health is that, even if you have not used prescription antibiotics for many years, chances are your gut may still contain them, compliments of your local supermarket, butcher shop, and meat processor.

    The problem does not stop with chemical additives either. To the catalog of risks, add the common American diet with its emphasis on fried foods, rich foods, fats, stimulants, and sugars. These substances are all irritating to the digestive organs and are sometimes deadly to the digestive flora that processes them.

    It is, in short, difficult to escape the long arm of food contamination. One recent study, reported at the Digestive Disease Week conference in 2002, tells us that even the tops of soda cans sold at the grocery stores are highly contaminated (those sold from vending machines are the safest).

    We are what we eat.

- **Medical drugs**—Clearly, medical drugs are a lifesaving benefit and a critical part of everyone's health care. We cannot do without them.

    At the same time, most prescription drugs and many nonprescription drugs trigger negative reactions, many of which are localized in the gut. The next time you purchase a drug, read the inventory of side effects printed on the label or box. All too frequently you will find nausea, constipation, diarrhea, heartburn, and indigestion included on the list. Nonsteroidal anti-inflammatory drugs such as aspirin are especially culpable in this regard. These agents are known to cause inflammation of the stomach and intestinal lining, which, in turn, reduces the population of friendly flora in the gut, eventually contributing to gut ailments such as leaky gut syndrome. The decision concerning whether or not to take an aspirin a day to thin the blood and prevent heart attack should be evaluated with this fact in mind and, of course, after consultation with your physician.

· **Alcohol, cigarettes, and unwholesome lifestyle factors—** Alcohol is a known killer of intestinal flora, and a major cause of acidity, stomach rawness, and inflammation of the intestinal lining. Cigarette smoke is carcinogenic, punishing to the mucous lining of stomach and intestines, and a major source of toxins.

Other lifestyle factors that take a toll on the gastrointestinal tract include insufficient sleep, lack of exercise, overweight, underweight, workaholism, and habitual use of street drugs.

· **Stress—**Chapter 5 is dedicated to the relationship between stress and digestive disease, and here it can simply be said that chronic feelings of tension, fear, worry, and depression produce major changes in the delicate balance of our intestinal ecology, all of which take their toll on the body. Within the digestive tract, for example, stress is known to alter stomach acidity, to reduce the population of helpful flora, and to interfere with the proper digestion, absorption, and assimilation of foods and vitamins. And that's just for starters. Though stress is often overlooked as an antecedent to diseases of the gut, it can be a primary cause of digestive distress for a number of people.

THE MANY BENEFITS OF PROBIOTICS

So what's the good news? Namely this: Though the depletion of helpful internal flora can result in significant health problems, champions of the probiotic revolution insist that, with the right choice of probiotic nutrients, given in the right amounts and at the right time, a great deal of the mischief enumerated in the list above can be rectified.

Here it should be said that not everyone agrees with the opinions of probiotic advocates. There are physicians, a number perhaps, who remain unconvinced concerning the healing properties of these substances, and who cite the lack of clinical data as reason for their skepticism. Moreover, enthusiasm for testing probiotics is minimal, although this lack of enthusiasm may be due less to the bona fides of probiotics, and more to the fact that major drug companies and universities, the major funding organizations for such procedures, have little to gain on a financial level from such studies, and rarely go out of their way to support them.

This said, it should also be stressed that a growing number of physicians are recommending probiotics to their patients, and are in agreement that friendly intestinal microorganisms curtail the growth of pathogenic bacteria in several critical ways:

1. Crowding out harmful microorganisms
2. Creating a more acidic environment in the intestines that discourages pathogen growth
3. Releasing substances such as lactic acid, hydrogen peroxide, and antibacterial agents (known as bacteriocins) that team up against harmful bacteria and produce a healthy equilibrium of gut flora
4. Improving the efficiency of digestion and elimination, thus increasing the speed at which noxious bacteria are removed from the gut

Because of these benefits, and because of the growing body of scientific evidence supporting probiotic's healing virtues, there are a number of physicians and gastroenterologists who routinely recommend probiotics for digestive ills, and who find that these powerful supplements bring many healing benefits. The interest in probiotics is immense. In fact, at the probiotic and alternative medicine–related symposia at the Digestive Disease Week conference held in 2002 in San Francisco, standing-room crowds showed up to learn more about the benefits of these powerful substances.

Some of the most evident and clinically established of these benefits include those discussed below.

Detoxification

According to an article in the *Journal of Applied Bacteriology* (1989) by Dr. Fuller of the AFRC Institute of Food Research in the United Kingdom, the healthy microbial environment in the human gut is thrown off balance by unfriendly forces such as medicines and poor diet. These substances make the body vulnerable to diseases and reduce the efficiency of food utilization. Dr. Fuller asserts that with probiotic treatment we reestablish the natural biological balance that exists naturally in wild animals, but which is altered in the human gut by the fashions of modern living.

Studies thus show that probiotic bacteria neutralize toxic metabolites, deprive pathogenic bacteria of the nutrients they need to survive, and actively produce antibacterial-type substances that kill off unfriendly invaders. The acidifying effect of probiotic bacteria, moreover, helps stem the proliferation of harmful putrefactive flora such as *Clostridia* and, at the same time, encourages the growth of friendly flora. The result of this interior housekeeping is that a great deal of harmful refuge is removed from the gut, the negative effects of medicines and poor diet on digestion are countered, and the digestive tract is made cleaner and more efficient.

Improved Bowel and Digestive Function

Probiotics are believed to stimulate peristalsis and increase the transit time of feces through the bowel, thus eliminating toxins more efficiently from the gastrointestinal tract and helping to restore regularity. Many stubborn cases of constipation can be relieved in a matter of weeks with a steady diet of probiotic foods, along with other natural remedies and supplements.

Likewise, even serious cases of diarrhea respond well to probiotics. Many patients undergoing tube feeding in hospitals develop intense cases of diarrhea. While there are many possible causes for this condition, recent data suggest that the administration of the probiotic bacteria *Saccharomyces boulardii* dramatically decreases diarrea in tube-fed patients. Many other studies testify to probiotic's antidiarrheal effects.

Finally, probiotic bacteria secrete enzymes that help break down foods into their essential components, a process that expedites the movement of wastes along the gastrointestinal tract. The result is improved digestion plus better assimilation of the carbohydrate-protein-fats nutrient groups.

Lowered Cholesterol

Though the jury is out on this one, there is much convincing evidence that regular consumption of probiotic foods lowers blood cholesterol levels. In trials at Oklahoma State University, research showed a decrease in the blood cholesterol levels of patients who regularly ingested *Lactobacillus acidophilus*. The conclusion reached at Oklahoma State, as reported by Dr. J. W. Anderson and Dr. S. E. Gilland in the *Journal of American College of Nutrition* (1999), was that the presence of *Lactobacillus acidophilus* "would make it possible for the organism to assimilate at least part of the cholesterol ingested in the diet, making it unavailable for absorption into the blood."

Disease-Fighting Resources

Probiotics appear to be useful in healing a number of specific digestive ailments. Dr. J. F. Columbel and colleagues write in the medical journal *Lancet* (1987) that yogurt containing the common probiotic *Bifidobacterium longum* reduces the side effects of many common medications. In Sweden, Dr. Mangell and colleagues studied the role of probiotics in healing *E. coli*–induced diarrhea in rats. Reporting their results in the journal *Digestive Diseases and Sciences* (2002), they tell us that pre-treatment with the probiotic *L. plantarum 299v* protects against *E. coli*–induced increases in intestinal permeability, thus fortifying the human body's intestinal barrier defenses.

Studies by Dr. Madsen and colleagues in the journal *Gastroenterology* (2001) likewise show that probiotic bacteria enhances bowel-barrier function and resistance to Salmonella infection. In Ireland, Dr. Fergus Shanahan writes in the journal *Clinical Perspectives in Gastroenterology* (2001) that "although probiotic research is at an early stage with regard to controlled therapeutic trials, there is encouraging preclinical and clinical evidence for its efficacy in treating Irritable Bowel Syndrome. . . . In humans, two studies using a nonpathogenic strain of *Escherichia coli* as a probiotic have shown the probiotic's equivalence with mesalamine in treatment of ulcerative colitis."

It is now common knowledge that the *Helicobacter pylori* causes ulcers and even cancer. Dr. Vilaichone from Thailand recently reported at the Digestive Disease Week in 2002 that *Lactobacillus acidophilus* has an inhibitory effect on the bacteria *H. pylori* in patients with stomach ulcers. Dr. Yan and Dr. Polk from Nashville, in a study presented at same meeting, demonstrated that *Lactobacillus* GG prevents programmed intestinal cell death in response to inflammation. Similarly, Dr. Silvia Resta-Lenert from San Diego at the same meeting reported that the probiotic bacteria *Streptococcus thermophilus, L. acidophilus, F. varius,* and *B. brevis* reduce the ability of *E. coli* to destroy cells in the intestines. (Can probiotics generate a similar inhibitive effect in cells from the rest of the body, helping prolong survival? Perhaps.)

Disease Prevention

Probiotics prevent disease as well as heal it. A group of investigators led by Dr. C. S. Pitchumoni gave *Lactobacillus* GG to 152 nursing-home patients undergoing antibiotic treatment, while a placebo was administered to 152 control subjects. At the end of the study, it was shown that the control group had a three times greater chance of developing diarrhea than the group taking probiotics. Presenting their results at the Digestive Disease

Week in 2002, the investigators stated that probiotic supplementation is definitely helpful in the prevention of antibiotic-induced diarrhea and that it should be considered whenever antibiotics are used.

Immune-System Booster

Studies show that, within the human immune system, probiotics promote increased production of infection-fighting cytokines and interferons, and boost the production of white blood cells. When used on a regular basis, they also elevate the levels of antigen-specific antibodies in the blood, and stimulate the destruction of harmful bacteria by phagocyte cells.

A recent study published in the medical journal *Lancet* (1999) associates low levels of the probiotic bacteria *Lactobacilli* in the vaginal tract of 4,718 young women with an increased incidence of HIV-1. Animal studies in Argentina indicate that mice fed foods containing *Lactobacillus acidophilus* and *Streptococcus thermophilus* undergo an increase in the production of macrophage cells, essential for resistance to infection. In a study reported at the annual Digestive Disease Week in 2002, Dr. Carol and colleagues from France reported that a probiotic combination of *Lactobacillus casei, L. bulgaricus,* and nonpathogenic forms of *E. coli* help mitigate the inflammation in Crohn's disease.

There is, finally, some indication that people whose immune systems are compromised by radiation treatment may profit from the immunological boost offered by probiotics. Dr. Urbancsek and colleagues, writing in the *European Journal of Gastroenterology Hepatology* (2001), state that based on their double-blind, placebo-controlled trial, use of the probiotic the *Lactobacillus rhamnosus (Antibiophilus)* is superior to placebo among patients suffering from radiation-induced diarrhea.

Antiyeast Qualities

A number of recent studies indicate that probiotic foods and supplements keep the spread of fungal diseases such as *Candida* under control. Clinical trials done in Europe and Japan show that *Bifidobacteria* probiotics inhibit the overgrowth of yeast, and manufacture substances that directly oppose and dramatically lower yeast populations.

Chapter 7 contains the specifics on *Candida,* and should be referred to if yeast infection is a problem.

Possible Anticancer Properties

According to the World Health Organization, many of the cancers found in women can be directly traced to faulty diet and nutrition. This is particularly relevant information in light of studies showing that probiotic flora neutralizes enzymes produced by harmful pathogens, and heals damage done by carcinogenic chemicals.

Recent research likewise suggests that cell-wall components of certain probiotic bacteria encourage the immunological housecleaning of malignant cells. Particularly interesting in this regard is an article published in *Cancer Research* (1993) profiling an animal experiment by Dr. Reedy and colleagues. Reedy's trial shows that the friendly strain of bacteria *Bifidobacterium longum* inhibits carcinogenesis in the liver and mammary glands, suggesting that probiotic's anticarcinogenic activity exerts a protective effect on other organs of the body besides the digestive tract.

Moreover, we know that, among societies where large amounts of probiotic foods are consumed, longevity tends to be high and cancer rates low. When considered in light of mounting evidence showing that diets heavy in fats and processed foods increase cancer risk, it is logical to conclude that the health and lifestyle choices we make in our daily lives do count, and that all of us retain a measure of control over whether or not we will someday develop certain deadly diseases.

TYPES OF PROBIOTIC BACTERIA

What are the actual bacteria in probiotic foods that do all this good work? Though researchers are frequently finding new types of probiotic organisms (for example, the *Lactobacillus rhamnosus VTT E-97800* discovered in Finland and not yet publicly available, or the *Lactobacillus casei Shirota,* used mostly in Japanese probiotics), a majority of strains are offsprings of several basic bacterial genera, the names and benefits of which are worth reviewing.

Here, in brief, is a list of the probiotic bacteria that are most useful in preventing disease and restoring digestive health. Probiotic supplements include many or most of these microorganisms, sometimes with more exotic or lesser-known species mixed in.

Lactobacillus acidophilus

A permanent resident of the small intestine, *Lactobacillus acidophilus* produces lactic acid and natural antibiotics such as acidolin, both of which inhibit the growth of harmful bacteria. *Lactobacillus acidophilus* is also credited with lowering blood cholesterol levels.

Lactobacillus bulgaricus

Lactobacillus bulgaricus is one of the essential ingredients of live-culture yogurt. Raising the acidic environment of the gut and killing off certain harmful organisms, it is a transient bacterium that passes swiftly through the gut and requires constant replenishment.

Streptococcus thermophilus

Like *Lactobacillus bulgaricus, Streptococcus thermophilus* is a transient organism that encourages an acidic environment, inhibits harmful bacteria, and is an essential ingredient in all brands of yogurt. It also helps produce the enzyme lactase, a primary ingredient in the digestion of milk.

Bifidobacterium bifidum and Bifidobacterium longum

The major natural bacterial inhabitants of the large intestine, these strains produce acid substances in the bowels that fight off colonizations by yeast, viruses, and harmful bacteria. They also manufacture highly important B vitamins, and assist weight gain in infants.

Bifidobacteria infantis

These bacteria are natural inhabitants of the intestines, forming the very foundation of a young child's digestive health. They acidify the intestines, help infants gain weight, and manufacture important B vitamins. Freeze-dried varieties are sometimes given to very young children to bolster their supplies of intestinal flora and relieve digestive problems. This strain also protects children from certain forms of diarrhea and dysentery.

Other Strains

Other types of probiotic bacteria you may find in commercial supplements include *Lactobacillus casei*, *Lactobacillus plantarum*, *Lactobacillus salivarius*, and *Lactobacillus rhamnosu*. There are a number of more unusual strains as well, all of which have their medical uses and their advocates.

ALL PROBIOTICS ARE NOT CREATED EQUAL

Remember, not all probiotic bacteria are the same, and neither are their effects. In a study reported at the annual Digestive Disease Week in 2002, Dr. Liam O'Mahony and colleagues from Ireland studied the effects of eleven different strains of probiotic bacteria on Salmonella infection in animals.

While most of the probiotic strains helped reduce Salmonella bacteria in the intestines of the infected animals, five of these strains also reduced Salmonella that had migrated into the body across the gut wall, and nine strains led to weight gain. Of the eleven strains studied, *B. infantis* UCC 35624 offered the best overall healing and protection.

PUTTING PROBIOTICS TO WORK FOR YOU

Who needs probiotics? Who stands to profit from them most? A thumbnail list of likely candidates includes the following:

- People who are chronically constipated
- People who suffer from chronic diarrhea
- People with high cholesterol
- People who are currently taking a course of antibiotics or undergoing radiation treatment
- People with unspecified but persistent digestive complaints such as gas, bloating, heartburn, and diarrhea. Probiotics may also be useful for people who suffer from skin diseases such as acne. In some cases, these rashes are secondary to gut infections.
- People suffering from chronic bowel problems or yeast infections, especially vaginal and urinary yeast infection. It is recommended that people in this category use probiotics under the guidance of a health-care professional.

A long list, yes, and with many more possibilities.

Be aware that, as in any new commercial field, regulation of claims made by manufacturers tends to be spotty. Many probiotic formulas remain undertested, and the promotional hoopla surrounding certain brands generates its share of half truths and unproven promises. The same is true with the quality control used to manufacture these products. It varies substantially from brand to brand.

Some probiotic supplements, for example, are poorly filtered, and arrive in the store with unwanted pathogens mixed in. In other instances, processing harms the integrity of the bacteria. A brand of yogurt may advertise itself with buzzwords like "natural" and "organic." But if it is not made from live active cultures, or if it is overheated, overpreserved, or watered down with jellies and sugars, it will deliver a minimum of nutritive value.

Likewise, some probiotics are subjected to violent spinning in the centrifugation process. This procedure can damage delicate microorganism chains. Still other probiotic products are manufactured in a satisfactory way, but are then shipped without adequate refrigeration, and the cultures die in transit.

Note that probiotic liquids are extremely potent when first manufactured, but that they are easily damaged by light, variations in temperature, and overhandling. Powders and freeze dried products tend to hold up better, though in some instances they are less potent than liquids.

A primary caution to take when purchasing a probiotic is to read the information on the package or bottle that tells you which strains are included. Check the product's selections against the listing of strains presented above. In general, the best probiotic brands include Lactobacillus bacteria such as *Lactobacilli acidophilus* and *bulgaricus,* and Bifidobacteria such as *Bifidobacteria bifidum* and *longum.* "A true probiotic," claims Natasha Trenev, president of the probiotic manufacturer Natren, "has to list species and strain, have the correct media, and contain the supernatent, which is the original growth media."

Another important feature to determine is whether or not probiotic supplements are housed and sold in a refrigerated climate. If not, it is probably best to avoid them—unrefrigerated bacteria die quickly at room temperature and above. A study carried out by the National Nutritional Foods Association of Newport Beach in California discovered that approximately 50 percent of the probiotic products vended in retail stores contain far fewer living organisms than are advertised on the labels, primarily because of lack of refrigeration. In a study presented at the annual Digestive Disease Week conference in 2002, Dr. Jeffrey Katz reported a wide range of bacterial composition and concentration among probiotics. According to Dr. Katz, 39 percent of the probiotic products he studied showed a significant variation between the concentration of live bacteria advertised on the labels and the actual amounts included in the products.

Another feature to check: Are the supplements properly packaged? It is good if the product comes in a bottle. It is even better if the bottle is darkly tinted. Dark glass protects delicate bacteria from direct light and heat and increases its life span. Probiotic products packaged in plastic should be avoided.

What about dampness control? The better brands of probiotics include a desiccant in their packaging to maintain internal dryness, as bacteria tend to die in a moist climate. People with food allergies will want to look for probiotic brands that are labeled as hypoallergenic, and that avoid the use of wheat or other highly allergic food substances.

Also check the expiration date on the package, and make sure you are purchasing a fresh batch. It is a good sign when the product features a guarantee of viability, and when the label assures you of a certain number of living organisms per gram in the mixture, measured as CFUs. The National Yogurt Association requires that active yogurt contain 100 million CFU per gram at the time of manufacture and 10 million at the end of shelf life. Since many of these bacteria die en route to the colon, these numbers may not be adequate to deliver enough bacteria alive to the colon to do the job. Some yogurts available in health-food stores carry much higher numbers than required. In general, 1 billion bacteria is adequate; 3 to 5 billion (or more) is better.

What about freeze-dried products? If prepared properly, these are fine, and do, in fact, increase shelf life. If refrigeration is not available, for whatever reasons, freeze-dried products make an excellent substitute.

Finally, there is the question of whether the addition of fructo-oligosaccharide (FOS) to probiotic products is a helpful or harmful addendum. A derivative of sugar fructose, FOS is found naturally in foods like Jerusalem artichokes, leeks, garlic, onions, and several grains. Proponents of FOS claim FOS adds valuable fiber to the diet, and encourages the growth of helpful *Bifidobacteria* in the colon. Some probiotics manufacturers intentionally add them to their products, and tout them as a valuable nutritional supplement.

Dr. K. S. Swanson and colleagues, writing in the *Journal of Nutrition* (2002), state that the supplementation of mono-oligosaccharides tends to have beneficial effects on microbial populations and systemic immune characteristics, whereas fructo-oligosaccharide supplementation decreases the concentrations of selected protein catabolites formed in the large bowel. The combination of the two enhances local and systemic immune function and decreases the concentrations of toxic compounds found in feces.

Similarly, writing in the journal of *Bone and Mineral Research* (2001), Dr. M. Tahiri from France concludes that intake of short-chain fructo-oligosaccharides increases intestinal absorption and the amounts of magnesium in postmenopausal women.

On the other hand, probiotic manufacturers like Natren claim that sugar-based FOS encourages yeast growth in the gut, along with the growth of *Klebsiella,* a pathogenic organism associated with a variety of diseases. They also claim that FOS is difficult to purify commercially (it is used in Japan as a low-calorie sucrose replacement in cakes and breads), and should be labeled as a chemical additive rather than as a natural supplement.

Where the truth lies is difficult to tell. Both sides make compelling arguments. In the long run, if the addition of FOS raises a red flag for you, there is an easy way around this. Simply opt for the conservative approach and avoid probiotic products that contain them.

A SAMPLING OF HIGH-QUALITY PROBIOTIC PRODUCTS

Since probiotics is a relatively new field, and since many health-conscious people are confused when they shop for these items, a description of seven popular commercial brands is presented below for your edification.

These seven brands are considered by many health practitioners to offer well-processed, carefully packaged products that contain a high density of fresh, live bacteria. The list below is not presented as a testimonial for these products, simply as an index of available and well-produced varieties. So shop with care, try them out, then stick with the brand that works for you. The Web sites, phone numbers, and addresses for these products are included in the Appendix.

1. **Allergy Research Group**—Allergy Research products contain *Lactobacillus acidophilus* and *Bifidobacterium longum* extracted from nondairy sources. Their nondairy origin makes them an excellent choice for people with milk allergies and lactose intolerance. Strict vegetarians will also find them useful.
2. **PB8**—A probiotic best-seller and winner of several awards, PB8 Pro-Biotic Acidophilus contains eight strains of beneficial bacteria per tablet. PB8 also puts out a nice line of probiotics for children.
3. **Natural Factors**—Another well-known and trusted manufacturer,

Natural Factors produces a fine line of *acidophilus* and *bifido* products containing a highly respectable 4 to 10 billion active cells. Natural Factors also produces a line of probiotics for children.

4. **D'Adamo 4 Your Type Probiotics**—D'Adamo probiotic supplements are specifically geared to different blood types, offering an interesting alternative to other brands. D'Adamo products are not centrifuged, which is good, and they include phytonutrients as well as bacterial flora.

5. **Natren**—Natren is one of the largest and most established sellers of probiotics. They manufacture a popular and reasonably priced line of flora supplements, along with associated products such as probiotic skin creams. Natren products are the probiotics you are most likely to find for sale at health-food stores.

6. **NutraCea**—A division of Nutrastar Inc., NutraCea markets the useful product Synbiotic-3. Each 500-mg capsule contains 4.5 billion live bacteria extracted from four different probiotic strains. The capsules are enteric coated to withstand corrosive digestive juices, allowing the maximum number of live bacteria to reach the colon.

7. **Custom Probiotic**—This company sells its Adult Formula CP-1 capsule containing five strains of probiotics with an extremely high bacterial count of 25 billion per capsule. This product is quite powerful and probably equally effective.

By way of an addendum, it can be added that Dr. W. Allan Walker, presenting at the annual postgraduate course of the American Gastroenterologic Association at the annual Digestive Disease Week conference in 2002, recommended the following probiotics, claiming they are both reliable and cost-effective:

- **VSL#3**—VSL#3 contains four strains of *Lactobacilli*, three strains of *bifidobacteria*, and one strain of *Streptococcus salivarius*. According to Dr. Walker, its high success rate at healing certain digestive disorders in double-blind, placebo-controlled trials has caused a great deal of positive buzz among digestive disease specialists.

- **Stonyfield Farm Yogurt**—The bacterial content in this brand of yo gurt is considerably higher than in most other commercial brands. And, as we know, the higher the concentration, the greater the chances that friendly bacteria will survive the digestive juices in the intestine, reach the colon, and make themselves at home on the colonic wall. Ideally, a brand of yogurt should contain at least 3 to 5 billion live bacteria to attain this lofty goal. Most available yogurts—with the exception of Stonyfield Farm—do not come close to this figure. Stonyfield yogurts are reputed to have 10 billion live bacteria at the time of manufacture, as compared to the National Yogurt Association's requirement of 100 million per gram. Stonyfield Farm also contains the powerful and unusual bacterial strains *L. casei* and *L. reuter*— an added plus.
- **Other probiotic aids**—Dr. Walker also suggests that patients use the probiotics Culturelle and 3 Actimel, along with kefir products in fermented milk form, and chewable tablet probiotics.

Finally, a last word of advice. As mentioned above, the claims for probiotics often exaggerate their own effectiveness. Despite what vendors may tell you, and despite the curative promise that these foods show in laboratory studies, probiotics are by no means a panacea for what ails you and should in no way be taken in lieu of medical treatment for serious digestive conditions.

Use these helpful supplements for the prevention of digestive disease and for the treatment of nagging but relatively minor ailments. But for serious digestive maladies, probiotics should be thought of as a useful support for conventional medical treatment, and *never* as a substitute for it.

chapter nine

Detoxification Techniques: A Clean Gut for a Clean Body and Mind

Internal-cleansing techniques are as old as medicine itself. Instructions for giving enemas can be read in the Eber Papyrus, an Egyptian document dating to 1500 B.C. In the Hindu Ayurveda, a medical system with roots tracing back to 4,000-year-old Vedic texts, water enemas and oil enemas are major constituents of an inner-cleansing procedure known as the "Five Procedures." Health-minded Greeks in ancient Athens regularly took the self-cleansing cure at the Aesculapian healing sanitariums located high in the cloud-covered mountains. Here a program of diet, fasting, purgatives, meditation, rest, and healing dreams was prescribed, both to cure disease and to calm the soul. The Greek physician, Hippocrates, whose caduceus staff is the symbol of modern medicine, recommended cleansing fasts for his patients, especially for stomach and gut problems. He was also an advocate of enemas for ridding the colon of toxins. So was Galen, one of the founders of Western medicine.

Detoxification therapy has been preached and practiced for thousands of years. Yet, like many nondrug-oriented procedures, it is rarely looked on today as a legitimate medical technique, and is conspicuously passed over in conventional healing programs.

In the absence of rigorously performed studies and FDA approvals, many medical researchers argue that any treatment, old or new, must automatically be considered ineffective until proven otherwise. All claims to its success should be labeled as "anecdotal."

Researchers will also tell you that we have medical methods today that improve on the old ways, and that make them outmoded. In the absence of rigorously performed studies and FDA approvals, a treatment is considered not effective. I once heard a colleague remark that we no longer need any type of detoxification procedures because "a good laxative gets the job done just as well."

Perhaps this is true, but most likely it is not. And, anyway, why use powerful laxative drugs when a wholesome regimen of fasting and herbs does the job just as well? Should we discard thousands of years of tradition simply because the pharmaceutical companies have a vested interest in not learning more about traditional, nondrug-based medical therapies? Should we throw the baby out with the bathwater? One could argue that such attitudes are not only biased and shortsighted, but are also potentially harmful to the health of a nation.

Why? Because at no other time in human history have detoxification methods been so needed as they are today. Consider, for example, the world as it existed 150 years ago. Our oceans were largely uncontaminated at this time, and our forests were mostly intact. The air we breathed was already compromised here and there by coal fumes and factory smoke, but it was still a good deal cleaner than the noxious yellow clouds that hover over most of the world's great cities today. In the absence of the internal combustion engine, languages of the world did not yet include terms we take so for granted today, terms such as "smog," "global warming," "toxic waste," and "greenhouse effect."

The foods we ate 100 years ago were whole foods. None of them were yet grown with chemical fertilizers or sprayed with toxins. None had their fiber pressed out at the food plant or the vitamins cooked away on the assembly line. None were treated with preservatives to increase shelf life at the supermarket.

Today, of course, as we know too well, the air, water, and food we take into our bodies are heavily freighted with pollutants of every kind—millions of them by official count. The result of this noxious bombardment is that our bodies are many times more contaminated than they were a century ago. Indeed, they are probably more contaminated than they have been at any other time in human history.

Moreover, as the situation worsens, we grow accustomed to bodily insults that were unknown to our recent ancestors. To accommodate the growing amounts of toxins in our air and earth, such as arsenic and lead, scientists continue to redefine what the "normal" and "acceptable" levels are for these poisons—as if the official act of deeming these substances safe makes them so. What's more, the fact that the human alimentary canal is the major intake and processing channel for these virulent substances means that over the years our guts take the brunt of all this pollution.

Is it any wonder, then, that by the time people in modern society reach adulthood they have eaten close to a pound of deadly heavy metals such as lead, mercury, cadmium, and aluminum, along with a good deal of arsenic, and at least 200 pounds of assorted toxic chemicals? Presently there are an average of 40 known carcinogens in our drinking water. There are 65 known carcinogens in our food, and 60 in the air we breathe. In the cellular tissue of a middle-aged woman or man, 177 different types of carbon-based chlorine substances can be found, many of them carcinogenic. Most men and women over the age of thirty-five in the United States are known to have detectable levels of the carcinogens DDT and PCB in their systems, although the federal government banned DDT-based pesticides in 1972.

A key problem with this abundance of pollution is that our bodies in general, and our digestive tract in particular, are not constitutionally built to process and eliminate the endless number of poisons found in contaminated food, air, and water. Many of these toxic substances thus linger for long periods in the body where they may contribute to the development of disease, and to a variety of mental-emotional conditions. It thus follows that any method that helps reduce the amount of toxins in our bodies and that cleans out the conduits through which these toxins pass is a welcome one.

Reenter detoxification.

How You Become Overtoxified

There are two ways in which the body can become overtoxified. The first is through the constant ingestion and inhalation of pollutants. On the list of contaminants we are likely to be exposed to within the next twenty-four hours are food preservatives, food flavorings, food colorings, emulsifiers, pesticides, agricultural fertilizers, certain medical drugs like antibiotics, air contaminants like automobile exhaust, cigarette smoke, smog, sprays, industrial fumes, plus heavy metals in the water and earth, chemicals from household cleaning fluids, workplace fumes, radiation, alcohol, street drugs, and all the other usual suspects that exert long-term destabilizing effects on the body's biochemistry.

The second way in which we become contaminated is by the production of toxins within the body itself. This process originates primarily in the digestive system, and is caused by factors such as infectious bacteria, yeast overgrowth, digestive disorders, food allergies, metabolism of medications, and perhaps also by a functional slowdown of the digestive organs themselves.

As people age, for example, peristalsis tends to become sluggish in the gut, and the transit time for wastes moving through the intestines slows to a crawl. As a result, toxins remain in the digestive tract for increasingly long periods of time. The longer they remain here, the more likely they are to reabsorb through the intestinal walls and enter the bloodstream. Once in the blood, these toxins are then transported to every part of the body, becoming that much more difficult to isolate and purge.

What physiological episodes actually take place when toxins reabsorb into the body? Once absorbed into the blood, the first location that many toxins travel to is the liver, one of the body's major cleaning and purifying organs. The liver makes a gallant effort to filter and detoxify this overflow. But it is already working overtime trying to perform its other functions, such as synthesizing proteins and regulating body metabolism, and before long it goes on overload. An extreme example of this process is when a person takes too much of a common over-the-counter medication such as acetaminophen. Large quantities of this chemical quickly produce an abundance of metabolites and toxins, forcing the liver into danger mode. In large enough doses, these "harmless" medications can literally kill us.

When such major overloads occur, unprocessed chemicals, heavy metals, and toxic metabolites begin to "leak" out of the digestive system and pass into the bloodstream. From there, they migrate to different cells throughout the body where they are drawn into the hair and nails, sucked up by fat cells, or absorbed into the bones. Once lodged in these "storage areas," the poisons remain until they are flushed or leeched out. In the meantime, they may cause cellular damage, trigger disease, and/or induce generalized feelings of fatigue, depression, and malaise.

So there we have it: Sluggish intestines, a colon that does not process all its wastes, a liver compromised by overwork, and different cells acting as storage repositories for poisons that should have been ejected long ago.

How to Tell When You're Overtoxified

The body is a miraculous instrument with an enormous capacity to absorb harmful influences. This means that, in certain cases, we may be toxified to the limit and still feel just fine. Or we may feel a few unpleasant twinges here and there but not recognize the origin of these sensations. What are the signs and response patterns that suggest overtoxification? How can we tell when its time to clean our internal house?

People who suffer from two, three, or more of the following symptoms, and have not been diagnosed by a physician as suffering from a specific ailment, should consider overtoxification as a possible culprit:

- Headaches
- Sinus congestion
- High blood-fat level
- Skin rashes and acne
- Bad breath

- Joint pains
- Constipation
- Cough and wheezing
- Fatigue
- Red eyes

- Dizziness
- Diarrhea
- Insomnia
- Indigestion
- Obesity

These symptoms are nonspecific, yes, and may result from a thousand possible malfunctions. But be on the alert when:

1. They appear in clusters and are not associated with a specific disease.
2. They come and go without apparent reason.
3. They linger without improvement and without apparent change.
4. No specific or satisfactory diagnosis can be made.

How do we go about protecting ourselves—and healing ourselves—from these symptoms once we identify their toxic roots? By taking a few days out of our busy schedules and applying a sound program of internal body detoxification. The following section describes how it's done.

BEGINNER'S GUIDE TO DETOXIFICATION TECHNIQUES

Knowledge is power. Learn as much as possible about detox strategies. Detoxification purges poisons from the body by neutralizing harmful substances, transforming them, or removing them directly from the system in the form of mucus, sweat, and wastes. The primary goals of detoxification are the following:

1. To remove toxins from the organs, specifically the organs of digestion and elimination: the stomach, intestines, kidney, and liver
2. To create conditions that allow the body to heal itself from the harmful effects of these toxins
3. To promote specific physical benefits including an improvement in the body's ability to assimilate food nutrients, the elimination of

potentially harmful bacteria and pollutants, and the facilitation of cell repair and maintenance

4. To increase a sense of wellness and well-being, both physically and mentally

Who needs detoxification? Basically, all of us. Even if we lived in a world without pollution, the day-to-day rounds of eating, breathing, digesting, and eliminating would leave their traces, depositing noxious residues in our body systems. As the years pass, the healthiest and fittest among us accumulate large amounts of these residues, and from time to time these residues need to be purged. Not to push the machine analogy too far, but, loosely speaking, periodic detoxification of the digestive tract is as important to body maintenance as a regular oil change and tune-up are to the life of a car.

Detox programs are helpful for a variety of situations. They aid in cleaning out unwanted bacteria and viruses left behind by infectious ailments. They speed up the rate of recovery from disease. They help people age gracefully. And they offer relief from the all-too-common sensations of fatigue and soreness, of feeling half alive, which in many instances are not caused by disease in particular but by an overload of litter and debris in body tissue.

Many health-conscious people, therefore, make a point of undergoing a detoxification program at least once a year, or even once a month. If the program is well balanced and does not overtax a person's system, it goes a long way toward restoring digestive function, increasing mental clarity, and promoting general feelings of well-being.

The methods described in this chapter feature several fundamental detox technologies including fasting, herbal cleaners, diet, sauna, and enemas. There are other options in this area, which, if you become an advocate of detoxification, you will no doubt discover for yourself.

If the thought of undergoing a detox regimen intrigues you, select a block of time on your calendar and set it aside as detox day or week. It's helpful if this time period falls on a weekend or, better, during a vacation. Most people find that they can work and detox at the same time without difficulty. Still, vacations make you more relaxed, and thus more respon sive to internal-cleansing techniques.

What physical reactions might you expect from a detoxification program? The first thing you should know is that there may be side effects, especially from fasting. Most are experienced during the first two or three days when the body is throwing off poisons at a ferocious rate, and almost all of them are minor. After this period, side effects usually pass. The possible reactions to detox include the following:

- Headache
- Unpleasant body odor
- Mucous drip and congestion
- Apathy or irritability
- Bad breath
- Nausea
- Fatigue

None of these reactions is serious. It is interesting to note, however, that sometimes symptoms from a past flu return during detox. If this occurs, do not panic. It is a positive sign—toxic substances that have been lingering in your body for years are finally being washed out. If you do feel unusually weak or dizzy during detox, or if these symptoms are severe and/ or continue for more than twenty-four to forty-eight hours, consult with your health-care provider.

Now for the good news. Once you complete a week or two of detox, there are a number of possible benefits awaiting you. These include increased energy, relief from sinus headaches and chronic congestion, sweeter breath, better skin, clearer thinking, stronger powers of concentration, heightened mood, larger and smoother bowel movements, and improved digestion—not to mention the favorable effects that detoxification brings to stubborn cases of chronic disease.

How long should a detox program last? If you are a beginner, limit the initial session to a week. After you get your sea legs and learn your body's tolerances, increase the time period to several weeks. It all depends on your needs and the detox strategy you adopt. Remember, undergoing detoxification does not mean that you must apply all the methods presented in this chapter all at once. You may, for example, wish to do a two-week cleansing program accompanied by only a three-day fast. You then spend the rest of the two-week period eating simple foods, taking saunas, and using cleansing herbs.

Each of the methods outlined below approaches detoxification from a different perspective and technique. Each is designed to clean different parts of the body and digestive tract. Some of these techniques, for example, clean the small intestines and the colon. Some flush out the liver. Some are designed to increase the flow of enzymes, bile, and digestive juices to heighten waste removal. Others allow the digestive system to rest, or force toxins out of the body through the sweat glands. Still others encourage the release of poisons from fat cells. Nature has provided many exit points in the body for the elimination of stubborn toxins. A good detox program takes advantage of them all.

Caution: Fasting should be done only if you are healthy and not suffering from a chronic disease. If you have heart problems, hyperthyroidism, blood-sugar abnormalities such as diabetes, mental disease, or any other type of chronic disorder, fasting may not be advisable. Consult with a qualified health-care professional before attempting any of the programs presented below.

Seven Great Ways to Detox Your System

1. Fasting

We go about our everyday lives working, playing, and, most of all, eating, eating, eating. In the process, our bowels rarely rest. Even when we are asleep, they bubble and churn away tirelessly. Eventually it becomes necessary to give these hard-working organs a break. Enter the fast.

Fasting, in a nutshell, is designed to reprogram the gut, to rebalance its energies, and to fine-tune many of the digestive and eliminative functions that become sluggish over time. Its benefits are many, not the least of which is a simple enhancement in well-being.

After going a day or two without eating, many people begin to feel sensations of buoyancy and inner peace. The absence of food in the gut allows the digestive system to recuperate. Energy is released to other parts of the body that would normally be used for digestion. Fasters often experience a unique sensation of total relaxation coupled with high levels of energy, plus a delightful keenness of the senses. While it's true that some fasters become tired and lethargic, most tend to remain invigorated, and a few people become positively exuberant.

Preparation. Several days before you begin to fast, eat simple foods; take smaller portions at each meal; drink plenty of liquids, especially water; and give yourself lots of time to rest. Prepare yourself mentally. You are about to take a holiday from an event you have participated in every day of your life, three to six times a day, namely, eating. This is no small undertaking. Treat it with the respect and mental preparation it deserves.

Methods of fasting. There are three basic types of fasts:

1. Water fasts
2. Juice fasts
3. Single-food fasts

Since no nutrients are taken in during a water fast, a water fast is more demanding than a juice fast. On the other hand, water flushes out the system better than juice, and tends to bring faster healing results. Single-food fasts are less purifying than liquid fasts, but are easier to practice, and many people believe they are safer as well.

All three methods are effective. The one you finally choose depends on your mental preparation, your degree of toxicity, and your physical health. In general, water fasts are better for people in excellent health, juice fasts and single-food fasts for people whose state of health is not at its peak.

Here's a game plan for all three.

How to perform a water fast.

1. On the first day of the fast, drink two glasses of water as soon as you get up in the morning, and drink two more an hour later. Take no solid food during the day.

2. Drink a full glass of water at mid morning. Drink another at lunchtime, another in the early afternoon, then another in late afternoon, early and late evening, and then before going to bed at night.

3. Prepare to urinate frequently. Each time you urinate, large amounts of toxins are being washed out. Urination is good. Just remember: Your bladder will be working overtime during a water fast. Plan your hourly comings and goings at work and play accordingly, with knowledge of where to locate a rest room kept firmly in mind.

4. If hunger gets the best of you, dine on a clear soup such as bouillon or miso soup. If you have an irresistible craving for solid food, eat a bit of banana or some applesauce.

5. While fasting, alternate times of rest with periods of activity. Gentle activity (not vigorous) amplifies the benefits of fasting by raising metabolism, oxygenating the blood, and speeding up elimination through urination and sweating. Walking, light stretching, light calisthenics, deep breathing, and household chores all get the juices flowing. Try to perform a half hour's worth of physical activity every day. Just don't push it. If you feel tired, rest. Use your discretion. Each of us has different needs in this area.

6. Drink only pure water. Distilled water is best due to its absorbent properties. Bottled water, filtered water, and fresh spring water are also excellent. Avoid tap water.

7. While fasting, supplement the cleaning process by taking a multivitamin and mineral every day, plus an additional 1,000 mg of vitamin C two times a day.

Reminder: Before beginning a water fast, always consult with a health-care professional who is experienced in fasting therapy. High-water-intake detox fasts should not be undertaken by people on fluid restriction.

How to perform a juice fast.

1. A few minutes after getting up in the morning, and every four hours thereafter, drink a glass of fresh juice. Supplement the drink

with four to five glasses of water taken at intervals throughout the day.

2. Make every effort to drink fruit and vegetable juices that are extracted from a juicer. If possible, use unsprayed, organic produce. Celery-carrot and celery-apple-parsley-carrot vegetable combinations are excellent, and all juice well. For fruit juice, try extracted grape juice, watermelon juice, and orange juice, either juiced singly or in combination. The apple-pear combination is also hardy. So is a combination of banana, apple, and grape. The following juices all provide refreshment and nutrition.

Juice one for fasting

1 yam

2 pears

2 oranges

Juice two for fasting

4 carrots

1 apple

½ bunch parsley

Juice three for fasting

1 yam

2 red grapefruits

2 pears

Juice four for fasting

1 honeydew melon, without rind

2 pears

1 lemon

Juice five for fasting

1 yam

2 lemons

2 cooked beets

1 onion

2 stalks celery

1 inch fresh ginger, skinned

3. If you do not have access to a juice extractor, the next best option is to use a commercial organic juice. The purer the juice, the better the detox.

   Note: If you are fasting on strongly acidic fruit juices such as lemon, orange, or grapefruit, drinking large amounts as soon as you get up in the morning can trigger indigestion and cramping. Let the first juice of the day be vegetable rather than fruit.

4. Avoid all solid foods while fasting, if possible. If your hunger gets the best of you, eat soft or juicy fruits such as bananas or mangoes. The more watery, the better. Vegetables such as cucumbers and celery are also good. Miso soup, clear vegetable soup, herbal teas, and bouillon make excellent stomach fillers. Another superb source of gut-friendly nutrition is to eat yogurt. Be sure to pick a brand made from live-culture bacteria.

5. As with a water fast, it is helpful to alternate rest periods with periods of activity. Paced physical activity amplifies the benefits of fasting by raising metabolism and speeding up the elimination of toxins through urination and sweating. Gentle exercises such as walking, stretching, and swimming are recommended. Practice them for about a half hour every day, depending on your health and tolerance. If you feel too tired to exercise, don't worry about it. Do what your body tells you is best.

6. Supplement your juice fast with a good multiple vitamin every day, plus 1,000 mg of vitamin C two times a day and a good combination probiotic (see Chapter 8).

Reminder: Before beginning a juice fast, always consult with a healthcare professional who is experienced in fasting therapy.

How to perform a single-food fast.

Besides juice and water, a third form of fast is gaining popularity these days—the single-food fast. Eating a single food gives the digestion a chance to rest, and allows the digestive tract to repair and readjust itself. The single-food fast also keeps the appetite at bay more effectively than liquid fasts and is generally the easiest of all types of fasts.

The concept behind this fast is simple: fasters dine exclusively on one type of food for a given period of time. Typical choices of single foods include watermelon, cantaloupe, melon, rice, grapes, and yogurt. After eating one food for three to seven days, fasters then gradually reintroduce other foods into their eating program. This is done slowly, adding two new foods one day (preferably soft), four new foods the next, and so on for about a week. After this time, normal eating patterns can be resumed.

The single-food fast, in other words, runs for approximately two weeks. During the first week, fasters eat only a single food; during the second week, they slowly reintroduce regular foods back into their menu.

One interesting option here is to make buttermilk the food of choice. Drink it several times a day, adding a teaspoon of honey for sweetening and an extra boost of nutrition. Use homemade buttermilk if possible or, if this is not available, a commercial variety made from live cultures. After four to seven days of an all-buttermilk diet, take another six to seven days to reintroduce new foods back into the diet.

Breaking the fast. After abstaining from food for the prescribed period of time, you will want to return to solid foods gradually. The day you break your fast, start by eating fresh, soft fruit accompanied by yogurt and an assortment of easily digestible, succulent vegetables. A large bowl of salad (lettuce, cucumbers, radishes, and tomatoes) with vinegar and light olive oil dressing, along with a glass of buttermilk, is also excellent. Eat a predominantly protein-based meal for supper, avoiding starches such as beans, potatoes, or grains. The next day, increase your intake of vegetables and fruits. Add some starchy vegetables, some bread, and some grains. On the third day, return to your normal eating patterns.

How long should you fast? Some people like to start off with a week's fast, but then end up cutting it short after a day or so. Others intend a two-day fast but enjoy the experience so much that they continue on for days. There are no absolutes rules.

In general, three days is a good goal to set in the beginning. After you become accustomed to fasting and learn your tolerances, you can, with your physician's go-ahead, increase this time accordingly. Any fast that runs longer than a week, however, is serious business, and should be done only under the watchful eye of a licensed health-care professional.

Finally, note that most healthy individuals can get along without solid food for two weeks and perhaps longer without experiencing any serious adverse consequences. Adequate hydration must *always* be maintained while fasting, however, and is a vital part of the process. Always drink plenty of liquids while on a fast.

How often should you fast? A snappy one-day or two-day clean-up fast can be undertaken once a week (for example, a juice or grainless diet). Longer fasts are best practiced once or twice a year. Some people make a point of fasting on their birthdays each year to help align the physical readjustments that fasting brings with their body's natural biorhythms.

2. Detoxifying with Food and Diet

After a round of fasting, many people continue to detoxify their systems with a diet of easily digestible foods that also contain toxin-fighting properties. Foods that fit this bill include the following:

- Cruciferous vegetables such as cauliflower, kale, turnips, Brussels sprouts, broccoli, and bok choy all expedite the self-cleansing process. Eat a serving of cruciferous vegetables at least once a day and preferably twice when on a detox diet.
- Foods replete with B vitamins, such as whole-grain breads, and vitamin C–rich foods such as cabbage, oranges, grapefruits, and peppers specifically help eliminate toxins generated by infection. Both food groups are useful for people recovering from antibiotic use.
- Foods rich in sulfur such as garlic, red peppers, onions, broccoli, Brussels sprouts, and eggs help the body rid itself of food additives and preservatives, environmental pollutants, and harmful intestinal bacteria.

- Fat-soluble toxins such as heavy metals and chemical pesticides that lodge in fat cells are notoriously difficult to purge. The body has its ways of eliminating these poisons, however, specifically through the liver and kidneys. This process is catalyzed by a number of metabolic processes that convert fat-soluble toxins into water-soluble metabolites, which the body can then eliminate with ease. Vitamin C and vitamin E both help in the process.
- Even more effective as a protective mechanism is glutathione. Made up of three amino acids, it guards the liver from toxic overload and, at the same time, protects body tissue from free radicals. It is one of the most powerful anticarcinogens known. Glutathione is found in citrus fruits, most vegetables, and meat. It is also available in supplement form.
- Go heavy on the greens. Chlorophyll-rich green foods such as cabbage, lettuce, broccoli, kale, and parsley have a purifying effect on the gut and provide large amounts of vitamins. Chlorophyll-rich foods oxygenate the blood, build more blood, and speed up internal healing. Green leafy vegetables are rich in folic acid and essential vitamins and minerals.
- Eating legumes and whole grains that contain the trace mineral molybdenum can eliminate sulfite-based food additives and preservatives such as those found in dried fruit. Low molybdenum levels in people with allergies have been shown to trigger asthmatic reactions. Conversely, when molybdenum levels are increased, allergic symptoms decrease.
- For smokers, it has been found that curcumin, the ingredient in turmeric that gives this spice its yellow color, helps neutralize hydrocarbons and carcinogens generated by inhaled tobacco smoke. Smokers are urged to use this spice liberally in their food, or to take a capsule or two every day with meals. Most Indian dishes are spiced with turmeric.
- Avoid too much milk, cream, and butter, but eat plenty of yogurt and acidophilus products. These wonderful foods multiply the helpful flora in the gut, which, in turn, improves elimination. Yogurt also ap-

pears to reduce blood cholesterol levels. Be sure to eat yogurt made from live cultures. See Chapters 7 and 8 for details.

- Eat only organic, unsprayed fruits, grains, and vegetables. Organic milk and yogurt are available at many health-food stores and some supermarkets. Note that yogurt brands available at health-food stores are more likely to contain greater quantities of live cultures than those sold at regular grocery stores. Check the label.
- During detox, avoid processed foods, white breads, sweets, fried foods, fatty foods, and highly spicy foods. Stay away from coffee and alcohol. Keep it bland; keep it simple.
- For a week or two, try eating only when you are hungry. Forget about three meals a day. Eat ten times a day if you like, but keep the portions small, lean, and bland. Chew well, and eat only until you feel three-quarters full.

3. *Detoxifying Supplements and Foods*
The supplements discussed below are all useful for cleansing the digestive apparatus and reducing liver toxicity.

Psyllium husk powder. Psyllium husk powder is a safe and potent natural bulk-forming laxative. It is mentioned many times throughout this book, and with good reason. A form of fiber, psyllium swells and hydrates the feces, stimulating peristalsis and encouraging stools to pass quickly and easily through the gut. Psyllium powder also eliminates cholesterol from the body, and serves as a kind of "scouring pad" to remove debris and toxins embedded along the intestinal wall.

A main ingredient of commercial laxatives such as Metamucil, Konsyl, and Perdiem, psyllium can be purchased as a powder or husk at health-food stores. It is also available in capsule form. While fasting, consider taking a spoonful of psyllium powder dissolved in water every day to enhance the detox effects. Be sure to wash psyllium down with two to three glasses of water. Avoid taking any medications within one to two hours after taking.

Milk thistle. Containing a powerful flavonoid combination and the antioxidant silymarin, milk thistle is a first-line herbal medicine for boosting liver function, regenerating damaged liver cells, improving liver ailments, and heightening the liver's ability to remove toxins. It is also a mild laxative.

Lab studies show that silymarin has a neutralizing effect on a number of toxins, including carbon tetrachloride, alcohol, and many industrial pollutants. Whereas the amino acid glutathione helps rid the body of many fat-soluble toxins, silymarin prevents this important substance from being depleted too quickly, thus promoting detoxification in yet another way. Dr. Bean in *American Clinical Laboratory* (2002) testifies to silymarin's healing properties, reporting that its beneficial effects are best seen in patients suffering with alcohol-induced cirrhosis of the liver. Many other studies testify to its detox powers. Milk thistle can be taken in fluid extract form or in capsules and tablets. It should not be taken during pregnancy or while breast-feeding.

Bentonite clay. Eating clay may sound far-fetched, but some people have been doing it for centuries, primarily because clay, and bentonite clay in particular, which comes from weathered volcanic ash, has amazing powers to absorb bacteria and to rid the body of unwanted contaminants. It also contains generous amounts of trace minerals such as thallium and ruthenium, which help absorb nutrients and throw off toxins.

Healing-wise, people tout bentonite for its ability to improve regularity; to relieve chronic constipation, diarrhea, and indigestion; and to increase the healing time for ulcers. Dr. Shen from Taiwan, in *Environmental Technology* (2002), recommends the use of bentonite clay to remove dissolved organic pollutant matter from water. He also suggests that clay may function as a recyclable medium for the absorption and combustion of organic pollutants. This finding supports the concept that, when taken in oral form, bentonite clay is, in fact, likely to prevent harmful effects in the gut.

Bentonite clay comes in a liquid suspension form. Take a tablespoon before each meal with two glasses of water, and another before going to bed at night. Bentonite clay is sold in some health-food stores and on the Internet. See the Appendix for details.

Probiotics and yogurt. Probiotic formulas provide strains of friendly digestive bacteria that help in beefing up digestion. These flora speed up elimination time, and help rid the body of a variety of unwanted toxins, especially stubborn yeast and infectious bacteria that cling tenaciously to the gastrointestinal tract. Use only yogurt with a high concentration of live cultures, or probiotic products. Consult Chapters 7 and 8 for specifics.

Black walnut hulls. Walnut hulls remove toxins, fatty materials, and certain parasites from the intestinal tract. It is available in 500-mg capsules. Take two capsules two to three times a day.

Flaxseed. As a gentle laxative and as a method for bulking up feces and eliminating toxins from the colon, flaxseed is a proven winner. Flaxseed oil is especially useful as an intestinal lubricant and as an overall detoxifier and antioxidant. Indeed, many health-care professionals consider it to be one of the best of all daily tonics for health and regularity. According to Dr. Fanich and colleagues from George Washington University, as reported in the *Journal of Renal Nutrition* (2001), flaxseed protects against structural and functional kidney damage in chronic renal diseases in humans. The journal *Urology* (2001) reports that Dr. Demark-Wahnefried and colleagues from Duke University Medical Center have shown that flaxseed supplements, when taken with a fat-restricted diet, improve the biology of prostate cancer. They suggest that further studies be made to determine the benefits of this regimen against prostate cancer.

Grind flaxseeds to a pulp in a coffee bean grinder or food processor, and take a spoonful or two twice a day. Use it on salads or baked potatoes. Flaxseed oil can be purchased at any health-food store. Keep it refrigerated; otherwise, it quickly turns rancid.

Licorice root. A wonderful overall internal cleanser, licorice is an antioxidant, liver protector, and potent detoxifier. In Chinese medical formulas, it is added to many mixtures to balance other herbs and increase their potency. Dr. Wang and Dr. Nixon report in the journal *Nutrition* *and Cancer* (2001) that licorice is known to have anti-inflammatory, antiviral, antiulcer, and anticancer activities. People with high blood pressure should not take the commercial form of licorice but should use the DGL variety instead. Do not use this herb for more than six weeks at a time. It should not be used by patients with irregular heartbeat, high blood pressure, or chronic liver or kidney disease. Persons over sixty years old should generally avoid use.

Garlic. Good for what ails you, garlic is an antioxidant, blood cleanser, and natural antibiotic, and helps lower blood fats. Garlic is useful for constipation and can be used for overall digestive cleansing. It may be taken as dried powder (500 to 1,000 mg), fresh cloves, or in garlic oil (8 mg a day).

Cayenne pepper. The heat in cayenne induces sweats that help eliminate body poisons. Cayenne pepper also increases metabolism and immune-system defenses and helps protect against stomach ulcers. Use as a spice in cooked food. Capsules in varying strengths are available for use as supplements.

Burdock root. A staple food among the Chinese and Japanese, burdock root is a blood purifier and antifungal, kills infectious bacteria in the gut, strengthens the liver, and purifies the blood. Try cooking a piece of fresh burdock root, which can usually be found at Japanese and Korean grocery stores. It's delicious. Do not use during pregnancy.

Ginger root. Besides its strong powers as a gut healer, ginger helps the body sweat and throw off toxins. The fresh variety has greater cleaning powers than the dried root.

Dandelion. Long used as a blood purifier, dandelion stimulates the body's ability to eliminate toxins on a cellular level. It is also an excellent tonic for the liver and is believed by some doctors to enhance white blood cell production, which in turn helps fight off infection.

Vitamin C. Vitamin C is a powerful antioxidant. Ample supplies are a must if the body is to successfully clean house. Take 500 to 1,000 mg a day.

Vitamin E. Vitamin E protects cells from destruction by free radicals. It also shields lung tissue from air pollutants, and its powerful antioxidant properties are believed to slow down the aging process in general.

Vitamin B complex. B vitamins help the liver perform its intricate detox work. They also fortify the immune system and improve digestion. B vitamins are best taken as part of a vitamin B complex.

Zinc. Zinc has strong antioxidant and healing qualities, and helps strengthen the immune system.

Copper. Copper aids overall body detoxification. Take it with zinc to enhance zinc's effects. Copper and zinc are included in most multivitamin formulas.

Choline. Choline is an essential component of cell membranes and is contained in compounds that move fat and bile from the liver, enhancing fat metabolism and cleaning the liver.

Tried-and-true traditional detox strategies. Try any of the following traditional Ayurvedic detox methods:

- Boil a teaspoon of shredded fresh ginger and three cardamom seeds together in a cup of water. Let the brew boil down to a half cup, then add a half cup of warm skimmed milk, plus a half teaspoon of honey. Drink as a detoxifier every day before breakfast for two weeks straight. During fasting days, drink it without adding milk.
- Cut up one onion and blend it into a juice using a blender or juicer. Drink a teaspoon of the mixture three times a day for two weeks. Another simple way to achieve internal detoxification is to drink a

freshly made combination of onion juice (two teaspoons), ginger juice (one teaspoon), and honey (two teaspoons). Take three table-spoons twice a day for two weeks. The inner-cleansing and detoxify-ing powers of fresh onion juice are legendary. These mixtures probably won't taste as bad as you think they will.

- The Hamdard drug company in India markets a powerful combina-tion blood detoxifier and cleanser based on Ayurvedic concepts. Known as Safi, it is a very popular remedy in India and is available in Indian grocery stores or on the Internet (see Appendix). Take one teaspoon in the morning with a glass of warm water.

- Baidyanath, along with many other drug companies in India, market the legendary Ayurvedic medicine for general detox known as Chyavanprash. Take a teaspoon two times a day with warm milk or water. You will find it at most Indian grocery stores.

- Neem leaf, or Azadirachta, is treasured in India for its strong internal and external cleansing properties. It is used extensively in Ayurvedic medicine to enhance digestion and detoxify the liver. For diabetics, studies show that neem helps lower and balance blood-sugar levels. Several studies document this herb's antimicrobial properties. Stud-ies by Dr. Sai Ram, for example, published in the *Journal of Ethno-pharmacology* (2000), and those of Dr. A. Vanka published in the *Indian Journal of Dental Research* (2001), show that neem leaf has strong purging and inner-purifying qualities throughout the body.

- For acne relief and skin purification, grind neem leaves into a paste and apply to the skin. Neem leaves can also be used to clean bacte-ria in the mouth. Dr. K. Almas, reporting in the *Indian Journal of Dental Research* (1999), recommends chewing neem sticks every day for oral hygiene and for ridding the saliva of unwanted bacteria. Dr. T. Venugopal and colleagues report in the *Indian Journal of Pedi-atrics* (1998) that children using neem chewing sticks for oral hy-giene are less likely to develop dental caries. Interestingly, students in India typically place neem leaves between the pages of their books to protect against paper-chewing insects.

- Detoxify your skin by applying a cinnamon or clove oil massage.

Both oils have antibacterial properties and are widely used in aromatherapy. Use these oils as a room freshener or in candle wax to detoxify the air.

4. Enemas and Colonics

When we enter the realm of enemas and colonics, we tread on controversial and shaky ground. First, we will discuss the difference between these two methods.

An enema involves the injection of liquid into the anus using a tube attached to an enema bag. The goal is to clean the lower part of the colon. Some people apply enemas with plain water. Others add lemon juice or olive oil to the water to further stimulate purging activity. Still others prefer commercial forms of enema fluid such as Fleets enemas. Still others prefer flushing fluids that are taken by mouth—for example, Golytely, CoLyte, and NuLytely, all of which require a doctor's prescription.

A colonic is a considerably more involved purging technique that must be administered by a trained professional at a colonic center, and that requires the use of special mechanical equipment to flush liquids far up into the colon, and then to reverse the flow and wash out wastes and impaction.

All about enemas. Enemas are primarily recommended for stubborn cases of constipation and for occasional internal flushes. When employed under the direction of a health-care professional, they are an efficient method of self-cleansing. They can also be self-applied, which makes this therapy available to everyone.

Generally speaking, enemas should be used only when necessary. Each time an enema is administered, the injected liquid does all the work, forcing the intestinal muscles that promote peristalsis into inactivity. When a person uses enemas too frequently, dependence may result (just as it does with habitual use of laxatives), and the muscles responsible for peristalsis soon lose their motivation and vitality. Enemas are thus recommended for occasional treatment of constipation or to add further detox power when fasting. Except in certain selected cases, they should by no means be used on a regular basis. Enemas containing phosphorus should not be used by patients suffering from renal failure.

A note about coffee enemas: A method developed during the 1930s by Dr. Max Gerson, coffee enemas were used at Gerson's clinic to treat various forms of cancer, apparently with some success. The theory behind the treatment is that coffee dilates the bile ducts and blood vessels, encouraging the excretion of cancer-produced toxins by the liver plus the dialysis of toxic products across the wall of the colon.

Today, a number of people use coffee enemas as a self-cleansing measure. Though the effectiveness of this method has not yet been substantiated in clinical studies, anecdotally speaking, users claim relief from a range of problems including insomnia, heart palpitations, fatigue, headaches, and a host of other woes. Coffee enemas have many advocates, some of them in high professional places.

If you intend to use coffee enemas as an adjunct to a detox program, be aware that there are cautions involved. For instance, too many enemas applied in a short period of time wreak havoc on the body's fluid balance. It is thus recommended that you use this technique with the supervision of a trained health-care specialist, at least in the beginning.

All about colonics. Champions of high colonics will inform you that over time the colon wall becomes caked with layers of poisonous debris and feces that literally clog up the digestive passageways the way sludge clogs a drain.

In my own practice and from my own observations, I have seen little evidence to back up this claim, and I consider the notion that most people's colons are narrowed with pounds of layered fecal remnants to be patently incorrect. What's more, colonic procedures are extremely invasive, and the centers where they are administered are rarely monitored by local health agencies for practice and sanitation. Colonics are known to deplete the digestive tract of much valuable flora, and bacterial and viral reinfection from poorly cleaned colonic equipment is always a lurking problem.

If you intend to take colonic treatment, it is recommended that you do so at a center with spotlessly clean equipment and a proven track record. Note that when undergoing colonic treatment, depleted intestinal flora should be continually renewed with probiotics and live-culture yogurt. Any good center will guide you in the use of these substances and will prescribe other appropriate supplements.

5. *Saunas and Steam Baths*

Presently, many countries including Germany, Finland, and the United States are conducting medical tests to study the effects of saunas and steam baths on chronic disease. These techniques are reputed to help chronic constipation and to calm irregularities in irritable bowel syndrome. Research is still in progress, though the consensus so far is that high-heat environments do indeed generate many health benefits. For example, the *Journal of the American College of Cardiology* (2002) reports that Dr. Kihara and colleagues studied twenty patients with congestive heart failure. Their findings showed that two weeks of sauna bath treatment significantly improved bloodflow, cardiac function, and clinical symptoms. Also, the *American Journal of Medicine* (2001) reports that studies by Dr. Hannukesela and Dr. Ellahham show that sauna bathing lowers blood pressure in patients with hypertension, and provides breathing relief to asthma and chronic bronchitis sufferers. According to this study, saunas also alleviate chronic pain and improve joint mobility in patients with arthritis.

One interesting case in Canada, as reported in the *Journal of Alternative Complementary Medicine* (1998), tells of work done by Dr. Krop with a patient debilitated for many years by working with chemical solvents. Undergoing sauna treatments and hydration therapy, the patient soon showed marked improvement. Eventually she was able to discontinue her medication entirely and return to her place of work (and presumably perform different, less toxic tasks). The heavy metals and toxins embedded in her tissue, it appears, were flushed out by the water and high heat, and her system received the cleaning and decontamination it had so long needed.

Two types of baths.

Two types of artificial high-heat environments are appropriate for detox—the dry heat of the sauna and the wet heat of the steam bath.

Though steam baths seem hotter than saunas to many people, this is due to the heavy precipitation in the air of a steam room, and in reality, saunas generate considerably higher temperatures. For this reason, saunas also tend to produce deeper sweating. Nonetheless, the restorative benefits of both methods are established, and both are excellent ways to relax the muscles, improve skin quality, stimulate circulation, and purge the body of toxins. Some health-care professionals believe that saunas also shorten the course of a cold or flu, and increase immunity to disease.

How does artificial heat help? When we enter a high-heat environment, our neurotransmitters stimulate our approximately 2 million sweat glands, causing them to pour out as much as a liter of perspiration. In this sweat are harmful bacteria, lactic acid, chemical toxins, excess salt, and a good deal more. Indeed, during a fifteen-minute sauna bath, the sweat glands may excrete as many heavy metals as it takes the kidneys to void in an entire day and night, for which reason many refer to the skin as the "third kidney." For people who are fasting, saunas and steam baths are especially helpful; they enhance metabolism and complement the detoxifying effects of the fast itself.

Do saunas and steam baths pose possible safety hazards? A few. Though some studies suggest that high heat lowers blood pressure, people with hypertension are nonetheless advised to consult a physician before entering a steam room. For some people, the dry heat of a sauna irritates the nasal passages. Others find that hot steam causes eye and skin irritation. People suffering from unstable angina and a history of heart attack or severe heart-valve malfunction should avoid saunas entirely.

While taking saunas and steam baths, users may also become slightly dehydrated. Drinking plenty of water is recommended, both before the bath and after. In general, it is wise never to remain in a sauna or steam bath longer than fifteen minutes at a time. And a last piece of practical advice: Do not jump into cool water immediately after a sauna bath, especially if you suffer from cardiac problems of any kind.

6. Dry Brush Massage

A useful, if little known, method of detoxification is provided via a daily brushing of the skin with a stiff bristle brush. A hairbrush is the ideal tool for this job, preferably one made of natural bristle. A loofah mitt or plastic bristle brush, however, will get the job done in a pinch.

Begin the brushing at the feet, stroking in an upward direction on the ankles, calves, and thighs. Move up the hips, then to the arms, and finally to the trunk. (Applying downward strokes in the trunk area is preferred by some. Others advise brushing in the direction of the heart.) If possible, have a partner finish off the treatment by brushing your neck and back. If a second person is not available, do the job yourself with a long-handled bath brush.

Brush your body this way until your skin feels refreshed and starts to take on a red glow. The best time to apply bristle brush treatment is in the morning, either before or after a shower. Try taking alternating hot and cold showers, then dry-brush your entire body.

Medical benefits of dry bristle brushing include improved circulation, enhancement of muscle tone, spreading out of fatty deposits, and improved skin quality. Brushing removes layers of dead skin, which, in turn, unclogs pores and improves elimination. Brushing also stimulates circulation, which likewise speeds up elimination of wastes. Dry brush massage on the abdomen is reputed to help relieve chronic constipation.

Finally, dry brushing simply feels great, especially after a bath or shower. Done with vigor, it promotes sensations of inner warmth, raises mood, and makes you tingle all over. Nothing feels better than being clean, both inside and out.

7. Assorted Detoxification Techniques

The auxiliary detox techniques described below are all recommended.

Exercise. Regular exercise stimulates circulation, strengthens the muscular and cardiopulmonary systems, encourages weight loss, aids digestion, improves sleep and mood, increases the body's ability to detoxify, and helps lower LDL (the bad cholesterol) and raise HDL (the good cholesterol).

Conversely, people who remain inactive for long periods of time, besides weakening and growing stale, build up stores of free radicals, which potentially produce a variety of diseases. Working out for as little as a half hour a day, at least four days a week, produces profound detox effects for every organ in the body.

For detailed information on exercise and its benefits to digestion, consult Chapters 5, 6, and 10.

Bathing your toxins away. Daily bathing is essential for purifying mind and body and for washing away surface contaminants that might otherwise enter the pores. Water temperature is important. For people who feel internally warm or hot a good deal of the time, lukewarm baths are best. People on the cold side are better served by warm or even hot baths. Try rubbing and massaging mustard oil or olive oil on your skin after each bath. In general, one bath a day is recommended. Too many daily baths dry the skin and deplete energy.

Caution: People with diabetes and other neurological problems should check the water temperature with a thermometer before stepping into a steamy hot bath, and not just rely on touch technique.

Body massage. Swedish massage, along with related systems such as Touch Point therapy, Therapeutic Touch, Craniosacral therapy, Foot Reflexology, Shiatsu, and others, is far more than just a feel-good indulgence. Besides inducing deep relaxation, relieving musculoskeletal pains, and increasing blood circulation, massage stimulates the lymph glands, which help drain wastes from tissue cells. Massage likewise increases the production of digestive juices, saliva, and urine. It also helps remove salt, nitrogen, lactic acid, and inorganic phosphorus from the system. Massage, in short, promotes self-cleansing as well as physical rehabilitation and mood enhancement. Include it in your detox regimen whenever you can.

Water. Every form of detoxification mentioned in this chapter is improved and aided by steady and regular water intake. At least eight glasses a day is the recommended dosage, though some people insist on ten. Water washes out the gut, enlarges the feces for smooth bowel movements, fights constipation, and speeds up toxin elimination through sweat and urine. Do not neglect this important resource as a front-line aid for internal cleansing.

Caution: High water intake detox systems should not be undertaken by people on fluid restriction.

chapter ten

The Age-Defying Gut: Choosing a Diet and a Program That Are Right for Your Age

Aging is a relative matter. That is to say, every one of us is aging all the time, every minute of the day and night. An infant ages and a teenager ages just as surely as a one-hundred-year-old person ages; we all grow older with each tick of the clock.

The difference between the aging of someone younger than age twenty-five and someone older than twenty-five is simply that the younger of the two is still growing into full physical maturity, while the person in their middle twenties is at the peak of a developmental curve that is just now beginning to make its descent.

Mercifully, the downward slope of this curve is very long, very gentle, and very gradual. Certainly, there are many sixty-five-year-olds who feel as right and fit today as they did in their twenties, the reason being that growing older does not necessarily mean growing more infirm. It means, rather, that our bodies are changing, and that our physiological processes are gradually becoming more sensitive to influences that tended not to bother us when we were very young. People who are conscientious about their health take note of these changes and strive to make the corresponding adjustments.

What actual changes take place in us as the years pass? A variety. Some are external and obvious, some internal and subtle, some begin early in the aging game, and others appear at a very advanced age. All of them transform us in one way or another, altering the way we see the world and the way the world sees us.

Over the decades, for instance, our hair tends to thin and gray, and our skin develops wrinkles. Memory weakens a bit, although the thinking process frequently appears to become sharper, deeper, and more focused as time passes. Inside the body the arteries of the cardiovascular system thicken and narrow after age thirty-five. Blood cholesterol and fatty deposits build up in the heart, lowering its ability to pump blood. The breathing apparatus loses some of its elasticity, breathing passages stiffen, and the lungs take in less air with each breath. Within the kidneys and bladder, urination becomes more frequent as both of these organs grow smaller with age. In men, the prostate enlarges; in women, the urethra shortens and becomes less flexible.

Sexual energy wanes gradually over time as well, a process that starts to become apparent in a person's forties and fifties as levels of sex hormones decrease in the blood. For men, the testes grow smaller, sperm production lessens, and sperm motility slows. For women the vagina and breasts shrink. Sexual activity tends to be less frequent in those over age forty, although in many reported cases the degree of pleasure and satisfaction derived by both partners increases as the years pass.

There are, of course, many other physical hallmarks of aging that take place in the nervous system; in the bones, skin, muscles, and joints; in vision and hearing; in mental capacity; and so forth. Yet in few parts of the body is aging more evident than in the digestive system.

INSIDE THE AGING GUT

Why is aging more evident in the digestive system? For one, our digestive processes are constantly busy. While many organs perform only on demand, the digestive organs are active most hours of the day and night. As the years pass, this incessant wear and tear takes its toll.

Genetics also plays a role. Some people are simply predisposed to developing stomach problems as they age. Most important, as the years pass, many people compromise the health of their gastrointestinal tract with poor diet, stress, lack of exercise, and questionable habits of living. Over time, the effect of these abuses is felt throughout the gut.

In which ways does the gut start to show its age? As people enter the weight danger zone between the ages of fifty-five and seventy-five, their bodies lose lean muscle mass, and weight tends to increase, especially if the diet has been heavy on fats and sugar. Saliva production in the mouth also decreases with age, as do digestive enzymes. Gastric mucosal blood-flow is also reduced over the years as is the ability to assimilate and transport nutrients. Vitamins and minerals may not absorb as well as they once did in an aging gut, and production of gastric acids slow. The taste buds decrease in number and size, and the ability to recognize sweet, sour, salt, and bitter tastes is diminished. In some older people, intestinal peristalsis becomes sluggish, resulting in chronic constipation. This is quite a list. And there are many more age-related changes that could be cited.

What exactly are the biological causes of this relentless decline of living tissue? And the big question: Is this decline inevitable? To understand aging on this deeper level, we must journey to the realm of the biochemical, and gaze for a moment through the eyepiece of an electron microscope. Here in the molecular world, we discover that a frantic struggle is continually taking place between the body's immunological system and the invading forces that wish to use our bodies for their own purposes. Foremost among these invaders are molecular structures known as *free radicals*.

A free radical, in brief, is a short-lived, highly reactive molecular fragment joined to an electron that is not paired up with a companion electron, and which becomes unstable as a result. Like everything else in nature, these unstable molecules seek completeness and equilibrium, and so they go in search of another electron. Roaming the vast cosmos of the infinitesimally small, they eventually meet up with a stable molecule, whereupon they immediately steal one of its two bonded electrons. In the process, they make the attacked molecule into a free radical as well.

Before long, this process of give and take generates something akin to a chain reaction, one molecule making the next into a free radical, and the next, ad infinitum. What is the result? A person's cells, DNA, and protein cells are all damaged, and many begin to function with lowered efficiency. The long-term effects of this atomic thievery, most scientists now believe, accelerate the aging process.

Free radicals are a natural consequence of human biochemistry and have their designated place in the biological scheme of things; however, when too many of these molecular events are produced all at once, they work decidedly in our disfavor. This process of internal corruption is encouraged by certain lifestyle habits, many of which can be tempered and even avoided entirely. On the list of free-radical triggers are smoking; stress; poor nutrition; overuse of alcohol; eating fried, charred, and barbecued foods; breathing air pollution and pesticides; and frequent contact with environmental contaminants such as toluene and benzene found in household cleaning products and paints.

Because the digestive system gradually weakens when besieged by free radicals and becomes more vulnerable over time (first on an invisible cellular level, then directly in our physical functioning), digestive diseases largely unknown during youth begin to show themselves as a person moves into early middle age. Typical ailments of the aging gut include ulcers, constipation, diverticulosis, acid reflux, gallstones, leaky gut, cancer, and others.

Fortunately, many of the degenerative changes that take place in the gastrointestinal tract as we age are not inevitable. A majority of them can be prevented, delayed, and even reversed with improved nutrition, exercise, and tender loving care. The rest of this chapter will show you how.

EATING RIGHT TO STAY YOUNG

Perhaps the number one resource for people who wish to slow down the effects of aging on their digestive system is antioxidants. Found primarily in fruits and vegetables, antioxidants are molecular structures that inhibit harmful oxidative reactions within the body's chemistry. Once ingested, antioxidants seek out free radicals and deactivate them before they have time to work their mischief.

In limited numbers, free radicals perform valuable services for the body, a fact that is not always made clear by champions of antioxidants. When kept down to a reasonably sized population, they produce energy for the body through oxidation and help kill off dangerous bacteria. It is only when free radicals are allowed to multiply unchecked that they become dangerous to the integrity of healthy tissue cells. This is where antioxidants come in.

In general, antioxidants are nature's combined sanitation and police department. They are designed to keep the body's free-radical population under control, to keep the process of oxidation in its rightful balance, and to assure that nutrients are properly absorbed and assimilated. However, antioxidants can only work effectively if enough of them are present and accounted for in the body at any given time. Unfortunately, many people who are middle aged and older become careless about diet and simply do not ingest enough of these helpful compounds at each meal. The result is that the free-radical population is allowed to increase out of hand, and the symptoms of aging soon speed up.

There are three ways to keep the free-radical population under control:

1. Avoid the habits of living that encourage free-radical production. This includes smoking, excessive use of alcohol, poor nutrition, and breathing polluted air.
2. Eat more antioxidant-rich vegetables and fruits.
3. Take supplements that have antioxidant properties.

Let's have a look at the definite steps we can take to ensure that all three of these criteria are met. We begin, as usual, with our most important aid: diet.

An Antioxidant-Rich Diet

Antioxidants are primarily found in fruits and vegetables, which are rich in the antioxidant vitamins C and E, as well as beta-carotene (which the body converts into vitamin A). If you eat these foods in great enough abundance, an adequate daily intake of antioxidants is assured. Also important are foods that contain antioxidant nutrients such as selenium (found in grains, meat, and dairy products), flavonoids (found in legumes, green tea, citrus fruits, berries, and onions), certain amino acids (found in garlic, nuts, liver, fish, eggs, and onions), and coenzyme Q_{10}.

Currently, it is recommended that active, aging people eat at least five servings of fruits and vegetables every day and, better yet, six or seven. This may sound like a lot of servings, but simple tricks can help. For example, add some banana and apple slices to your cereal at breakfast. When you're thirsty, drink a glass of orange or grape juice. At lunch, make a large salad, or slip a slice or two of tomato and some greens into a sandwich, finished off with a piece of fresh fruit. For dinner, eat at least two and preferably three vegetable servings with the main course.

Antioxidant-rich fruits such as berries, red grapefruit, prunes, apricots, oranges, and red grapes make excellent between-meal snacks. So do high antioxidant vegetables such as fresh cauliflower buds, cabbage chunks, and pieces of tofu.

The following is a list of twelve foods and food groups that are fabulously rich in antioxidants.

1. **Green leafy vegetables**—Fresh green leafy vegetables such as kale, cabbage, bok choy, endive, spinach, watercress, beet greens, parsley, and the like provide lavish amounts of the antioxidants lutein, folate, and beta-carotene, plus a hefty supply of vitamin C. Make it a practice to eat a salad containing these greens at least once a day.

2. **Whole grains**—Brown rice, wheat, barley, and millet contain vitamin E and, hence, antioxidants. Avoid processed white bread. It provides few nutrients and has very little antioxidant capacity.

3. **Red fruits**—Typical red fruits include grapes, strawberries, raspberries, red grapefruit, and tomatoes (yes, tomatoes are a fruit). All of these fruits are rich in lycopene, vitamin C, and beta-carotene. Red grape juice has four times more antioxidant capacity than orange juice or tomato juice, and is often recommended as a protective nutrient for the cardiovascular system.

4. **Citrus fruits and juices**—Grapefruits, oranges, lemons, and limes, either in fruit form or juice form, carry large stores of vitamin C and antioxidant-rich bioflavonoids. They also contain stores of potassium and folic acid.

5. **Soy products**—Tofu, tempeh, and other soy-derived products are endowed with plant estrogen and plenty of antioxidants. Soybeans contain isoflavones, nutrients that some researchers believe contribute to the low levels of breast cancer among women in Japan where lavish amounts of tofu are eaten every day.

6. **Prunes**—Prunes contain an abundant source of "oxygen radical absorbance capacity" (ORAC). Strong ORAC is reputed to raise the antioxidant power in the blood and to slow aging symptoms. Other foods with a high ORAC rating include raisins and berries.

7. **Chili**—The much-maligned hot chili contains large amounts of vitamin C. Some people believe its endorphin-raising qualities also help elevate mood.

8. **Blueberries**—Blueberries contain some of the highest antioxidant levels in all the human cuisine. Animal studies show that a half cup of blueberries a day helps reverse the effects of failing memory.

9. **Garlic**—Fresh garlic contains vast supplies of antioxidants and is used by health-care professionals to fight infection and treat cancer. Garlic also provides useful phytochemicals—plant substances that protect against cancer, dementia, and heart disease.

10. **Turmeric**—Scientists are excited about the role turmeric may play in anti-aging defenses. Interestingly, in India, where almost every cooked dish contains turmeric, the prevalence of Alzheimer's disease is very low.

11. **Tea**—Though green tea is touted as *the* high antioxidant player, black tea contains approximately the same amounts of free-radical fighting substances as its green relative. Harvard researchers found that a cup of black tea a day substantially reduces the chances of heart disease. Other studies suggest that green tea has preventive effects on both chronic and lifestyle-related diseases (including cardiovascular disease and cancer).

In the prestigious journal *Annals of the NY Academy of Sciences* (2001), Dr. Sueoka and colleagues from Sitama Cancer Center Research Institute in Japan report on the positive benefits of green tea. Based on their data, green tea is one of the most significant cancer preventives available to us today. Cancers that can be thwarted include cancer of the skin, lung, oral cavity, esophagus, stomach, colon, pancreas, and breast. The researchers also report that people who drink ten cups of green tea a day experience a significantly decreased risk of cardiovascular disease.

12. **Other foods high in antioxidants**—Other strong sources of antioxidants include peas, cauliflower, yams, beans, broccoli, carrots, Brussels sprouts, alfalfa sprouts, squash, beets, bell peppers, onions, corn, eggplant, melons, peaches, plums, apricots, fish oils, and seeds.

For maintaining a healthy, young-at-heart digestive system, also consider taking the following dietary steps:

- Go very easy on high-cholesterol foods, and keep daily dietary-fat intake below 30 percent. These substances clog arteries, encourage obesity, and are anathema to the health of men and women over the age of forty.
- Avoid fried foods. Frying, especially deep frying in fat, creates free radicals. Fried foods are notoriously hard on the digestion.
- In the summer, go easy on barbecued meat. Eating charred food causes free-radical production in the body. Note that the delicious black crust on burned steak and chops is carcinogenic.

- Avoid heavy alcohol use. Alcohol is a notorious producer of free radicals, and is corrosive to both the liver and the stomach. The prevalence of chronic alcoholism in this country is 10 percent among men and 3 to 5 percent among women.
- Exposure to radiation, even for short periods of time, encourages massive production of free radicals. If you are presently undergoing radiation treatment, or if you have undergone it in the recent past, it is strongly advised that you increase your daily antioxidant intake, both through food and with supplements (discussed below).
- Avoid large doses of caffeine. If you are a coffee drinker, keep your daily quota down to a cup or two a day. Or consider switching to herbal teas. Coffee is known to encourage free-radical production.
- Eat less at each sitting. As we age, digestive acids in the stomach thin out, and the body is forced to toil that much harder to break down its food. The less we eat at each meal, therefore, the less strain we place on our stomachs and our hard-working livers and intestines. Eating less also keeps weight down, another boost to longevity.
- When dining, eat slowly, chew your food thoroughly, avoid drinking liquids with your food, and don't rush. Studies show that people who habitually eat when they are angry, rushed, and anxious digest food poorly and tend to develop functional digestive disorders such as chronic constipation or diarrhea.
- Avoid eating prior to and immediately after exercising. Also avoid eating when you are walking, talking animatedly, driving a vehicle, and at least two hours before going to sleep at night. As we age, these behaviors can have devastating effects on our digestion.

Antioxidant Supplements

Think of antioxidant supplements as an insurance policy. Take the right ones and, statistically speaking, your chances of living a long and healthy life increase. However, do not look on antioxidant supplements as a substitute for a sound diet. This is a profound mistake and should be avoided. In order for supplements to work properly, they require a selection of nutritious foods to support their chemical processes. A nutritious diet *plus* selected antioxidant supplements is the best of all combinations.

First-class antioxidant supplements include those discussed below.

Vitamins A, B, C, E, and Beta-carotene

While a good multivitamin provides the minimum daily requirement for antioxidant vitamins such as A, C, and E, some people boost the antioxidant effect by taking each of these vitamins separately in capsule form. In general, 5,000 IU of vitamin A, 1,000 mg of vitamin C, and 300 to 500 IU of vitamin E are recommended as age retardants, while for acute sickness even higher doses of vitamin A may be prescribed on a short-term basis. According to Dr. Pandey, writing in the *American Journal of Epidemiology* (1995), and Dr. Zheng, reporting in the same journal (1995), intake of vitamin A supplements both prevents certain types of cancer and has a positive effect on general longevity. Talk to your doctor before taking high doses of vitamin A.

It should also be added that for the aging gut, a solid vitamin B complex helps in the production of red blood cells, and provides protection against kidney stones, muscular atrophy, circulatory system disease, digestive disorders, and mental deficits. Vitamin B also fights depression, a problem that appears with increasing frequency as we age.

Though B vitamins are not antioxidants per sé, they help support free-radical-fighting mechanisms in the body. For example, elevated blood levels of the amino acid homocysteine appear to stimulate the production of free radicals, and high amounts of this substance are linked to several diseases of aging, including osteoporosis, stroke, heart attack, and Alzheimer's disease. Vitamin B, it turns out, helps convert homocysteine to methionine, thus lowering the amount of homocysteine in the blood and, with it, the risk of disease.

By the time Americans turn sixty-five, approximately 35 to 55 percent have developed chronic gastritis, a condition that is related to low production of stomach acid. As a result, the gut may not properly absorb important vitamins and minerals such as calcium, folic acid, iron, and vitamin B_{12}. Substantial helpers in this regard are calcium, vitamin B complex supplements, and hydrochloric acid (HCl) tablets, all available at any health-food store. Do not take HCl if you suffer from ulcers or heartburn. See "Gastritis" in Chapter 16 for further steps you can take to avoid age-related gastritis.

Finally, for bone loss associated with aging, vitamin D and calcium supplements are highly beneficial. These supplements should be taken together, as vitamin D helps absorb calcium.

Selenium

An important but often neglected trace mineral, selenium is a potent antioxidant with substantial anti-inflammatory and immune-boosting virtues. Once in the system, selenium works in cooperation with vitamin E to prevent the formation of free radicals and to discourage damage to cell and tissue structure. Selenium is often packaged with vitamin E in supplement form.

People with cancer and heart disease are commonly found to have low levels of selenium in their bodies. Selenium deficiency can also trigger seizures. Conversely, studies suggest that selenium supplementation strengthens the body's immune defenses and helps fights arthritis, cataracts, and digestive cancers such as cancer of the stomach and colon.

A dosage of 50 to 200 mg a day of selenium is usually adequate for preventive purposes. Be careful not to exceed these limits, as 1,000 mg of selenium a day or more can promote toxic effects. As with most other trace minerals, a little selenium goes a long way.

Coenzyme Q_{10}

The mitochondria, a granular structure found in every cell of the body, contains enzymes responsible for converting food to energy. One of the most important of these enzymes is coenzyme Q_{10} (CoQ_{10}).

CoQ_{10} is synthesized within healthy young people in generous supplies. But as people approach middle age, production of this substance begins to decline and, with it, levels of immune-enhancing antioxidants drop too. In people with a low CoQ_{10} count, digestive ailments such as cancer, heart disease, and obesity are more likely to occur. However, a true deficiency state has not yet been established.

CoQ_{10} is extremely well tolerated and produces almost no known negative side effects. Many people over the age of forty routinely take a 30- or 60-mg capsule a day to assure heart health and to build up needed reserves of age-fighting antioxidants.

Many studies have been done on this powerful nutrient, with much evidence to show that, besides retarding the effects of aging, it curtails the symptoms of specific diseases. An eight-year study of 424 patients by Dr. Langsjoen and associates, as written up in *Molecular Aspects of Medicine* (1994), shows that cardiac patients treated regularly with CoQ_{10} report a statistically significant increase in cardiovascular function. At the end of this study, 43 percent of subjects were able to stop taking from one to three of their regular heart medications.

CoQ_{10} also appears to help people with diabetes. T. Kishi and colleagues, as reported in the *Journal of Medicine* (1976), notes that out of 126 diabetic patients, more than 8 percent were tested as deficient in coenzyme Q_{10}.

Other areas in which coenzyme Q_{10} appears to help include blood pressure regulation, heart function, angina, cancer, weight loss, and even periodontal disease, all potential problems for a person old enough to start receiving solicitations from the American Association of Retired Persons.

Carnosine

A peptide composed of the amino acids alanine and histidine, carnosine is found in muscle and bone tissue throughout the body. When added to the diet or taken as a supplement, it is reputed to fight the *H. pylori* infection, helping heal ulcers and possibly relieve the symptoms of stomach cancer.

Most of the research on carnosine has been done in Russia, and studies are spotty and inconclusive. One interesting Russian study, however, published by Dr. Boldyrev and colleagues in the journal *Bioscience Reports* (1999), reports that when added to a standard diet, carnosine modifies the development of several senile characteristics in rats. The beneficial effects of this protein on test animals were observed by Dr. Boldyrev and his colleagues on both behavioral patterns and physical longevity in test subjects.

Dietary carnosine is found in meat and fish. In supplement form, 150 to 500 mg should be taken twice daily. Carnosine usually comes as part of a zinc-carnosine complex.

Lycopene

A form of carotene synthesized mainly from tomatoes, lycopene is a powerful antioxidant. In several clinical trials, it was shown to generate some anticancer effects, especially in cases of prostate cancer. In one study of lycopene, male subjects who ate 6.5 mg of lycopene a day showed less risk of developing prostate cancer than subjects who ate little of this substance. Similar improvements were noted with breast cancer and cancer of the gastrointestinal tract. Dr. Kohlmeier, as reported in the *American Journal of Epidemiology* (1997), found a significant correlation between a high daily intake of dietary lycopene (primarily through tomatoes) and a lower chance of heart disease.

Alpha Lipoic Acid

Because of its strong antioxidant effects, alpha lipoic acid is sometimes touted as a "fountain of youth" drug. Though one must take such phrases with a grain of salt, studies show that alpha lipoic acid does, in fact, provide many health benefits. For example, it helps control hypertension, protects the liver against hepatitis, improves metabolism of blood sugar, enhances detoxification, and increases the flow of blood to the peripheral nerves, helping damaged nerve fibers regenerate. Dr. Ford, writing in the journal *Metabolism* (2001), states that alpha lipoic acid lowers cholesterol levels and improves intestinal blood flow.

Alpha lipoic acid also appears to work well in concert with other antioxidants. Dr. Berkson in the journal *Medical Klin* (1999) tells of three patients with hepatitis C who were treated with a triple antioxidant therapy including alpha lipoic acid. At the end of the session, the patients improved enough to resume a normal life and no longer required liver transplantation. Writing in the journal *Chemical and Biological Interactions* (2001), Dr. Arivazhagan and colleagues report that alpha lipoic acid reverses the age-associated decline in the body's antioxidants, and therefore may lower the increased risk of oxidative damage that occurs during aging. They also concluded that alpha lipoic acid enhances the activities of mitochondrial enzymes and antioxidant status, thereby protecting the mitochondria against the aging processes.

The recommended maintenance dosage of alpha lipoic acid is between 50 to 100 mg a day. In people with diabetes and liver problems, administered amounts can be as high as 300 to 400 mg a day or more. People who have diabetes should consult a health-care professional for guidance before taking large doses.

Ginkgo Biloba

The ginkgo craze started some years ago in Japan where it had long been known to increase the power of short-term memory and to turn back the mental effects of aging. Today, ginkgo biloba is one of the most widely taken supplements in the world. When staying late at the office, or when a quick burst of mental energy is required, many people turn to ginkgo in lieu of caffeine.

One of the major benefits that ginkgo affords is an improvement of blood and oxygen flow to the brain. This increase appears to improve a spectrum of age-related problems, including headache, dizziness, tinnitus (ringing or buzzing in the ears), male impotence, and memory loss. Dr. Cohen from the University of California in San Francisco found ginkgo to be 84 percent effective in treating sexual dysfunction caused by antidepressants.

Ginkgo is also a powerful free-radical fighter, a mild mental stimulant, and a concentration enhancer. It is documented to be helpful in dementia, even the dementia caused by Alzheimer's disease. Finally, ginkgo appears to help prevent the development of certain retinal disorders, including diabetic retinopathy and age-related macular degeneration. Include ginkgo in your supplement regimen.

The usual dosage of ginkgo is 50 to 80 mg standardized to 24 percent ginkgo. Take 40 to 80 mg, two to three times a day.

Fenugreek Seeds

Studies by Dr. Gupta and colleagues, in the journal of *Journal of Association of Physicians of India* (2001), report that fenugreek seeds provide antioxidant properties and improve insulin resistance, both of which are anti-aging aids. Mix equal amounts of fenugreek seeds and onion seeds, and take one teaspoon with a glass of warm water shortly after waking up in the morning.

Other Sources of Antioxidants

Other supplementary sources of antioxidants among herbs and foods, all available at health-food stores, include the following:

- Chaparral
- Shiitake mushrooms
- Thyme
- Peppermint
- Purslane
- Milk thistle
- Pearl barley
- Oregano
- Sage
- Seaweed and kelp

To give you an idea of the correlation between tradition and science, I refer you to a study by Dr. Ohsugi and colleagues from Japan. The authors studied the active-oxygen scavenging activity of seventy traditional herbal medicines and tonics used in China and Japan from the standpoint of their anti-aging potential. Writing in the *Journal of Ethnopharmacology* (1999), the authors state that a vast majority of these medicines showed scavenging activity to varying degrees, lending credence to the widely held belief that traditional medicine has scientific merit.

OTHER AIDS TO A YOUNGER GUT

Exercise

Numerous studies confirm that exercise is effective in postponing mortality and enhancing longevity. Conversely, people who do not exercise as they age are several times more likely to develop cardiovascular problems than those who work out on a regular basis.

According to several studies, physically fit people are less likely to die of cancer than those who rarely or never exercise. One study reported in the *Journal of Medicine and Science in Sports and Exercise* indicates that physical fitness provides a substantial measure of protection against cancer mortality. Studying more than 25,000 male adults over a ten-year period, investigators found that men with the highest levels of fitness had a 55 percent lower risk of cancer death than men who did not exercise. A moderately fit person in this study ran twenty to forty minutes three to five times a week. Subjects with the greatest amount of fitness performed exercise at the recreationally competitive level. The study also found that nonsmokers who were the most physically fit had the lowest risk of dying of cancer.

Exercise is nourishing for every part of the mind and body including the gastrointestinal tract, which requires regular physical movement for several reasons: (1) to keep its muscle tissue toned and flexible, (2) to increase blood circulation, and (3) to stimulate a harmonious flow of bowel contents and digestive juices. An inactive, non-exercising person is prone to sluggish bowels and chronic constipation as he or she ages.

In general, daily exercise profits every part of the body including the digestive system. Exercises that are especially helpful for long-term gut health include those discussed below.

Stretching

As we approach middle age, our muscles and tendons tighten up, 30 to 40 percent of our muscle mass atrophies, and stiffness sets in. That is, stiffness sets in unless we keep our limbs and torso flexible.

Touching toes, upward and forward stretches, windmills, push-ups, halfway knee bends, torso twists, and sit-ups all provide that needed extension, as do regular rounds of stretch-oriented calisthenics. Walking, rowing, lifting, raking leaves, and housework are all good. Your stretch quotient profits too by consciously extending your reach when performing daily activities. For example, consciously exaggerate your stretch as you reach for the sponge or the car keys. Stretch your arms and legs when you get out of bed. Bend over a bit further when putting on your shoes, and so forth.

The more you stretch, the more limber you become, and the more this limberness impacts positively on digestion. Stretching also speeds up healing, increases circulation, and moves the blood to areas of the stomach and bowels where it is most needed.

Strength Exercises

Strength exercises improve our ability to lift and carry and perform strenuous tasks. Weight exercises are most effective in this category, preferably in a program tailored for your age and state of health. For people who have osteoporosis, weight-bearing and resistance exercises are especially recommended. A local gym or personal trainer can be helpful in this area. A strong body means a strong gut.

Endurance Exercises

Walking, jogging, stair stepping, calisthenics, and sports that stress long-term exertions are good. So are rowing, hiking, and swimming.

Endurance improves heart rate, helps us to breathe deeper, and quickens circulation. Do, however, pace yourself, and do not push yourself beyond comfortable limits.

Aerobic Exercise

As we age, our breathing becomes increasingly shallow, and the body's ability to process oxygen is lessened. One method of staving off oxygen depletion is the regular performance of aerobic exercise (the word "aerobic" means "use of oxygen").

Aerobic exercise raises the heartbeat to its maximum sustainable level (MSL) per minute, and keeps it there for a measured period of time, say five to ten minutes, depending on your exercise goals and degree of fitness. Reaching this maximum level stimulates circulation, strengthens the cardiopulmonary system, improves endurance, oxygenates the system, and wakes up every organ in the body. Aerobics help exercisers maintain their weight, another plus for longevity and gut health.

How do you determine your personal MSL? Start by subtracting your present age from the number 220. That is, if you are fifty years old, subtract 50 from 220. This gives you a maximum sustainable heart rate of 170. If you are sixty years old, subtract 60 from 220, giving you a maximum sustainable heart rate of 160. Once you know your MSL, you then monitor this count by doing the following:

1. First, take your pulse for thirty seconds while exercising.
2. Count the number of beats during this thirty-second period. Double this number, and you have your current heart rate for that moment.
3. Compare this number to your MSL.

For example, suppose you determine that your MSL is 160. The next time you work out aerobically, take your pulse after exercising for five to ten minutes. Let's say you get a reading of 98 beats per minute. This means that your heart is presently beating at approximately 60 percent of its maximum sustainable level (98 is slightly more than 60 percent of 160).

Assuming that 60 percent of your maximum sustainable heart rate is your goal—an exerciser's goal can vary from 60 to 75 percent in this regard—you are now right on target. Continue exercising at this plateau for five to ten minutes, then gradually slow down and cool off.

Repeat your aerobic workout at least four times a week. In a week or two, you will feel brighter, more relaxed, and more fit. Jogging, fast walking, rowing, dancing, swimming laps, and group aerobic exercises are all aerobically based.

Tips for Exercising as You Age

- Before beginning any exercise program, be sure to schedule a complete physical examination. While at the doctor's office, consult with your health-care provider concerning the type of exercises best suited to your age and physical condition.
- Warm up at the beginning of each exercise session, and cool down at the end. Avoid sudden exertions, and pace yourself. Easy does it.

Sudden changes in workout intensity can cause muscle spasms and overtax the heart. Pushing too hard for too long is harmful at any age.

- Avoid working out for more than an hour at a time. Thirty- to forty-five-minute sessions are fine, especially for people over age fifty. Forty-five minutes of workout time, four times a week, will soon make you thoroughly energized, fit, and trim.

- Increase the intensity of your daily workouts, but do it slowly. As a rule of thumb, people over age forty should increase the intensity of their fitness activity by approximately 10 percent a week.

- Exercises that strengthen and tone the aging gut include sit-ups, toe touching, windmills, and torso twists. If you have back trouble, note that approximately 80 percent of back problems are caused by weak abdominal muscles. For a complete set of powerful gut-toning yoga exercises, consult Chapter 6.

- For people over fifty, yoga and tai chi offer ideal workouts. Both systems place an emphasis on stretching and toning, neither system jars or jumbles the organs, and both make the health of the digestive system a high priority. Consult Chapter 6 for specifics.

- As you grow older, consider substituting gentle workouts for more strenuous forms of exercise. Jogging, for example, pounds the joints and over time contributes to skeletal problems. Instead, try fast walking on a treadmill or outdoors. If you have a history of falls, avoid exercises that compromise balance or that place you in precarious postures and positions.

- Environmental extremes during exercise are also less tolerated as we age. Be sure the workout room is warm and well ventilated. Avoid cold workout environments whenever possible.

- Consider taking up swimming for overall body health. Swimming exercises every muscle and joint in the body without impact or strain. When all is said and done, swimming is probably the best of all exercises for people over age fifty.

Tips for Maintaining an Aging Gut

- As we age, our gastrointestinal equipment and especially our bowels accumulate large amounts of toxins, residues, and debris. An excellent way of flushing these substances out of the system and rejuvenating the delicate membranes and cells of the digestive tract is with periodic detoxification. Consult Chapter 9 for easy-to-apply detox techniques.

- Along with death and taxes, one of the unalterable realities of modern life is stress. Over time, the pressures of worry, anxiety, and depression reduce the alimentary tract's effectiveness, and eventually make it sick. Fortunately, there are a number of steps that can be taken to lower the stress levels of day-to-day life, and to take the psychic burden off body and mind. Consult Chapter 5 for exercises and techniques that help.

- One of the gastrointestinal problems faced by many people over age sixty is lack of adequate hydration. A gut that does not receive adequate amounts of water to process food and wastes tends to produce dry stools and sluggish peristalsis. The remedy here is an easy and pleasant one. All of us, and especially people over age forty, are advised to drink at least eight glasses of pure water every day (unless you are on fluid restriction). Start by drinking a full glass immediately after awakening. This will jog your elimination system and promote regularity. Have one or two glasses mid morning, one at lunchtime, several in the afternoon, and several in the evening. A majority of seniors do not drink enough water, and many suffer from some degree of dehydration.

- Keep your weight down. As we age, excess weight stresses the heart, slows digestion, encourages high blood pressure, and puts undue pressure on the muscular and skeletal systems. Statistically speaking, obese people have the shortest life spans, while people who maintain weights appropriate to their size and body structure live the longest.

- Avoid eating too much at each meal. Though overeating is the source of much fun-poking and is rarely thought of as a true health hazard, it is, in fact, according to the findings of many clinical studies, an identifiable cause of early human death. According to studies in the *Journal of American Geriatrics Society* (1999), for example, Dr. Roth and colleagues from the Gerontology Research Center at the Johns Hopkins University in Maryland maintain that dietary caloric restriction in animals is the most reliable and reproducible means we have of slowing down the aging process and prolonging life. Results of studies by Dr. Verdery and colleagues from the Arizona Center on Aging in Tucson, as reported in the *American Journal of Physiology* (1997), similarly show that caloric restriction increases good HDL levels of cholesterol in monkeys. Investigators suggest that caloric restriction leads to beneficial effects on body composition and glucose metabolism, and may prolong life by decreasing one of the main causes of human mortality, atherosclerosis.

  When you eat, in other words, pace yourself and try not to overstuff. One good trick is to eat until you are three-quarters full, and then leave the table. Within twenty minutes, you will feel full, minus that bloated feeling in your gut.

- Finally, there are the simple lifestyle considerations that play such an important part both in the health of the gut and in one's overall body integrity. Smoking, drinking, drug habits, working too hard, lack of sleep and rest, a negative outlook on life, and burning the candle at both ends all take their toll.

We live longer when we live better. Strive to stay happy and healthy.

chapter eleven

Inflammatory Bowel Disease (IBD): Crohn's Disease and Ulcerative Colitis

I nflammatory bowel disease (IBD) is a blanket term for a condition of chronic inflammation in the bowels. While inflammation in the bowels may occur for a variety of reasons, IBD is generally described as "idiopathic," which means that its causes are largely unknown. IBD takes two forms: Crohn's disease and ulcerative colitis.

The cause of each ailment is not entirely known and seems to vary from person to person; this makes treatment especially difficult. In fact, many experts believe that Crohn's disease may be not one disease but several, while ulcerative colitis may have at least two subsets.

One current theory, relatively well substantiated in medical literature, is that IBD is triggered by the immune system's attempt to fight off some form of toxin, virus, or bacteria in the fecal stream. The inflammation that results becomes self-perpetuating in predisposed people, especially those with a hyperpermeable (leaky) gut.

Other possible causes of IBD include overuse of anti-inflammatory and antibiotic drugs; reduced blood supply to the intestinal tract; food allergies;

and intense conditions of stress. While evidence for stress as a cause is debated for humans, it has been shown that among cotton-top tamarin monkeys placed in captivity, most develop colitis. Conversely, monkeys living free in the jungle almost never contract this disease. A genetic factor also enters the picture, and specific genes predisposing people to IBD have been identified. The population groups most likely to develop IBD include children, teenagers, young adults and people from fifty to seventy years old. Neither Crohn's disease nor ulcerative colitis is contagious.

At present there is no medical cure for inflammatory bowel disease, other than removal of the entire colon and rectum in cases of ulcerative colitis. No wonder, according to a report by Dr. Hilsden and colleagues in the *American Journal of Gastroenterology* (1998), alternative and complementary medicines are used by a majority of patients suffering from IBD.

CROHN'S DISEASE

While the inflammation in Crohn's disease can strike anywhere along the gastrointestinal tract, it is most commonly centered in the small and the large intestine. In a few instances it appears in the stomach, the esophagus, and albeit rarely, the mouth.

The inflammation in the small intestine is usually in the lower section, the ileum, although upper sections can occasionally become inflamed as well. This virulent inflammation tends to penetrate deep into the many layers of the intestinal lining, causing rawness and pain, and sometimes a thickening of the intestine that may block the movement of digested materials through the gastrointestinal tract. Abnormal passages (fistulae) may occur between loops of the bowel or between the intestines and the bladder, skin, or genital organs.

The symptoms of Crohn's disease differ among individuals, and according to the part of the intestinal tract under siege.

ULCERATIVE COLITIS

Ulcerative colitis is a form of IBD that affects specifically the lower gastrointestinal tract (colon and rectum), causing inflammation along the superficial layers of the colon lining. Eventually, discrete clumps of cells in these inflamed areas die, and sores or ulcers form along the colon that bleed and leak quantities of mucus and pus into the gut.

The symptoms of ulcerative colitis tend to come and go according to mysterious rhythms. Once a person contracts the disease, the symptoms tend to return. Like Crohn's disease, colitis can trigger complications in other parts of the body, such as arthritis, eye problems, hepatitis, blood clots in veins, sores on the skin, and an increased predilection for cancer.

A Word of Warning

If you suffer from either Crohn's disease or ulcerative colitis, seek medical help immediately. When used as adjuncts to conventional treatment, natural remedies are certainly helpful for these ailments. But use them only as adjuncts, and in consultation with your physician. Crohn's disease and ulcerative colitis are serious ailments: do *not* attempt to cure yourself of them with natural remedies alone. If medical treatment is delayed, the conditions may worsen severely and surgery may become necessary.

HERBAL AND NATURAL REMEDIES

Some people report relief from the following treatments. Again, such remedies should be used as supplements to conventional treatment, and not on their own.

Probiotics

There is a great deal of excitement these days in the medical profession over the emerging role of probiotics and prebiotics in the treatment of IBD. In their findings published in *Digestive Disease and Sciences* (2000), Dr. Guslandi and colleagues report that treatment with the probiotic *Saccharomyces boulardii* (1 g per day), when applied with conventional medication (such as mesalamine), resulted in only 6.26 percent of relapses in patients suffering from Crohn's disease. Among patients treated with mesalamine alone, 37 percent of patients experienced relapse. *Saccharomyces boulardii* is already being used in mainstream medicine for treatment of relapsing pseudomembranous colitis.

In the Netherlands, Dr. Henri Braat reports that the probiotic *Lactobacillus rhamnosus* suppresses inflammatory responses and may be beneficial in maintaining remission in Crohn's disease. Dr. Guandalini has shown that *Lactobacillus GG* is effective in treating pediatric Crohn's disease. Several studies document a potential role of *Lactobacillus plantarum* in treating IBD as well.

Just as with antibiotics taken for infection, it should be pointed out, a given probiotic is not equally suitable for all individuals. IBD is probably several diseases, and thus individual patients may respond in different ways to different probiotic treatments.

The research findings of Dr. Shibolet and colleagues, published in *Inflammatory Bowel Diseases* (2002), show variable responses to probiotics by mice in studies of various models of colitis. It is likely that in the future some specific and unique combinations of probiotics will be found to have specific responses with different types of IBD. One probiotic preparation gaining increasing popularity is VSL#3, a potion containing three strains of *Bifidobacteria*, four strains of *Lactobacilli*, and one strain of *Streptococcus salivarius*. Each packet of VSL#3 contains 450 billion bacteria (the dose is one to two packets per day). The preparation is known to enhance gut barrier function, and is effective in treating pouchitis. It is also used for the prevention of postoperative recurrence in Crohn's disease.

Reviewing the literature on probiotics in the journal *Inflammatory*

Bowel Diseases (2000), Dr. Shanahan states that probiotic therapy in animal models and in humans with ulcerative colitis is reasonably promising, and finds compelling the circumstantial evidence for biotherapeutic modification of the enteric flora in Crohn's disease.

Aloe Vera

The old tried-and-true extract has a solid reputation for treating IBD. Its anti-inflammatory qualities keep redness, soreness, and inflammation under control, coating and soothing raw tissue. For everyday use, aloe in capsule form is best. Take three or four capsules in the morning and two at night. A word of warning: Aloe vera can have a laxative effect on some people. If your inflammatory condition is already causing diarrhea, wait until the condition clears up before using this remedy.

Fish Oil

Cogent evidence suggests that the omega fatty acids in fish oils are a useful therapeutic agent for the management of IBD. Recent studies indicate that the marine fish oil supplements EPA and DHA help reduce colitis and exert an anti-inflammatory effect on intestinal tissue. Dr. Arslan and colleagues in Norway have shown that seal oil (10 ml three times a day) has beneficial effects in cases of IBD, particularly on joint pains associated with the ailment. Dr. Almallah and colleagues in Britain, writing in the *American Journal of Gastroenterology* (1998), show in a double-blind, randomized controlled study that the administration of fish oil extract (EPA, 3.2 g; DHA, 2.4 g) daily for six months produced clinical benefits in patients with colitis. The findings by Dr. Greenfield and colleagues, published in *Alimentary Pharmacology and Therapeutics* (1993), show that evening primrose oil, a related substance, also provides some symptomatic relief in ulcerative colitis.

For patients taking steroids, there is some indication that fish oil can reduce the required dosages of these highly toxic drugs. Omega-3 fish oil capsules are available at any natural foods store. Take three or four

1,000-mg capsules a day. Enteric-coated capsules are better tolerated by IBD sufferers than are the non-enteric kind.

Butyrate

Butyrate is a major fatty acid that feeds and nourishes the epithelial cells lining the colon. Dr. Wachtershauser and Dr. Stein, writing in the *European Journal of Nutrition* (2000), state that butyrate plays a critical metabolic role in maintaining the mucosal barrier in the intestine, and that in the process it helps prevent the gut from becoming leaky. Butyrate has also been shown to assist in wound healing and to reduce intestinal inflammation. Wachtershauser and Stein conclude that the addition of supplemental butyrate to the diet may be an appropriate way to alleviate symptoms of inflammatory bowel diseases and to enhance healing in people who have been operated on for an IBD condition. Butyrate enemas can be used to treat both Crohn's disease and colitis. See the Appendix for information on finding and ordering supplies.

Other Herbal Remedies

Alfalfa, slippery elm, fenugreek, devil's claw, Mexican yam, tormentil, ground flaxseed, and other herbs are all reputed to reduce gut inflammation, soothe internal gastrointestinal membranes, and ease certain symptoms of IBD. The study by Dr. Hong and colleagues, published in *Journal of Ethnopharmacology* (2002), concludes that the polygalae root can be helpful in treating experimentally induced colitis in mice. Dr. Rodriguez reports in the journal *Phytotherapy Research* (2002) that enemas prepared from the stem bark of *Myracrodruon urundeuva,* popularly known by its Portuguese name *aroeira,* are effective for healing experimentally induced colitis in rats. Tryptanthrin, a natural product derived from the medicinal plant *Polygonum tinctorium,* has been studied extensively in experimentally induced colitis in mice. While all the mice treated with tryptanthrin in one study survived, 90 percent of the control mice died; the observation suggests that tryptanthrin may provide effective therapy for colitis sufferers.

Ayurvedic medicine has been somewhat successful in its use of herbal potions to treat IBD. The *Cordia myxa* fruit, for example, has been shown to alleviate experimental colitis in rats. As reported in *Plant Medicine* (2001), Dr. Gupta and colleagues in India looked at the effects of gum resin of *Boswellia serrata* (300 mg three times a day), used as an adjunct to conventional sulfasalazine therapy in patients suffering from ulcerative colitis. The gum resin induced remission in 70 percent of the patients, while only 40 percent of the patients who used the sulfasalazine alone experienced remission. All these herbal potions can be purchased at any good health-food store or from a supplier of Ayurvedic medicines.

Chinese Medicine

Numerous Chinese herbal medicines, including *wei tong ning,* have been tried or are recommended for IBD, with varying degrees of success. Drs. Chen, Nie, and Sun studied the effect of Chinese herbal medicines on intractable ulcerative colitis. Reporting the results of their double-blind study (1994), the investigators concluded that a therapeutic regimen using *jian pi ling* tablets was effective in helping 86 percent of patients. Studying patients with ulcerative colitis, Drs. Zhou, Yu, and Gu compared the effects of supplementary retention enemas using quick-acting *kuijie* powder with the effects of conventional sulfasalazine treatment alone. They found that the additional *kuijie* was effective in helping 98 percent of patients, as compared with 71 percent of patients helped when treated with sulfasalazine alone.

Folate

For persons suffering from colitis who fear their condition may become cancerous, growing evidence indicates that folate, or folic acid, protects against this. Dr. Choi and Dr. Mason report in the *Journal of Nutrition* (2000) that folate deficiency encourages cancer, whereas folate supplementation beyond the daily requirement produces a protective effect. A recent study demonstrates that colitis patients who use folate for at least

six months reduce by 28 percent the risk of acquiring colon cancer. Dr. Lash
ner and colleagues, in a 1997 study reported in *Gastroenterology,* comment
that "daily folate supplementation may protect against the development of
neoplasia in ulcerative colitis." Folic acid supplements are available at any
health-food store. Most multivitamin preparations contain low amounts of
folate. I recommend taking at least 1 mg per day.

Arginine

Numerous experts, including Dr. Perner and Dr. Rask-Madsen, in their article "The Potential Role of Nitric Oxide in Chronic Inflammatory Bowel
Disorders," published in the journal *Alimentary Pharmacology and Therapeutics* (1999), discuss the potential benefits of the amino acid arginine in
treating inflammatory bowel disease. Dr. Becker and colleagues, in the *Journal of Pediatrics* (2000), report low arginine concentrations in the colons of
premature infants before the onset of colitis. Dr. Amin and colleagues, in
the same journal (2002), state that arginine supplementation prevents the
development of colitis in children. The same may be helpful for adults.
Try a daily supplement of arginine and see for yourself.

Vitamins and Minerals

Make a conscious attempt to eat properly and to supplement your meals
with a good selection of multivitamins. Nutritional deficiencies are common in IBD patients, especially those suffering from Crohn's disease,
even when the disease is in remission. Common deficiencies among IBD
sufferers include zinc, magnesium, selenium, folic acid, and vitamins A,
E, and B complex. When present in the body in the right amounts, these
nutrients can help maintain intestinal structural integrity and generate antioxidant and wound-healing functions. Many experts routinely recommend vitamin supplementation and multivitamin-mineral combinations
for IBD sufferers.

There is a high incidence of osteoporosis among IBD patients, and calcium supplementation can help in this regard. For patients taking corti-

costeroids, a combination of calcium and vitamin D supplementation is strongly recommended. Iron-deficiency anemia is also common among IBD patients. Although oral intake of iron is known in some cases to trigger relapse, intravenous iron therapy has proven useful in replenishing iron deficit and rebuilding iron stores. Talk with your physician or healthcare professional about this.

Fiber: Maybe Yes, Maybe No

Evidence shows that a high-fiber diet can help against colitis. Dr. Bamba and colleagues, in the *Journal of Gastroenterology and Hepatology* (2002), demonstrate that germinated barley not only modulates the composition of bacteria in the colon, but produces significant clinical improvement as well. This is especially true in patients who suffer from ulcerative colitis and are intolerant of conventional treatment. Dr. Kanauchi, in the *Journal of Gastroenterology and Hepatology* (2001), reports that the beneficial effects of germinated barley may be due in part to the increased butyrate production that barley generates. Dr. Ben-Arye, reporting results of a random controlled study, as published in *Scandinavian Journal of Gastroenterology* (2002), suggests that wheatgrass juice is an effective and safe adjunct treatment for patients suffering from ulcerative colitis. Green tea has likewise been shown to have healing benefits for experimental colitis in mice. as reported in the *Journal of Nutrition* (2001).

If you have a family history of IBD but do not yet have it yourself, eat preventively and take in plenty of fiber-containing fruits, vegetables, and grains. Fiber can sometimes irritate the gastrointestinal lining, so if you are already suffering from active colitis, get your fiber in juice form instead; especially good are juices made from leafy vegetables. Crohn's patients showing a potential for intestinal blockage may also benefit from a low-fiber diet; they should avoid popcorn, corn, raw broccoli, spaghetti, squash, and raw cauliflower. Again, what is good for one IBD patient may be detrimental for another.

Exclusion Diets

Some researchers believe that IBD is related to food allergies, especially allergies to wheat, dairy, corn, and highly processed foods containing stabilizers and suspending agents. If you suspect that this is at the heart of your IBD, eliminate suspect foods from your diet and note any improvement. The literature on this subject is controversial. A study by Dr. A. M. Riordan and colleagues, published in the journal *Lancet* (1993), shows that people suffering from Crohn's disease and using elimination diets reported fewer relapses than patients using conventional treatment alone. IBD sufferers are also advised to avoid spicy and highly seasoned foods, especially when the symptoms of IBD are acute.

More Tips

Eat plenty of fresh cultured yogurt to build up friendly flora in your gut. Regular daily supplements of the amino acid L-glutamine is also known to reduce gut permeability, relieve symptoms, and rebuild gut-wall cell structure. Dr. E. Kaya and colleagues, in a study published in *Diseases of the Colon and Rectum* (1999), have shown that glutamine enemas are effective in treating experimental colitis in rats. So far, however, studies in humans with IBD are not encouraging. Get plenty of exercise and always avoid stimulants such as tobacco and coffee.

FIGHT STRESS

As it does in so many ailments, stress may both contribute to the development of IBD and worsen the symptoms once the condition appears. Research shows that colitis patients frequently develop a worsening of symptoms when placed in stressful situations. Dr. Shaw and Dr. Ehrlich, reporting in the journal *Pain* (1987), state that ulcerative colitis patients doing relaxation exercises reported less pain and took fewer medications than those not receiving antistress treatment. Dr. R. Richard Waranch, in

Advanced Therapy of Inflammatory Bowel Diseases (T. M. Bayless and S. B. Hanauer eds., 2001), suggests a five-step program of stress management consisting of problem assessment, education, increase in healthy behaviors, positive thinking, and frequent use of relaxation techniques. He further proposes mood therapy to enhance stress management skills. In the same book, Peter Nielsen, a former Mr. Universe and an active IBD patient, emphasizes the role of fitness therapy in managing this complex disorder.

In short: Let go and relax.

chapter twelve

Treating Ulcers

Ulcers—manifestations of what is technically referred to as "peptic ulcer disease," found in the stomach and the duodenal portion of the small intestine—are often considered the quintessential ailment of our time. Indeed, for years the very name was synonymous with notions of pressure in the workplace and trouble at home. Responsible for $5.65 billion in health-care costs yearly in the United States, ulcers are traditionally attributed to undue stress, as well as to poor diet, malnutrition, and a number of other influences. There is no question that those suffering from ulcers more commonly face stressful life situations and that their ulcers take longer to heal. Yet it was only in the early 1980s that scientists started to take a closer look at a common bacterial resident of the stomach known as *Helicobacter pylori.* More probing revealed that *H. pylori,* in fact, was often the cause of ulcers that had long been attributed to other factors. With proper antibiotic treatment, it was discovered, most ulcers can be alleviated, and in many cases entirely cured and their recurrence prevented.

Ulcers can appear during the teen years, but most ulcer sufferers begin developing symptoms between the ages of twenty and fifty-five. For reasons not wholly understood, males used to contract the ailment twice as often as females; more recently, the occurrence is almost equal. People with blood type O suffer from ulcers more frequently than do those with other blood types.

As a rule, ulcers should never be ignored, not only because of the havoc they bring to the digestive system and to lifestyle in general, but also because when left untreated they can lead to life-threatening complications. As many as 10 to 20 percent of Americans will develop an ulcer during their lifetime.

The symptoms of ulcers include:

- Nausea and/or vomiting
- Heartburn
- Burning pain in the upper abdominal regions. In the case of duodenal ulcers, the pain tends to come when the stomach is empty (between meals; at night and early morning), and it is usually relieved by eating. In contrast, patients with gastric ulcers develop pain when they eat, making them reluctant to eat and causing weight loss.
- Abdominal discomfort
- Traces of blood or bleeding in the gastrointestinal tract
- Dark, tarry stools

Symptoms, it should be pointed out, are poor predictors of an ulcer diagnosis. Most people with ulcer-like symptoms usually do not have ulcers.

LIFESTYLE CONCERNS

While many ulcers can be traced to bacterial causes, other factors can and do increase the likelihood of their developing and worsening. Many studies have been carried out to determine the relationship between ulcers and stress, and in a majority of these trials stress has proven to be a significant exacerbating factor. Ulcers are associated with increased life difficulties such as financial and marital conflicts. A twenty-year prospective study showed a link between psychological problems like hostility and malad-justment and the subsequent development of ulcers. People who suffer from ulcers are cautioned to slow down, relax, practice relaxation exercises and meditation, and fashion a lifestyle that emphasizes rest, recreation, and removal of major stressors. Not surprisingly, hypnotherapy has been shown to be beneficial for the healing of ulcers.

Smoking is a major irritant of the stomach lining, and smokers are known to suffer duodenal ulcers more frequently than do nonsmokers. When ulcers occur among smokers, they are even slower to heal. Excess alcohol is a culprit too. Like tobacco, alcohol irritates the stomach lining and can make a bad case of ulcers far worse. Avoiding indulgence in both these habits is imperative for ulcer sufferers.

Nonsteroidal anti-inflammatory drugs such as aspirin, when taken fre-quently, can have a harmful effect on the stomach lining, and over time can cause ulcers. One study showed that people who took aspirin on a daily basis to thin their blood and reduce risk of stroke and heart attack developed ulcers six times more often than non–aspirin takers. Aspirin is particularly corrosive when taken in conjunction with alcohol. (Hangover victims who habitually douse the aftereffects of alcohol with aspirin should be aware of this.) Ulcer sufferers are cautioned to avoid carbon-ated drinks, black tea, and coffee (particularly in the morning). Coffee may increase acid secretion, and is associated with increased incidence of *H. pylori* infection, which in turn is responsible for most ulcers. Coffee in-take is more likely to cause ulcerlike symptoms rather than ulcers them-selves. High intake of fruits, vegetables, and fiber, as well as vitamin A supplementation, has been linked to a decreased risk of ulcer formation.

Avoiding bad habits and substances will help significantly in alleviating the pain of ulcers, and in some cases will help prevent them as well.

HERBAL AND NATURAL REMEDIES

Ulcers are serious business and should be attended to by a physician. As mentioned, if untreated they can turn cancerous; in general they should not be left untreated. Use the following methods as adjuncts to conventional treatment. Do *not* try to cure your condition with these substances alone. These treatments may be especially helpful if symptoms persist despite a documented healing of an ulcer, or in cases where symptoms suggest an ulcer but none is found on testing.

Vegetable Juices

Since some foods irritate ulcers, ulcer sufferers may receive adequate nutrition, as well as soothe the stomach lining in a digestible and delicious way, by drinking homemade vegetable juices. Using a juicer, try a combination of carrot and celery. Or just plain carrot. Cabbage juice alone or mixed with other vegetable juices is credited by many for soothing ulcers and helping them heal.

Raw Cabbage

Eating plenty of raw cabbage is believed to stimulate the same healing qualities produced by cabbage juice. Include liberal amounts in your daily salads; a plateful three or four times a day yields best results.

Helpful Herbs and More

The following are useful supplements for ulcer sufferers:

- Licorice
- Citrus seed extract
- Aloe vera
- Slippery elm
- Alfalfa (supplements and sprout form)
- Ginger (raw or in tea)
- Fennel
- Juice from cooked barley
- Guar gum

Yogurt and Probiotics

Yogurt and related soured-milk foods are excellent for treating ulcers. Not only are they easy on the digestion, but the friendly bacteria help heal and soothe gastrointestinal lesions. See Chapters 7 and 8 on yogurt and probiotics for detailed information.

Vitamins and Minerals

Vitamins A and E are known to promote the healing of mucous membranes in the body, especially along the gastrointestinal tract. Zinc, manganese, and copper are also recommended for ulcer sufferers.

Dietary Measures

While controversy surrounds the question of what ulcer sufferers should or should not eat, and while the dairy products once integral to the anti-ulcer diet are now frowned upon by many doctors, the consensus among healers is that people suffering from ulcers should eat sensibly and carefully but at the same time avail themselves of a wide variety of foods. Most vegetables are fine for ulcer patients, especially leafy greens and potatoes. Cooked rice and barley are good and should be eaten frequently. Creamed soups, fish, and cream of wheat all have a soothing effect on the gut.

As far as fruits, try those you like and determine your own tolerance. Citrus may produce too much acid; others—especially papayas—may prove useful. As a rule, meats and grains are well tolerated. Unless your doctor tells you otherwise, a general high-fiber diet is best.

Avoid large, heavy meals. Eat slowly, chew thoroughly, and make mealtime as pleasant as possible. Although little scientific testing has been done in this area, it is plain common sense that the more relaxed and content we are while eating, the better our digestive tracts will like us for it.

chapter thirteen

Treating Intestinal Gas

L ike death and taxes, all of us experience bouts of gas at one time or another, burping it out or expelling it through our rectums. Never mind
that emitting gas around others is a social gaff or that most cultures
throughout time have looked on this practice with repulsion and sometimes
even censure (in ancient Rome it was against the law to break wind in public). The truth is that this often joked about and much snickered at bodily
process goes with the territory of being human and alive.

Some people, it is true, hold stubbornly to the belief that, if they can
avoid eating gas-producing foods like cabbage and soft drinks, they will
become gas-free. But this is a patently wrong assumption. We all pass gas
whether we want to or not. It is a natural and inevitable by-product of eating and digesting. The only thing to worry about in this regard is if you do
not pass gas. *Then* something may be wrong. But such a condition almost
never occurs. Don't be alarmed.

Technically known as *flatus,* and medically described as "the formation
of air or gas in the intestines due to the fermenting action of bacteria on di-

gesting food," intestinal wind is composed of an amalgam of different gases, primarily nitrogen, carbon dioxide, hydrogen, methane, and oxygen. (Methane is sometimes present, although only in about a third of the world's population.) The proportion of these gases and their concentration is highly variable. For example, studies report the nitrogen content to be as low as 11 percent in one person's gas and as high as 92 percent in another's.

These gases, interestingly, are entirely odorless, and are not likely to offend anyone. It is actually the sulfur emitted by the bacterial fermentation of foods in the colon, coupled with hydrogen gas (forming hydrogen sulfide) that produces the room-clearing smells. Other compounds that can also contribute to smell include food components and metabolites, volatile amines, and certain fatty acids.

The degree of odor in flatus varies, a phenomenon due mainly to the fact that each of us produces a slightly different internal mixture. Some people generate more methane gas, while others are hydrogen makers. Both gases are odorless. Still others manufacture large volumes of hydrogen sulfide, a gas that clouds the area with strong odors. The notion that only people who are sick or who have poor digestion produce putrid-smelling gas is a popular misconception. Odor is rarely related to disease or even to the type of foods one eats. There are a few exceptions to this rule. Intestinal blood passed in feces has a unique and offensive smell. Pancreatic disease can lead to malodorous gas. But, in general, foul odor is a benign phenomenon, if a malignant one socially, and is rarely related to our health or eating habits.

The mixture and components included in intestinal gas likewise differ among human beings, depending on a number of variables. These variables include age, ethnicity, diet, environment, and habitat. For example, people who live at high altitudes and, even more so, astronauts who travel outside Earth's atmosphere, produce a gas that is richer in carbon dioxide than those who live at sea level.

What physiological processes actually cause flatus? Or in common parlance, farting—that familiar low, bubbling, Bronx cheer we know so well? Two characteristics: volume and velocity. For example, if you build up a great deal of gas (volume) and expel it from the rectum at high speeds (velocity), you have a very loud fart. If you take a small amount of gas and expel it at a very slow speed, you have a quiet or even noiseless fart.

Oddly, people suffering from enlarged hemorrhoids are believed to have louder flatus than others. This strange phenomenon, if it is really true, is probably due to the fact that the anal sphincter muscles and the outlet in people with large hemorrhoids are tighter than those of non-sufferers. This tighter opening produces more obstruction, which causes the expelled gas to meet more resistance, which in turn causes a particularly loud sound. Perhaps.

How often do the ordinary Joe and Jane pass gas on any given day? More often than we might think. Reports suggest that the average adult passes flatus eight to fifteen times a day. There are also those on the Vesuvian end of the graph, a few of whom are known to break wind as many as fifty and even a hundred times a day. And there are those who pass gas only once or twice a day. In general, up to twenty-five times a day is considered within the normal range.

Passing gas can also be an entirely unconscious event. Sometimes we know we're doing it, but just as often we don't. Nor is gas a respecter of gender—men and women discharge at more or less the same volumes, and at the same rates.

How much gas is actually passed at each break of the wind? Volumes for the rectal excretion of gas vary enormously, from 500 to 1,500 ml per day, with the average falling somewhere in the 700-ml mark. Dr. Steggerda, writing in the journal *Annals of the New York Academy of Sciences* (1968), describes a study in which a diet featuring 51 percent pork and beans increased subject's gas-passing from a meager 15 ml per hour to a whopping 176 ml per hour. According to the world's foremost flatus expert, Dr. Levitt from Minnesota (who proudly carries the label of the King of Farts), a typical gas-passer produces an average of 16 to 64 ml of gas every hour of the day.

Young people often complain that older folks pass gas more often than they should. Their observation is understandable, but not entirely accurate. Older people do not produce more gas than younger people. They simply pass smaller amounts more frequently. Decades of wear and tear on the aging rectum make this organ more rigid and less compliant than in the young. Plus, the anal sphincter weakens with age. This double whammy forces older people to expel gas at inopportune times and places, making them the butt of jokes by those who will someday, if they but knew, be in a similar situation.

In sum, as far as intestinal gas, burping, and flatulence are concerned, all of us are the usual suspects. What then is the problem with gas? Usually there isn't any. That is, not until levels of gas build up such volumes that unpleasant and persistent symptoms take place inside us such as bloating, burping, intense flatulence, ongoing discomfort, and sometimes unremitting pain.

When this happens, what can we do to help others and ourselves? Many things, a number of which are simple and natural. Before we learn what these methods are, however, some basic education concerning the ins and outs of this ubiquitous and bothersome condition are in order.

SYMPTOMS OF INTERNAL GAS

The following are the most common and obvious symptoms of gas:

- Flatulence
- Belching
- Abdominal bloating
- Stomach pain

Contrary to popular opinion, burping and flatulence do not necessarily go together, and many gas sufferers report flatulence alone, or burping alone, as their major complaint. Let's look at these symptoms one at a time in the following sections.

Flatulence

Although flatulence is often the object of merriment, and sometimes of outhouse humor, too much gas is no laughing matter. Occasionally, it can be the sign of a serious underlying disease. More often, it is simply the body's way of telling us we're eating too many gas-producing foods, swallowing too much air, and/or making unwise lifestyle choices such as smoking, overeating, or drinking too much alcohol.

Belching (or Eructation)

Though considered gauche in Western culture, burping is a normal and even expected post-meal response in many parts of the world. To *not* belch at least once after a meal in some cultures is as an insult to the culinary skills of the chef.

Belching occurs when air in the stomach rises up the esophagus and passes out the mouth. This upward expulsion is usually caused by swallowed air, although it can also be due to overrelaxation of the lower esophageal sphincter muscle triggered by foods such as tomatoes, onions, and alcoholic beverages. Sometimes, belching results from eating too much too fast.

The familiar sound of the burp is produced by the movement of swallowed air echoing in the food pipe as air is moved up and out. A little burping during the day is normal and nothing to worry about. In cases of indigestion or nausea, belching can sometimes clear the system of internal gas and relieve symptoms of pressure and/or indigestion.

Constant burping for more than a few hours at a time, however, is abnormal, and is usually caused by stress and anxiety. If this condition continues for more than a day or two, seek a physician's advice. Recommended ways to combat belching include chewing food slowly (not gulping), eating and drinking slowly, avoiding chewing gum, limiting intake of carbonated and alcoholic beverages, and clenching a pencil between the teeth.

Abdominal Bloating and Distention

Does the presence of bloating, a feeling of fullness and swelling in the abdomen, indicate the presence of too much abdominal gas? Sometimes, but not always. During gassy spells, our abdomen may feel full and protuberant. Then we belch and a sense of relief follows, clearly indicating that the discomfort was caused by gas.

In some cases, however, bloating, especially chronic bloating, is due to a specific disorder, such as irritable bowel syndrome or functional dyspepsia, and has little to do with gas. Or the bloating may be caused by poor motility in the digestive tract. Many people with excessive gas, moreover, do not experience any bloating at all, which means that the two symptoms, gas and bloating, are not synonymous. Note, finally, that for reasons not entirely understood, women tend to suffer from bloating far more frequently than men.

Stomach Pain

Sometimes gas moves into the chest area, stretching the nerve endings in the esophagus, and producing chest pains. At other times, excess air gathers in the stomach, producing sharp, jabbing pains. In still other cases, feelings of intense discomfort are felt in the lower abdominal regions. All these pains can be due to simple gas.

Many stomachaches, however, are not necessarily caused by gas, but by other concerns such as irritable bowel syndrome, ulcers, stress, sensitive stomach, gallbladder problems, and more. A stomachache per se, in other words, is not necessarily a sign of gas. Note that if any type of pain in your stomach or bowels is unusually severe, something may be wrong. Seek a physician's advice right away.

WHAT CAUSES GAS?

There are two major reasons we get gas: (1) fermentation caused by intestinal bacteria and (2) swallowed air. Let's look at both causes in the following sections.

Intestinal Bacteria

Most intestinal gas is caused by foods that are only partially broken down in the stomach and small intestine. These half-digested (and sometimes undigested) substances continue on into the colon where billions of intestinal bacteria now get into the act.

Ravenously fond of the sugars and carbohydrates found in intestinal wastes, these bacteria feed on the half-digested residues, breaking them down further, and fermenting them, a great boon to digestion. In the process, the fermentation generates volumes of carbon dioxide, hydrogen, methane, and oxygen. As much as 90 percent of the flatus that is passed rectally is manufactured by these bacteria.

Of the three nutrient families that comprise the human diet—proteins, fats, and carbohydrates—carbohydrates lead the list of gas-producing foods. Fatty foods, which many people assume are first-rank gas producers, pale in comparison to carbohydrates and their by-products.

Primary examples of high gas-forming carbohydrates are Brussels sprouts, onions, soft drinks, chickpeas, garlic, and coffee. Think also of prunes, cabbage, eggplant, and broccoli. Then there are soybeans, cauliflower, nuts, alcoholic drinks, and dairy products. The list goes on.

There are also differences in gassiness levels between varieties of the same carbohydrates. Italian onions, for example, produce two to three times more gas than their Dutch counterparts. Moreover, foods that contain large amounts of soluble fiber, such as bran and fruit, are also great gas builders, as are many of the sugars found in carbohydrates. Legumes, for instance, contain the sugars raffinose and stachyose, which many people cannot break down in their intestines, and so they pass practically intact into the colon where the gas-making bacteria have a field day on them. Hence, the gassiness of beans.

One persistent misconception about carbohydrates and gas is that fruit juices produce no flatus because they contain no fiber. The fact is that fruit juices are loaded with sugars. Many of these sugars go down easily, reach the colon undigested and unabsorbed, and are then attacked by a horde of gas-producing, fermenting bacteria, generating volumes of gas. It is not only the fiber in fruit that leads to gas, but the unabsorbed sugars they contain as well.

Finally, keep in mind that individual digestive response is also a significant variable in gas production, and that the vegetables and fruits mentioned above do not affect every person's colon in exactly the same way. For example, two people may eat the same-sized portion of baked beans. The first person reacts by manufacturing vast amounts of flatus. The second person produces only small amounts. Some people are simply gas makers; some are not.

Swallowed Air

The stomach does not manufacture air on its own. Air must first be taken in through the mouth, usually while swallowing food and drink, and sometimes while breathing anxiously when stressed and excited.

Once in the stomach, most of this air is sent back up the air tube and released through belching. Occasionally, a tiny bit ends up working its way down through the digestive tract where it is ultimately emitted as flatus. As a rule, no more than a tiny percent of all swallowed air is ever passed through the rectum. The main manufacturer of intestinal gas *by far* is bacterial fermentation.

The Gassy Goods Hit List

The foods listed below are all known to generate plentiful and sometimes excessive amounts of intestinal gas. Some of these foods cause extra fermentation and gas release in the colon. Others are resistant to digestive enzymes or have an especially slow transit time through the bowels. Here's the lineup:

- Apricots
- Bananas
- Beans
- Bran
- Bread
- Brussels sprouts
- Butter
- Cabbage

- Carbonated drinks
- Cauliflower
- Celery
- Cheese
- Coffee
- Cream
- Eggplant
- Eggs

- Garlic
- Honey
- Ice cream
- Milk products
- Nuts
- Onions
- Peanuts
- Peas
- Popcorn
- Potatoes
- Prunes
- Raisins
- Soybeans
- Sugar
- Wheat germ
- Wine

This list may seem to leave few foods for you to eat. But, in fact, there are many low-gas items to choose from. Foods that produce low to moderate amounts of gas include apples, asparagus, avocado, barley, berries, cantaloupe, cucumber, peppers, fish, fowl, meat, olives, okra, rice, tomatoes, and zucchini.

The catalog of gas-producing foods, incidentally, is not ironclad, and, as mentioned, different foods affect different people's stomachs in different ways. Some individuals, for instance, find that nuts produce significant burping and intestinal gas. Others tolerate nuts easily. The same is true for apples, asparagus, citrus fruits, cauliflower, bread, carrots, raisins, and sauerkraut—some people become desperately flatulent from these carbohydrates, while others remain gas-free.

If you love grains but find them high in gas and difficult to digest, know that rice produces less gas than any other grain. It is also among the easiest of all foods to digest, and is invariably kind to people with touchy stomachs.

Food Preparation

Besides the food itself, different methods of cooking, processing, and food preparation can also cause gas problems. Eatables that are panfried or deep-fried are almost always troublesome in this area. The problem lies in the fact that such foods move particularly slowly through the stomach and intestines, fermenting longer and thus emitting more gas. Foods doused in gravies, foods covered with hot sauce, and creamy desserts—you know the drill—all are culpable in this regard.

On the list too are artificial sweeteners, such as mannitol, that are added to many sugar-free chewing gums and cough lozenges, and that generate hydrogen gas in large quantities. In many cases, fructose, a natural sweetener added to many foods, passes through the small intestine into the bowels largely undigested, also producing hydrogen gas as it goes.

Refined flour products are also on the list. Long heralded as being easy on digestion and almost gas-free, it is now believed that refined wheat flour and refined oat flour can both increase gas levels and spawn flatulence. The same is sometimes true for whole oats, whole-wheat products, and corn.

Note, finally, that just about all dairy products (except yogurt) are included on the gas-producing roster, mainly because they may generate lactose intolerance. Triggered by a chronic inability to digest the sugar lactose, which is found in most milk-product derivatives, lactose intolerance produces stomach cramps, diarrhea, and volumes of intestinal wind (see Chapter 7 for more information). Those who suffer from this common ailment, or who experience gassiness and flatus whenever they eat dairy products, are advised to keep their consumption of these foods to a minimum, and/or to eat lactose-free dairy products, available at most supermarkets.

A Brief Word to Vegetarians

From the list of foods presented earlier, you can see that most gas-producing eatables are in the carbohydrate family. From a dietary perspective, this means that vegetarians are often more gassy than meat eaters. There is nothing wrong with this, of course; just beware of the illusion, not at all uncommon, that because you avoid meat you also avoid flatulence. The truth is quite the opposite.

As a consolation prize, vegetarians tend to pass gas more quietly than omnivores, and their gas smells less. Vegetarians are also constipated less frequently than omnivores, and their stools are larger, softer, and more bulky (all that fiber). Finally, vegetarians tend to have fewer problems with hemorrhoids and anal fissures than meat eaters due to the ease with which vegetable and fiber wastes are passed.

WHEN GAS IS MORE THAN JUST A NUISANCE

Can gas be serious? Most of the time, no. Most of the time, it is a natural by-product of swallowing air and/or bacterial fermentation in the bowels. Nothing to worry about.

The time to worry is when intestinal gas becomes excessive, persistent, and measurably painful. When these conditions occur, a physician's advice is your best course, especially if the problem is accompanied by other gastrointestinal complaints.

What possible ailments does excessive and painful gas signal? Since gas is a "normal" phenomenon, it is often difficult to establish a direct relationship between its external cause and its internal effect. Nonetheless, the medical disorders discussed in the following sections can all contribute to painful gas buildup.

Hiatal Hernia

A hiatal hernia takes place when the hole (or hiatus) in the diaphragm, where the esophagus passes into the stomach, becomes enlarged and a segment of the stomach protrudes upward through the gap.

The causes of hiatal hernias are often difficult to pinpoint, though the symptoms are quite recognizable. They include heartburn, vomiting, regurgitation of food, and, most specifically, stomach acid that rises up the esophagus and into the throat, accompanied by burning and discomfort. Other related symptoms include belching, bloating, and intestinal gas. Bear in mind that most people with a hiatal hernia never experience problems or symptoms of any kind directly associated with this condition.

Diverticulosis

Diverticulosis is a digestive condition in which small pouches or sacs, known as diverticula, develop along the colon wall. These pouches form in colonies at the weakest parts of the wall, varying in measurement from pinhead size to marble size.

Although considered a normal part of the aging process by experts in the West, this disorder is uncommon in cultures that eat a predominantly vegetarian diet, and it is thought by many experts to result from lack of adequate fiber in the diet.

It is also theorized that chronic gas suppression—"holding it in"—contributes to the development of diverticulosis. According to the theory, when gas is habitually prevented from exiting, it backs up into the upper rectum and sigmoid colon where it exerts pressure on surrounding tissue. Over time, this pressure weakens the intestinal wall, contributing to the development of diverticula. For more information on diverticulosis, consult Chapter 16.

Other Disorders That Cause Excessive Gas

People who experience chronic burping and gas may be developing upper gastrointestinal disorders such as acid reflux or peptic ulcer disease.

People suffering from celiac disease have difficulty digesting the proteins found in gluten and develop gas when they eat gluten-containing grains such as wheat or barley.

Parasites and infectious diseases of the stomach such as *Giardia* are famous for causing abdominal bloating and gassiness. An ailment known as Meganblase syndrome produces frequent belching, severe air swallowing, and an enlarged bubble of gas in the stomach that sometime becomes so painful people think they are having a heart attack. The symptoms of this somewhat rare ailment usually abate when sufferers force themselves to belch.

Chronic and ever-increasing amounts of burping or intestinal gas can also be associated with a variety of maladies caused by intestinal obstruction, or a slow, malfunctioning gut. Included on this list also are gastroesophageal reflux disease (GERD), Crohn's disease, ulcerative colitis, internal hernia, and colon cancer.

Note that gas by itself is rarely a symptom of any of the above ailments, and is almost always accompanied by other gastrointestinal complaints, especially in serious disorders.

What can physicians do to help patients overcome persistent gas? First, they will want to clinically rule out serious disease. Diet will be reviewed, eating and drinking habits looked at, and a physical exam given, complete with blood tests, abdominal X rays, and probably a hydrogen breath test as well.

When patients report bloating and abdominal distention along with gas, doctors look for inflammation or obstruction in the abdomen. In patients over age fifty, or in patients with a history of colorectal cancer, a colonoscopy is usually appropriate. For inordinate amounts of belching, an upper GI series or upper endoscopy may be ordered.

If nothing serious is discovered after the examination and tests are complete, doctors may then prescribe a low-gas diet and/or nonprescription medications such as simethicone, activated charcoal, lactase supplements, or a digestive aid such as Beano. Or doctors may simply suggest that patients eat more selectively, eliminate gassy foods from their menus, exercise regularly, and cut down on the stress and tension in daily living.

TREATING GAS THE NATURAL WAY

Since intestinal gas by itself is rarely dangerous, feel free to sample and experiment with the natural remedies presented below at your leisure, either in sequence or several at a time. A best-bet approach is to combine one or two of the herbal methods presented here with dietary measures plus a physical treatment such as self-massage. In most cases of ordinary flatulence and/or excessive burping, it is a given that two or more of these measures used in combination will help bring relief.

Dietary Treatments for Gas

Slowing down one's inner gas-making machine is generally a no-brainer. Simply find the foods that give you gas, and don't eat so many of them.

Begin by making note of the gas-producing foods listed on page 251 that cause you trouble. Then put yourself on an elimination diet, keeping a record of your progress. Start by eliminating one category of gas-producing food from your table for several days (like sweets or cruciferous vegetables). Keep written records of the results. If the gas does not subside, return these foods to your menu, and eliminate another category of gassy items. Continue doing this until you experience a noticeable decline in gas levels. Once you identify the culprit foods, steer clear of them. Or at least reduce your daily intake.

Dr. Levitt from Minnesota, the self-styled King of Farts, tells in *Digestive Disease and Sciences* (1979) of a man who broke gas on an average of thirty-four times a day. Using an elimination diet, this man settled on a low-lactose and low-wheat product diet. Within a few weeks, he had reduced his number of daily eruptions by half.

Besides eliminating gassy foods from your table, there are other simple dietary measures that dramatically help curb gas, including the following:

- Avoid drinking liquids with your meals, especially carbonated beverages. Liquids thin digestive enzymes in the saliva and stomach, and reduce their ability to break down foods. More food then goes undigested, producing a greater number of food lumps in the gut. These lumps ferment and make gas.
- If you are lactose intolerant, use lactose-free milk products, or add an over-the-counter lactase enzyme to your dairy foods. These enzymes help digest lactose, reducing gas and stomachaches, and allowing you to enjoy your ice cream in the process. Also try taking acidophilus tablets with your meals three times a day.

  Some people do not know they are lactose intolerant. If you have suspicions, try cutting back on dairy products for a week or try using lactase enzymes, and see if your gas declines dramatically. If it does, you may have lactose intolerance. See Chapters 7 and 8 for more information.
- Avoid carbonated and/or fermented food and drink. On the list here are carbonated water, seltzers, soda, beer, ale, apple cider, canned whipped cream, and carbonated medications such as Alka-Seltzer and bicarbonate of soda.

- Avoid chewing gum and sucking on hard candies—both cause you to swallow air. Sipping liquids from a straw is contraindicated for the same reason. Avoid lying down or sleeping immediately after you eat.
- With regard to eating slowly and chewing well, during the turn of the century, a gentleman named Horace Fletcher (1849–1919) developed and promoted a popular eating system. Though Fletcher's program covered many areas of nutrition, it is best remembered for a technique known as Fletcherism. In a nutshell, Fletcherism calls for chewing food so thoroughly that it turns into a semi-liquid before it is swallowed. Fletcher believed that refining food in this way leads to better digestion, and hence to better overall health. Does it work? No one knows for sure, and no recent clinical trials have tested it. Nonetheless, some people swear by this method, and it is easy to do. Why not give it a try and see how it affects your gas?
- Calcium channel blockers taken for high blood pressure slow down digestive activity in the gut, and trap air in the bowels. The same is true of narcotic drugs (heroin and opium addicts are notoriously constipated). If you use calcium channel blockers and are experiencing uncomfortable levels of gas, talk to your doctor about using an alternative medication.
- If, like most people, you find that beans give you gas, try preparing them in the following way. First, boil the beans for two to three minutes, then allow them to soak for six to twelve hours in cold water. Rinse thoroughly, being sure to discard the soak water (it contains the indigestible carbohydrate residues that you want to eliminate). Cook the beans in fresh water until they are soft and tender. (Try adding a dash of baking soda to beans while they boil.) This method reduces their gas quotient considerably. Note that canned beans are often precooked (check the label), which makes them easier to digest than the uncooked kind. Another trick for bean lovers is to eat beans in the form of sprouts. Sprouting lowers beans' gas-producing tendencies, and makes them easier on the digestion.
- For cooking and degassing beans, some people prefer a product called Beano. Beano is a food enzyme dietary supplement that eliminates gas

In beans, as per its name, as well as in onions, broccoli, whole grains, and other gas-producing foods. It is added to food after it is cooked and ready to eat. Dr. Kagaya and colleagues report in the *Journal of Gastroenterology* (1998) that Beano helps reduce intestinal gas in test subjects by as much as 30 percent. Dr. Ganiats and colleagues show similar findings, as reported in the *Journal of Family Practice* (1994).

- If you smoke, quit. Smoking, especially pipe smoking, is one of the most common causes of air swallowing and, hence, of gas.
- Try this experiment. Cut down on foods that are particularly high in fiber for two weeks. Then gradually reintroduce these foods back into your diet one at a time. Sometimes your body needs a short vacation from high-fiber foods to eliminate excess gas.
- If you think you suffer from flatulence more often than others, try keeping a list, noting the number of times you pass gas each day. Perhaps you are high on the scale. Or, surprisingly, you may be well within the normal range of daily emissions. Passing gas is such a vivid and visceral event that we sometimes exaggerate its frequency.
- Take extract of gentian root a half hour before eating. Gentian root is believed to stimulate production of hydrochloric acid and other digestive juices, which help fight gas and also boost appetite. Take the gentian root plain or, better, take it mixed in a commercial product such as Angostura bitters or one of the many European bitter products available at health-food stores.

Herbal and Medicinal Treatments for Gas

The following carminative (gas-reducing) herbs and medicinals are all useful against intestinal gas.

- **Chamomile tea**—A wonderful relaxant, chamomile tea soothes the digestive tract and reduces gas in the process. Drink a cup at night before going to bed.
- **Ginger**—Purchase fresh ginger root, cut off about an inch's worth of root, peel it, slice it into several pieces, boil it in three cups of wa-

ter for about twenty minutes, and drink immediately. Ginger is an antispasmodic and a specific for just about every digestive ailment we know of, gas included. Add some honey to the boiling water and you have a delicious warming tea as well.

- **Papaya leaf**—Papaya leaf contains papain, a digestive enzyme that breaks down even the toughest foods, including meat. Take it as a tea or in capsule form. While you are at it, eat a fresh papaya or two when gas strikes. Papaya is an excellent digestive aid in general. Or try chewing papain or bromelain tablets after each meal.
- **Fennel**—Fennel is a staple in India where it is used to calm angry stomachs and reduce flatulence. Try eating a handful of fennel seeds next time you're gassy. At Indian restuarants, it is common practice to offer fennel seeds instead of mint candy after dinner.
- **Peppermint tea**—An old favorite, peppermint tea is an excellent specific for relieving the pain of overeating. It also helps absorb gas and relieve bloating.
- **Sage**—Dried sage leaves brewed as a tea help flatulence. Chewing the leaves promotes similar results.
- **Golden seal and myrrh**—According to Dr. Dolara in the journal *Planta Medicine* (2000), myrrh has anti-*E. coli* and anti-*Candida* properties. Mix equal parts of golden seal and myrrh, and then brew as a tea. Take half a cup twice a day for gas.
- **Activated charcoal**—An old favorite, people have taken this highly absorbent powder for centuries to reduce stomach wind, especially hydrogen gas. Today, commercial charcoal comes as an odorless, tasteless, highly refined powder in either tablet or capsule form. Two to four capsules or tablets a day usually do the trick. Hall and colleagues gave activated charcoal to a group of subjects, along with portions of beans. They then checked their gas levels. Reporting their results in the *American Journal of Gastroenterology* (1981), investigators found that subjects who took the charcoal had far less flatus than those who did not. Results from other studies of charcoal, however, have not been as consistent as these.

Caution: Once in the digestive system, activated charcoal absorbs everything in sight along with the gas—vitamins, nutrients, and chemical medications included. Always take this supplement separately from meals and medications. Also, prolonged use can cause constipation, and even if you take precautions, over time activated charcoal deplete nutrients from your system. Use it on occasion and sparingly.

Ayurvedic Remedies for Gas

Pour several drops of rose water into a glass of water and drink the liquid three times a day. Another Ayurvedic recipe designed to encourage belching (and hence evacuation of air) calls for mixing a half teaspoon of carbonate of soda mixed with a half teaspoon of sugar. Take twice a day.

Other potent Ayurvedic specifics for flatulence include the following:

- Take a half of a handful of *Aloe barbedensis* leaves (Ayurvedic name: kumari), grind them in a mortar and pestle (or a blender), then mix the pulp with two to three teaspoons of ghee. Take the mixture twice a day until gas levels decrease.
- Mix the following herbal ingredients together: one part saffron, two parts fresh ground black pepper, three parts fresh pulped or shredded ginger, three parts fresh or dried mint leaves, four parts celery seeds, five parts Ruta graveolens seed (Ayurvedic name: sitav), and twenty-five parts honey. Mix thoroughly, and take a half teaspoon two to three times a day until gas levels diminish.
- Boil eight ounces of milk down to four ounces. Add 180 grains of powdered root of long pepper (Ayurvedic name: pipli). Boil this mixture for several minutes, then add a teaspoon of sugar. Let the mixture cool. Take a teaspoonful two to three times a day until flatulence levels decrease.
- Neem leaves are an excellent choice for calming gassy stomach and relieving bloating. Take the leaves in powdered capsule form. Neem

leaf is also an antimicrobial and is an excellent herb for aiding the digestion and improving the skin. In fact, in India, neem is used for just about every ailment.

Note that Ayurvedic herbs can be purchased at most Indian food markets, health-food stores, Indian pharmacies, and/or directly from suppliers on the Internet. See the Appendix for names and addresses.

Hands-on Methods for Reducing Gas

Along with teas, medicinals, and dietary changes, hands-on physical methods are an excellent way to relieve flatulence and bloating. Try the following:

Yoga

There are several standard yoga postures used for expelling gas and discouraging its production. See the following postures (asanas) in Chapter 6. All are excellent for relieving wind:

- Eka Pada Pavanamuktasana (one leg to chest gas-reducing posture)
- Hasta Pada (forward bend holding the ankles)
- Sitting Twist
- Uttanasana (forward bend from a standing position)
- Yoga Mudra (sitting position)

Here's another fast and easy yoga posture that helps purge gas. Lying flat on a hard floor, pull your knees tightly up to your chest. Remain in this position for several minutes, rocking gently back and forth. Then stand up, take a few deep breaths, lie down again, and repeat the rocking movements. Chances are you will feel the results immediately.

Self-Massage

Use this method on yourself or ask a partner to do it for you. Place both palms on the stomach and, applying moderate pressure, massage in a circular, clockwise direction (the direction that food moves when passing through the digestive system). Some people are extremely sensitive to pressure in the abdominal regions, so be sure not to press too hard. If performing this massage for someone else, take your cue from him or her.

Massage the stomach area for five to ten minutes. Some drops of massage oil scented with peppermint or sweet fennel (both used in aromatherapy to aid digestion) make the rubbing smoother and deeper.

Heat

Applying external heat to the abdominal area often helps relieve stubborn cases of flatulence. Wet heat works best for some people (a hot-water bottle or hydroculator does the trick). For others, dry heat is preferred (a heating pad). For still others, soaking in a hot bath for fifteen to twenty minutes, or even in a hot sitz bath, relieves the pressure. See the Appendix for information on obtaining professional quality dry and wet heating pads.

Caution: People with diabetes and other neurological problems should not use this method.

Daily Exercise

Exercise, exercise, exercise. It doesn't matter which form you choose—aerobics, jogging, tennis, bicycling, swimming, dance, tai chi, or yoga. All of these methods fight gas and help keep you in shape as part of the bargain.

Walking is an especially pleasant way to aid digestion. Or try climbing stairs. Run on a treadmill. Swim in a community pool. Stretch and move vigorously. Work around the house or around the yard. The goal is to stay as active as you can. If your job keeps you chained to a desk, stand up frequently, stretch, breathe deeply, and walk around. Even small breaks help.

Stress Avoidance

Perhaps it is a cliché to blame every ailment, including gas, on stress, but studies show that this is not far from the case. Stress, we know, produces specific digestive symptoms including stomachaches, indigestion, gas, bloating, and a condition known as hypomotility where the movement of food is slowed and stalled in the intestine. Lesson? If troubled by gas and other stomach symptoms, relax more, unwind more, and enjoy more. Your digestive tract will be accordingly grateful.

chapter fourteen

Natural Remedies
for Constipation

In most cases, constipation is a symptom rather than a disease. This may be splitting hairs to some extent. Anyone who has suffered from stubborn constipation—and who among us has not?—considers it nothing less than a good ol' ailment.

Nonetheless, in a majority of cases, infrequent bowel movements and hard, compacted stools are secondary effects, the result of personal habits and harmful lifestyle choices. There is an old saying that what takes a long time to come stays a long time as well. This maxim clearly applies to constipation. There are many people who have suffered this affliction for years and not thought much about it, enduring it day after day, ignoring the discomfort it brings, shrugging it off as a normal side effect of living. These people tend to develop chronic conditions that are particularly difficult to cure.

Disregard, however, is just one of many possible causes. Constipation may, for instance, be due to nothing more complicated than a habitual tendency to postpone nature's call. After years of intentionally repressing the urge to defecate, nature simply stops urging.

Constipation can also be caused by prolonged physical inactivity, a condition endemic to many Americans. (Interestingly, in the language of many highly active hunting-and-gathering cultures, there is no word to describe constipation.) It can be a reaction to medications such as diuretics, iron pills, antibiotics, and muscle relaxants. It can also be a result of poor diet or of injurious personal habits such as narcotic drugs and long-term laxative use. Inadequate fiber intake; overconsumption of starches, refined sugars, and processed foods; and even negative mental states such as stress and depression, all can slow waste removal to a crawl. And, of course, in a minority of cases, constipation is the result of serious diseases such as diabetes, lupus, disorders of the thyroid or pituitary glands, and even cancer.

What all this means in terms of self-treatment is that there are many types of constipation, and that techniques that cure one person's condition do not necessarily cure another's. The good news, though, is that constipation tends to respond gratifyingly well to natural therapies, and that in a majority of cases, even chronic cases, natural remedies are all that are needed to remedy the situation. For example, one or two natural supplements are all that is necessary to get the digestive juices and the bowel waste flowing properly for some people. In other instances, a change of diet and bowel habit may be called for. In a few cases, an overall program of lifestyle modification is appropriate.

In most of these situations, improvement takes place within a matter of days or weeks. If relief does not come after giving these natural remedies a healthy try, and if more than three to four weeks go by without success, it may be time to seek a physician's advice. If the physician then determines the problem is "just constipation" and nothing more, a continued and extended trial of natural remedies may be warranted. Remember, a problem that has developed over decades of time may take several weeks or even months to resolve.

Important Things to Know About Constipation

Before deciding on the best course of natural treatment for simple constipation, we suggest that you become familiar with basic facts concerning the elimination process. Consider the following questions and answers.

What Physiological Process Actually Causes Constipation?

Once the food we eat is processed in the stomach, it is passed through the small intestine where most of its water and nutrients are absorbed, then down to the colon for further absorption, bacterial fermentation, and finally removal by excretion.

If too much water is removed during this process, waste residues thicken and harden more than usual, and their transit time through the gut slows down. This slowdown results in dehydration of stools and a prolonged contact of the feces with the colon wall, allowing more time for water to be extracted from the fecal matter and thus more time to harden. The result is a vicious cycle of slow transit, dehydration of waste, hardening, compacting, and finally chronic constipation.

The actual act of expelling fecal matter (as well as withholding it when defecation is socially inappropriate) is under voluntary control, utilizing abdominal and pelvic muscles in a well-coordinated fashion. At a subconscious level, however, the bowels are set to process food and wastes by a kind of "cruise control," the speed of this control differing for each person. Constipation occurs when this control mechanism is weakened, and/or when a discoordination takes place within the parts of the digestive machine.

How Do You Know When You're Constipated?

Constipation is a self-evident ailment with many obvious indicators. You will recognize it when you suffer from one or more of the following symptoms:

- Hard, small, compacted bowel movements
- A rubbing, abrasive pain when passing stools
- Infrequent bowel movements (two or fewer movements per week), and/or difficulty moving the bowels in a smooth and easy way
- A sense of incomplete defecation after toileting

- A bloated, full sensation in the abdomen much of the time, even between meals, and a sense of relief from bloating after defecating. These symptoms may also suggest constipation related to irritable bowel syndrome or spastic colon.
- A sudden change in normal bowel movement patterns, with uncharacteristically long periods of time between movements. (**Caution:** Sudden and persistent constipation or, for that matter, any abrupt alteration in bowel habit without prompt response to natural remedies may signal a serious problem and should always be evaluated by a physician.)
- Bleeding hemorrhoids. This condition is often associated with diarrhea as well as with chronic constipation.

How Many Times a Week Should the Bowels Move to Stay Healthy?

The answer to this frequently asked question depends on each person's individual age, constitution, lifestyle, and digestive vigor.

At least three movements a week is considered within the normal range of frequency by most gastroenterologists. Some people, however, produce such small and incomplete stools at every bowel movement that these movements constitute a kind of constipation, even though overall frequency is greater than three per week.

In general, active people eliminate more often than inactive, and people who eat plenty of fiber eliminate more frequently than those who do not. And while it is questionable practice, perhaps, to gauge overall health by the number of bowel movements a person makes in a week, many health-care professionals agree that the more formed movements a person has, the better it is for his or her health. Elimination is, after all, just that—the elimination of toxins and wastes. The faster and more frequently these materials are removed from the system, the less chance there is of stagnation and reabsorption of toxins. This does not mean that we should attempt elimination several times a day, or that diarrhea is better than constipation. Moderation is the key. Indeed, too many bowel movements a day can lead to loss of fluids and nutrients, as well as to an upset in the delicate balance of helpful bacteria in the colon.

What Is the Best Time of Day
for a Bowel Movement?

Peristalsis is most active in the morning, especially between the hours of 5:00 A.M. and 7:00 A.M. (in Chinese medicine, the life force is believed to be most concentrated in the bowels at this time). Digested masses of food have worked their way down to the colon from last night's supper by now, and are ready for prompt removal. This makes the hours before breakfast an ideal time for defecation.

In people with chronic constipation, however, due to the stimulatory effect of food on the colon, defecation immediately after breakfast may be more productive than defecation before. Indeed, bowel movements made after a meal are generally more productive than those made before the meal or at bedtime. Moreover, bowel movements taken later in the day and between meals tend to be less ample than morning stools, more difficult to pass, and often produce a sense of incomplete defecation. At the same time, never put off a persistent urge to defecate. Any time of day or night is a good time for a bowel movement. As a rule of thumb, when the urge comes, go.

Why Is Privacy Important for
Maintaining Regularity?

It is said that to successfully fight constipation, we must pay attention to the three Ps and the two Fs. The three Ps are (1) privacy, (2) position while toileting, and (3) peristalsis.

The two Fs are (1) adequate fiber intake and (2) adequate intake of fluids.

Privacy is ranked number one among the Ps—for obvious reasons. Nobody, no matter how extroverted, wishes to be stared at while answering the call of nature. Even before potty training, toddlers hide behind a sofa or curtain when making a bowel movement. The urge for privacy in the privy appears to be a natural and universal instinct.

Why is this so? Most likely because a person making a bowel movement requires a certain amount of quiet and concentration to get the job done. Human beings are simply made this way. Any sense of being spied on or bothered during this time interferes with the physiological processes of elimination. As doctors well know, success at moving the bowels is often as psychological as it is physical.

In my own practice, I often see privacy issues arising among caregivers and their patients. Often, the caregiver hovers over the patient, even when the patient attempts to toilet. Though the caregiver means well by this and only wants to help, the patient often becomes embarrassed and fails to pass a stool.

For this reason, it is important that patients and caregivers come to an agreement on toilet privacy. Caregiver and patient can, for example, agree that the patient is to be left alone in the commode for ten to fifteen minutes at each session. If a private bathroom is not available for the purpose, a curtain or divider can be put up to provide privacy.

How Important Is Position for Relief from Constipation?

Position is very important. The first thing to keep in mind about position is that the modern flush toilet, as efficient and sanitary as it may be, forces users to assume a body position that is intensely cramping, that cuts off the downward movement of feces in the colon, and that is basically a far cry from the way nature intended us to eliminate.

How *did* nature intend us to eliminate? In a word: by squatting. See, for example, how toddlers naturally assume the squatting position when they pass stools. Or how people from many rural cultures willingly adopt this posture, even when flush toilets are an option. If you have ever had occasion to squat in the woods yourself, or to use an Eastern-style squat-seal toilet, you too have experienced the ease and speed with which wastes are voided by assuming this position.

Why is squatting better, physically speaking? Normally the angle between the rectum and anal canal is approximately 90 degrees. This sharp angle prevents the easy downstream transfer of stool and the involuntary emission of gas. When a person sits on a modern toilet, this sharp angle is exaggerated and sharpened even more, interfering significantly with a free downward flow.

If one squats while defecating, however, the anorectal angle improves significantly, allowing an easy downward movement of stool. At the same time, the anal sphincters also relax, further facilitating the drop. Squatting likewise moves the pelvic muscles into positions that are far more conducive to smooth movements than the cramped, on-the-toilet position.

Of course, when I inform my patients of these rather arcane facts, they often retort by saying that squatting is too difficult, and that even holding this position for a minute or two is highly uncomfortable, to say the least. And, of course, they are right. But there is a way around this. Try it next time you sit on the commode. First, place a foot-high footstool under your feet. When you attempt to eliminate, bend forward as far as you can comfortably go, and notice the difference. Placing a pillow on your thighs to rest your arms makes the forward bend easier and more relaxed.

These few simple adjustments, I tell my patients, approximate the position of squatting and substantially facilitate bowel movements. This position is especially useful in cases of chronic constipation.

Are There Any Types of Toileting Positions You Should Always Avoid?

Perhaps the worst position anyone can assume for a bowel movement is sitting on the toilet with feet dangling in the air. It is far better to plant the feet firmly on the floor when defecating. In the dangling position, the already acute anorectal angle is further exaggerated, and the configuration of the abdominal and pelvic muscles becomes severely compromised. Feet on the floor, please.

What Part Does Habit Play in Regularity?

A large one. Choose a time of day for toilet activities, preferably shortly before or after breakfast, and stick to it. Even if the bowels do not respond at first, persist. Eventually, your digestive system will get the idea and re-program itself to fit the schedule.

Like the rest of us, our organs of elimination are creatures of habit. Accustom them to perform at certain hours of the day, and eventually they comply. Regularity then increases accordingly.

How Can You Tell If Your Bowel Movements Are Healthy?

Though many people find the job disagreeable, it is a good idea to glance at your stools for a moment or two before flushing to make sure they are in good order. The signs of healthy elimination are as follows:

- Stools should be relatively soft, about the consistency of toothpaste and about the length of a banana. If stools are thick, soft, and bulky, this is usually a sign you are eating many of the right foods.
- Healthy stools are often a dark-pumpkin color or a light brown. Stools that are consistently black and greasy-looking may be due to incomplete digestion. If stools are black, it is a good idea to examine them for possible signs of blood. Don't be alarmed. Most dark stools are perfectly okay. It just never hurts to check.
- Though stools usually have some odor, a strong sulfurous smell may indicate poor digestion. In general, the stools of meat eaters have a stronger smell more than those of vegetarians.
- Hard, scaly, pelletlike stools signal low fluid intake. Loose stools suggest poor digestion or stomach upset. Pencil-thin stools may indicate a blockage, slow peristalsis, or even cancer.
- Emitting gas while defecating is common and nothing to worry about. An overabundance of emitted gas at every toileting, however, is not normal.
- Contrary to popular opinion, if your stools float, this is not a sign of undigested fat. Stools float because of the air trapped inside them, or because of their high-fiber content. If your stools float, this is a good sign, or a neutral one at worst, and nothing to worry about.

Do Mental States Affect Bowel Regularity?

The mind-body interface plays a prominent role in bowel regularity, and should not be underestimated as potential sources of regularity problems. You may have noticed, for instance, that emotional upsets or shocks often cause instant diarrhea. Or that prolonged periods of worry and anxiety can be accompanied by sluggish bowels.

Dr. S. Dykes and colleagues report in the *European Journal of Gastroenterology and Hepatology* (2001) that as many as 60 to 70 percent of patients with intractable constipation show evidence of suffering from some form of psychological or psychiatric disorder. Their studies found that as many as one-third of patients demonstrated irrational attitudes of one kind or another toward food. The investigators recommend that constipated patients who suffer from mental problems should be provided with psychological evaluation before undergoing drastic treatment measures such as bowel surgery.

As discussed previously, the gut has a mind of its own, commonly known as the "little brain," and, in many ways, it functions autonomously from the brain. Biofeedback is thus routinely used by gastroenterologists in the treatment of constipation. Dr. S. R. Brown and colleagues in the journal *Diseases of Colon and Rectum* (2001) report that all patients in their studies who suffered from constipation benefited from biofeedback therapy and, as a result, avoided the need for a colectomy (the surgical removal of the colon). Dr. Brown and associates recommend that biofeedback be seriously considered as a safe and inexpensive treatment for all forms of chronic constipation. Biofeedback is also helpful, studies show, for constipation in people with limited disabilities, and for people with neurological disorders such as multiple sclerosis.

Can Simple Constipation Be Harmful?

Occasional bouts of constipation are harmless. But be careful: recurring constipation is the body's way of warning us that something is amiss, either in the gut itself or in a nearby organ. It also warns us that the food we are taking in is being improperly digested and assimilated, and that we should improve our eating habits.

In general, constipation is a sign that the vital energy released from nutrients is not being properly assimilated and distributed through the system, and that the sensitive and vital balance between the "brain" in the stomach and the "brain" in the head is out of equilibrium. No wonder constipation is so often accompanied by feelings of depression and fatigue, as well as by the normal side effects of abdominal bloating, distention, and discomfort.

A little constipation now and then is harmless. But too many instances over the long run are a danger signal that should not be ignored.

What Physical Signs Indicate That Constipation May Be Due to Serious Causes?

If a person's normal bowel patterns are suddenly and significantly altered, this can be cause for concern. So can blood in the stool, sudden unexplained weight loss, prolonged fever, pain in the lower abdomen, diarrhea in patients with a history of constipation, and constipation accompanied by abdominal distention and vomiting. All such symptoms including change in bowel habit should be taken seriously, and promptly referred to a physician. The older the person, the higher the risk for cancer.

A FEW MORE IMPORTANT THINGS TO REMEMBER ABOUT CONSTIPATION

When constipated, be careful not to strain during bowel movements. Chronic straining can cause bleeding hemorrhoids and hernias, tissue tearing, and painful anal fissures. On rare occasions, it can also trigger a vasovagal reaction, causing the heart to slow down or even stop. Rather than force the issue, use the natural remedies featured below.

Remember too that when you travel, when you alter your diet, when you undergo a severe emotional shock, or when you expose your body to sudden environmental change, constipation can often result. Next time constipation strikes, ask yourself: Have I changed any of my normal routines or habits lately? Have I introduced a new food or drink to my diet? Have I recently undergone a sudden shock or emotional trauma? If the answer is yes to any of these questions, you have probably discovered the cause of your irregularity.

Finally, in review: The most common causes of constipation are poor diet, dehydration, change of routine, and lack of exercise. By adding fiber to your meals, drinking at least eight glasses of water a day (unless, of course, fluid restriction is advised by your physician), cutting down on junk foods, reducing sugar intake, proper positioning during defecation, and increasing daily activity levels, a surprisingly large number of cases can be remedied without recourse to further treatment. Most cases of simple constipation require neither laxatives nor trips to the doctor. A majority of cases pass on their own in a few days. Just give it time and let nature take its course.

USING NATURAL LAXATIVES

Many members of the medical community regard over-the-counter laxatives with a suspicious eye, especially so-called "stimulant laxatives" such as castor oil, cascara sagrada, senna, bisacodyl, and phenolphthalein that work directly on the intestines. Although not definitively proven, I believe that, unless supervised by a physician, the long-term indiscriminate and chronic use of laxatives can be harmful.

Why? For several reasons. Many brands of stimulant laxatives irritate the lining of the colon, eventually causing "cathartic colon." This condition increases constipation rather than improves it, making the colon wall less responsive to the movements and stimulation of fecal matter.

Stimulant laxatives also sap the vigor of the digestive organs, and habitual use makes these organs "lazy." *Why bother?* the digestive organs metaphorically ask. *The laxatives are doing all the work for us.*

Eventually, under these conditions, the elimination system loses its ability to function properly without first being shocked into action by chemical stimulants. The result is laxative dependence, either physiological, psychological, or, in some cases, both. My advice: Except for occasional use in mild, short-term constipation, only use laxatives—especially stimulant and osmotic laxatives—under a physician's supervision.

Types of Natural Laxatives

The next time constipation occurs, why not consider trying natural alternatives before turning to drugstore remedies? Natural laxatives are easier on the digestive system than chemical laxatives. They are less expensive and are rarely habit-forming, even when used for long periods of time. Because they are derived from natural plant materials, the digestive system processes them easily, and side effects—especially dependence—are rare.

So what's the downside? Occasionally people feel gassiness and bloating from natural laxatives, especially when fiber-based laxatives like psyllium are taken in too large a dose. Mixing fiber-based laxatives with prescription medications can also slow the working of the medicine, a condition that is easily avoided by taking medications and laxatives several hours apart. Note that long-term use of fiber does not cause a nutrient deficiency, as is sometimes reported, if vitamin and mineral supplements are added to the diet on a regular basis.

Most natural constipation remedies are classed in the category of *bulk-forming laxatives*. Included in this category are the following:

- Bulk-forming foods
- Bran
- Psyllium seed husks and their commercial derivatives (such as Metamucil and Colon Cleanse)
- Malt soup extract (Maltsupex)

Let's review these substances one by one in the sections below.

Bulk-Forming Foods

Perhaps the best-known bulk-forming foods are prunes, both the fruit itself and the juice. For many people, a few prunes every day and/or a glass of prune juice is all that is needed to maintain regularity.

Boil five or six prunes together over a low heat for an hour, then drink the juice in the morning and eat the prunes at night. Stewed or boiled prunes are usually more helpful in combating constipation than the dried variety.

Other foods that build bulk and help move the bowels are rhubarb (stewed is best), figs, aloe vera, and sauerkraut. Also useful are high-fiber foods. More information on fiber and constipation is included in the discussion on dietary changes later in the chapter.

Bran

Wheat, rice, or oat bran can be purchased at most supermarkets or health-food stores today. Sprinkle it over your breakfast cereal. Or use it as a garnish for meat loaf and vegetables. If you eat bran by the spoonful, be sure to wash it down with at least eight ounces of water. Too much bran and too little water cause compaction rather than cure it.

An added advantage is bran's reputed cholesterol-lowering effect, especially oat bran. In addition, bran expands in the stomach, making eaters feel full more quickly and thus helping with weight control. Finally, the fiber in bran is reputed to help prevent colon cancer, diverticulosis, and gallstones. Not bad.

Psyllium Husk Powder

Most spectacular of the bulk-forming laxatives are the powder of psyllium seed husks, a pure fiber plant that produces truly astonishing results for many constipated people, sometimes within twenty-four hours.

Psyllium powder increases the size of the feces, which in turn stimulates the lining of the colon. It increases peristalsis, helping transport wastes out of the colon in record time. Even people who rarely suffer from constipation find that their bowel movements become larger, more frequent, easier to pass, and more satisfying with daily psyllium use. For some people, psyllium also helps relieve loose bowels and even diarrhea. It is especially effective for people who eat low-fiber diets.

Add a heaping teaspoon of psyllium seed powder to a glass of water, stir until the mixture starts to thicken, and drink. Follow immediately with a glass of water to wash down the mixture. This follow-up glass of water activates the effects of the psyllium, and prevents it from thickening in the throat and stomach.

Start by taking a teaspoon of psyllium powder husks every morning in a glass of water. If one dose per day does not help the constipation, increase to two or three glasses a day. Once the psyllium starts to take effect, you can cut back to a maintenance dose that works best for you.

Some people also like to mix psyllium powder with portions of bran. Try filling a glass with juice, then adding a spoonful of bran and a spoonful of psyllium powder. Mix thoroughly, drink down immediately, and follow up with a full glass of fresh water.

Note, finally, that while commercial brands of psyllium such as Metamucil are gratifyingly effective, purists insist that plain, unprocessed (and unflavored) psyllium sold under the name Psyllium Husks Powder is the most effective. On the other hand, unflavored psyllium tastes heavily glutinous, and must be stirred for what seems like hours before it thoroughly dissolves (make sure the water is cold, not hot). Another psyllium-based laxative, isabgol, is used widely in India and Europe, and has been shown to be of marked benefit, even when other commercial products produce inconsistent results. Isabgol is available in the United States at health-food stores and Indian grocery stores. Try the different varieties, and decide for yourself.

Malt Soup Extract

Malt soup is another helpful commercial bulk-forming laxative that exerts a naturally stimulating effect on the bowels similar to that of bran and psyllium.

While many people rate psyllium as more effective than malt soup, malt soup has an avid following, and some users find it easier to swallow. Like psyllium and bran, malt soup produces no side effects, and peristaltic activity in the bowels does not become dependent on it.

Caution: Bulk-forming laxatives can lead to bowel obstruction for the neurologically impaired and for bedridden patients with constipation. People with these conditions should use high-fiber laxatives only if supervised by a physician.

WHEN NATURAL LAXATIVES DON'T WORK

In most cases, natural laxatives do the job. But not always. When this route fails, a carefully individualized bowel regimen consisting of judiciously selected laxatives becomes necessary, usually with a doctor's supervision.

The first line of defense here is a high-fiber diet and high fluid intake, coupled with the use of mild osmotic laxatives such as Milk of Magnesia. In stubborn cases, a more effective laxative such as Lactulose may be recommended. (If Lactulose is used, remember to increase your water intake while using this preparation.)

Stool softeners such as Colace also remain in wide use in conventional medicine, though their efficacy is yet to be clinically established. Drinking mineral oil is of dubious value, and is considered outdated. Enemas and suppositories may help people at risk of impaction, and are a useful alternative for stubborn constipation. Polyethylene glycol solutions such as MiraLax, GoLytely, NuLytely, and Colyte are used in cases where all the above measures fail to produce the desired results.

Finally, be aware that laxatives, even natural laxatives that are considered mild for adults, can be strong medicine for children. Check with your physician before administering any type of laxative to a constipated child.

OVERCOMING YEARS OF CONSTIPATION WITH BASIC DIETARY CHANGES

A Crash Course on Fiber

The most direct and effective way to combat constipation is to add laxative-action foods to your menu, and to remove foods that have a binding effect. Specifically, this means the addition of unprocessed, high-fiber foods, and the subtraction of highly processed, low-fiber foods.

Fiber, as you may already know, is the nonmetabolized residue of plant tissue, the parts of the fruit or vegetable that pass through the body undigested, and that exit largely intact. You won't find this substance in meats, fish, or dairy products. It comes exclusively from the plant kingdom and is embedded to some degree in practically all vegetables, fruit, grains, and nuts.

There are two basic types of fiber: water-soluble fiber and water-insoluble fiber.

Insoluble fiber such as wheat bran is less susceptible to bacterial fermentation than the soluble varieties found in vegetables, pectins, and gums. Insoluble fiber likewise holds more water than soluble, and contributes more to stool bulk. Both forms of fiber are useful, and both are necessary.

Fiber's ability to relieve constipation is legendary, and with good reason. Fiber exerts a strong absorbent action in the gut, drawing local stores of water into the feces and swelling their size and weight. These stores add both bulk and softness to the stool, and help it to pass swiftly and easily through the digestive tract. Tests show that people who eat a high-fiber diet eliminate more frequently than those who do not. The stools of regular fiber eaters are large and full, and fiber eaters excrete more wastes at each bowel movement than non-fiber eaters.

The following foods in their fresh, unrefined, and unprocessed forms are all high in fiber, and should find a place on your menu if constipation is an ongoing problem. Sometimes, the addition of these foods alone causes immediate improvement for constipated persons. Some of the fruits on the list such as apples, moreover, may also bring indigestible sugars to the digestive tract, and act as mild osmotic laxatives.

Apples	Green beans	Peas
Avocados	Grits	Pineapple
Bananas	Kidney beans	Potatoes in their skins
Beets	Lentils	Prunes
Bran	Lettuce	Raspberries
Broccoli	Mangoes	Rolled oats
Cabbage	Okra	Strawberries
Carrots	Oranges	Tomatoes
Cauliflower	Parsnips	Walnuts
Celery	Peaches	Whole-wheat bread
Corn	Pears	

Eating Tips to Remedy Constipation

Note that when certain grains are heavily processed (such as polished rice and white bread), they lose a majority of their fiber, becoming soft and pulpy, without the all-important fibrous covering. These denatured substances tend to slog ponderously along inside the digestive tract, no longer stimulating the lining of the gut, and becoming part of the problem rather than the solution to it. To counteract the ill effects of commercial processing, incorporate some or all of the following dietary tactics into your daily eating:

- Substitute unrefined, unprocessed grains and nuts (in breads, cakes, rice, peanut butter, and so on) for the refined varieties.
- Eat whole-wheat bread and cereals instead of refined flour breads and cereals.
- Eat the skins and edible seeds of raw vegetables and fruits for added fiber.
- When cooking pasta, use whole-wheat varieties in place of pasta made from refined flour.
- Sprinkle bran and wheat germ over meat dishes, pancakes, cereals, spaghetti, and desserts. These sprinklings add a pleasant, crunchy taste to the food and increase fiber intake.
- Make it a habit to eat foods from cultures that include large amounts of fiber in their diets. Mexican, Chinese, Indian, and Middle Eastern dishes all fall into this category.
- Eliminate foods that cause constipation. These include coffee, tea, sugar, chocolate, fatty meat, fats in general, and fried foods. Most foods on this list are notorious for causing frequent indigestion, acid reflux, bloating, and flatulence as well.
- Increase your daily intake of fresh fruits and vegetables. The list on page 280 offers some best bets.
- Add a steady diet of live-culture yogurt and kefir to your menu. Both of these fermented dairy products add millions of friendly bacteria to the bowels. They are beneficial both for aiding digestion and for increasing ease of evacuation. See Chapters 7 and 8 for details.

- Eat foods that ferment quickly in the gut. A starter list includes sauerkraut, sauerkraut juice, cabbage juice, sourdough bread, miso, and pickles. Sample a drink made of half sauerkraut juice, half tomato juice, plus a squeeze of lemon. If it helps, drink it every other day. You can also make your own sauerkraut. Shred a head of cabbage, place it in a ceramic crock or large glass jar, fill it to the top with water, and add several tablespoons of salt. Close the jar and allow the cabbage to ferment in a warm, dark place for several weeks. Test the mixture every few days. Some people find that punching a few holes in the top of the cap allows air to circulate in the bottle, and prevents gases from building up from fermentation in the container.

- Keeping the colon well lubricated is one of the best ways we know to achieve regularity. Do it by including high-quality oils in your diet such as flaxseed oil, EPA fish oils, and borage oil, all of which are sold in supplement form. These oils keep the intestines lubricated and, at the same time, provide the body with essential fatty acids important for cellular health.

- Avoid cooking with cheap oils. If you cook with olive oil, always use extra virgin olive oil. It's more expensive, but far better for you, and more tasty as well. The difference will be apparent in everything you cook.

- Use recipes that include natural laxative foods such as garlic, rhubarb, bran products, kefir, pumpkin seeds, papaya juice, prunes, apricots, and ground flaxseed. All of these items can be purchased at any natural food store.

- Many people start the day with a cup of coffee to "get their bowels moving." Though coffee is a diuretic and a stimulant, overuse produces the opposite effect—constipation. Monitor your coffee intake; overuse takes its toll.

- Caffeine and theophylline are found in most types of black and green teas, and both flush fluids from the body by causing increased urination. To compensate, the body steals water from the intestinal tract, causing hardened stools and a slowdown of intestinal transit time. This flushing process appears to take place only in people who drink large amounts of tea. Again, moderation is the key.

- When getting up in the morning and before going to bed at night, eat a soft banana with a teaspoon of honey. Make sure you eat the banana on an empty stomach. Bananas and honey have a lubricating effect on the intestines, and are useful in any anticonstipation diet. Interestingly, bananas are also helpful for slowing down cases of diarrhea.
- A mixed drink of honey, lime, and water helps purify the digestive system. Mix two teaspoons of honey and the juice from half a lime in a glass of water. Think of this drink as an engine cleaner for your car. This concoction is also good for your heart.
- Some people have cured persistent and long-term constipation simply by changing their diets, and eating large portions of fiber-rich fruits and vegetables at every meal (including breakfast). Rule number one: Never underestimate the power of high-fiber fruits and vegetable taken with plenty of water to improve digestion and elimination. For many people, a simple change in diet is all that is needed to restore regularity.

The Easiest Cure of All

A friend of mine has suffered from intermittent constipation since adolescence. Tiring of laxatives and other extreme measures, he overheard a conversation one day in the supermarket. A woman, he learned, had totally eliminated her constipation simply by drinking two glasses of water every day before eating breakfast. What the heck, my friend figured, so he tried it. Now he rarely, if ever, suffers from constipation.

This does not mean that every case of chronic constipation is cured by drinking water in the morning. It does mean that for certain people lack of adequate hydration is a major cause of uncooperative bowels. For such people, irrigating and stimulating the bowels with several glasses of water upon awakening and then drinking several more glasses throughout the day is sometimes all that is needed to reset the liquid balance in the gut.

Why not give it a try? For the next several weeks, drink eight to ten glasses of water a day. Take at least two glasses between meals, and two before breakfast. You may be pleasantly surprised. For some people, warm water is more stimulating to the gut than water cooled to room temperature.

Caution: Drinking ten glasses a day of coffee or soda or even juice is not the same as drinking water. Far from it. Large quantities of these liquids have diuretic effects that cause increased elimination of fluids through the kidneys, reducing the water left over for gut irrigation and resulting in constipation.

EXERCISE—LAXATIVE NUMBER ONE

Individuals who perform regular exercise are rarely constipated. Exercise works—especially for constipation. So add it to your to-do list if you have sluggish bowels. The following exercise systems are all excellent for stimulating the gut, increasing peristaltic activity, and improving digestion. Add any of them to the other healing modalities and you won't be disappointed.

Yoga

Many of the stretches and lifts in yoga are specifically designed to tone the gut, and to increase circulation in the organs of digestion and evacuation. While the information in Chapter 6 provides a selection of yoga methods for general digestive health, the following yoga exercises are specific for constipation, and serve as an excellent introduction to this powerful method of body toning and rehabilitation.

- Lie on your back with your legs straight. Relax for several minutes, then sit up, keeping your legs flat on the floor. Place your right leg over your left leg as far to the left as it will go, being careful not to strain. Hold this position for twenty to thirty seconds, then slowly bring your leg back to the starting position. Repeat the same movement with the left leg. Perform ten repetitions, five times to one side, five to the other.

- Lie on your back with your legs straight. Relax. Inhale deeply. Pull your right leg up to your chest, pressing your knee against your abdomen with both hands, and keeping your left leg flat on the floor. Press firmly for ten seconds, exhale, bring the leg down, and repeat with the other leg. Perform three repetitions with each leg.

  Next, inhale and pull both knees against your chest. Press for five seconds, exhale, and bring your legs down to the floor. Repeat as many times as you like. This exercise is remarkably helpful for constipation and for abdominal troubles of any kind.

- Sit on the floor with your back straight and your legs extended. Bend forward and try to touch your right foot with your left hand. This stretch should be firm but not painful. If you have difficulty reaching your foot, be sure not to force it. A gentle stretch is all that's necessary. Hold the stretching position for ten seconds. Then return to the starting position, bend over again, this time touching your left foot with your right hand. Alternate sides until your back and abdominal regions feel well stretched and pleasantly tired.

- Stand straight with your legs spread approximately a foot apart. Bend over and touch your right foot with your left hand. Hold this position for five seconds, return to the standing position, then reverse, touching your left foot with your right hand. Repeat until pleasantly tired.

- From a standing position, raise your arms straight over your head with palms pressed together. Rotate your trunk to the right as far as it will comfortably go. Hold for five seconds, return to the original position, then twist to the left. Do five twists to each side.

- Do ten sit-ups in the morning and ten at night. Sit-ups can help against constipation, though they should be done in moderation. If you have never done sit-ups, start with just a few and build gradually.

- Lie on your back for several minutes with your legs together. Place your hands under the small of your back. Slowly raise your legs into a shoulder stand, supporting your lower back with both hands. In the final position, your legs and torso should be nearly perpendicular to the floor. Your hands should be locked into the base of your back, your chin pressed against your chest. Remain in this posture for several minutes, feeling the blood flow down your legs, filling your abdomen with warmth and a sense of well-being. This is one of the best of yogic postures for constipation and for problems of the lower organs in general.

Other Useful Exercises for Constipation

Relaxed walking is extremely helpful for constipation, especially if it is done in the early morning when peristalsis is most active. Though not a yoga exercise per se, walking acts on the body much in the same ways, stimulating blood flow, increasing oxygen intake, raising metabolism, and reducing stress. Taking a walk immediately after getting up in the morning and then before going to bed is standard practice in Indian culture.

Regular calisthenics and aerobics are also helpful for maintaining regularity. Whether it is running, swimming, or sports such as tennis and basketball, any invigorating activity that provides physical stimulation is recommended.

Whatever exercise you enjoy, however, be regular about it. This is the key. Try to exercise at least four times a week for a half hour to an hour each time. When you get up in the morning, run through a few stretching exercises to get your blood flowing and to tune up your gastrointestinal system, just in time for your morning elimination.

Most of all, keep active. A moving, breathing, vigorous gut is a happy gut.

REGAINING REGULARITY WITH MASSAGE AND ACUPRESSURE

The sigmoid colon, located where the lower colon begins its descent into the rectum, contains several sharp angles, and food residues tend to get trapped in its curves. This blockage causes an impediment to the downward flow of fecal matter, with constipation resulting.

Direct massage applied to the sigmoid area can help. Massage increases peristalsis, stimulates enzymatic activity, and helps free trapped wastes. Does massage for constipation sound far-fetched?

Consider that Dr. Kenefick from the United Kingdom, in a study reported at the annual Digestive Disease Week convention in San Francisco in 2002, tells us that sacral nerve stimulation by massage alters neuromuscular function, and can help a number of forms of constipation. Likewise, Dr. Mimidis and colleagues, in a Canadian study reported at the same meeting, demonstrated that, by using a mechanical vibrator on the abdomen, bowel function is substantially stimulated, even in severely constipated patients. So why not give massage a try?

First, find a friend or companion who is willing to be your massage partner. Stomach massage can be self-applied, although it is more effective when applied by another person. Staying passive while your lower abdominal areas are pressed and kneaded allows you to relax, enjoy, let go, and receive the full benefits that massage brings.

If you are performing the massage, begin by having the person lie on his or her back with the abdomen exposed. Place one hand on top of the other just below the navel. Rub the abdomen in a clockwise motion, following the direction that food moves through the digestive tract. Massage movements should be round, firm, slow, and deep. Oil applied to the skin helps the process along nicely (crushed garlic added to warmed olive oil is a traditional Ayurvedic mixture for enhancing the effects of stomach massage).

Next, place your palms directly on the navel, one hand on top of the other. Slide your hands briskly back and forth, applying firm, steady pressure. Continue this motion for several minutes.

Finally, with your palms placed directly over the navel, slide your palms from the navel down to the base of the groin, pushing inward as you go with a firm but comfortable pressure. Then return to the starting spot and repeat. Massage oil is especially recommended for this maneuver. It makes the job easier for the masseur, and more pleasurable for the recipient.

When the stomach massage is complete, follow up by stimulating the following acupressure points. Note that acupressure is best applied with the thumb. Push down on the designated acupressure point with firm but moderate pressure, making sure not to press to the point of pain. All acupressure techniques listed below can be self-applied.

- Press the point one and a half inches directly below the navel. Apply pressure for thirty seconds, stop, then press for another thirty seconds. This point is the most effective acupressure location on the body for healing stomach problems of any kind.
- Press the points on each foot directly below and to the outside corner of the nail on the big toe. Press twice for thirty seconds each time.
- Press the point on the sole of the foot, just below the ball of the foot and in line with the third toe, for thirty seconds.
- Apply firm, direct pressure to the solar plexus for thirty seconds. People with chronic constipation should stimulate this point several times a day.

TREATING CONSTIPATION WITH A VARIETY OF NATURAL REMEDIES

Herbal teas, vitamins, spices and herbs, mental exercises, and other tricks of the trade all help constipation. Complement the therapeutic programs above with one or more of the following techniques:

- A popular Ayurvedic remedy for constipation is to boil barley for several hours, strain off the water, and drink. For increased effectiveness, add a radish to the water and boil with the barley. You can also eat the barley as a side dish.
- Another Ayurvedic remedy for constipation calls for grinding up a small amount of nutmeg and mixing it into a glass of warm lemon juice. Drink twice a day. This remedy is especially useful for constipation accompanied by bloating and stomach distention.
- Every morning, on an empty stomach (before breakfast), drink a spoonful of olive oil mixed with a dash of fresh lemon juice. This simple method is believed to cleanse the blood and liver of toxins,

and to help lubricate the colon for easier passage of stool. A teaspoon of flaxseed oil each morning is also effective and can be taken in lieu of the olive oil.

- Take a teaspoon of blackstrap molasses every morning and night. This is an old but venerable remedy.
- Agar-agar, a form of commercially processed seaweed, is an excellent laxative, and can be taken as a supplement at all meals.
- A glass of buttermilk with breakfast is a tried-and-true old-timer that many people swear by.
- An effective laxative tea can be prepared from the following herbal ingredients: one part chamomile, one part senna leaves, one part anise seeds, one part angelica, and two parts borage flowers.

    Mix the ingredients together, and place a teaspoon of the mixture into a cup of boiling water. Steep, sweeten to taste, and drink twice a day.
- A helpful herbal concoction for constipation can be prepared from the following herbal ingredients: four parts buckthorn, four parts cascara sagrada bark, four parts calamus root, four parts fennel seed, and one part aloe vera.

    Mix the ingredients well. Place a quarter of a teaspoon of the mixture into boiling water, steep for ten minutes, then strain off the leaves. Sweeten to taste, and drink each night before retiring.
- A warm sitz bath each morning and night is an old and honored remedy for constipation. Sitz baths stimulate blood circulation and nerve action in the lower parts of the body, with a positive rebound effect felt in the digestive system. As an alternative, place a warm compress over your abdomen for twenty minutes, followed by a cold compress.
- A popular and effective Chinese aid for constipation is made in the following way: Soak one cup of rice in water until it is soft and glutinous (soaking overnight is best). Once the rice is soft, boil a handful of walnuts in water for ten minutes, then pour the rice, ground walnuts, and rice water into a blender, and grind to a pulp. Remove the mixture and boil it over low heat until it becomes thick and sticky.

Eat a portion of this tasty porridge every day for regularity. It makes an especially fine meal for breakfast.

- For a constipated child, add two teaspoons of rice bran syrup or honey to a cup of milk and have the child drink it every six hours. Children like the taste of this concoction and drink it willingly. If the child shows no improvement in a day or so, consult a physician.

- Mix a sprinkle of powdered nutmeg into a glass of hot water and add the juice of one lemon. Drink twice a day.

- According to Chinese medicine, peristalsis is most active in the early hours of the morning, especially between 5 and 6 A.M. Ironically, this is the same time recommended by Ayurvedic doctors for bowel movements. Is it a coincidence? Train yourself to use the toilet at these times every day, and see.

- Try this simple exercise in self-suggestion: Just at the moment you are about to fall asleep, quietly repeat the following message to yourself ten to fifteen times: "Tomorrow I will have a satisfying bowel movement."

Many cases of constipation are psychological and respond surprisingly well to simple autosuggestion. This phrase is best whispered at that sensitive time when we hover between waking and sleep. At this moment, our minds are especially vulnerable to autohypnotic suggestion.

WHEN CONSTIPATION BECOMES SERIOUS: VISITING YOUR DOCTOR

What should you do if none of the remedies presented in this chapter relieves your constipation? When and if this happens, visit your physician immediately and describe all of your symptoms. The doctor's job is to then play Sherlock Holmes, using his or her expertise to ferret out what's at the bottom of this stubborn condition.

In the process, doctors will ask you a battery of questions; the queries listed below are representative of what they may wish to know. Before you visit your physician, I recommend that you review these questions and make mental notes of the answers you will give. Preparation and knowledge on the patient's part go a long way toward helping a doctor make a successful diagnosis.

- Describe the constipation symptoms that are bothering you. Constipation means different things to different people. It is not unusual in my experience for patients to complain of constipation, then to define this constipation as *only* one bowel movement a day—a far cry from the three movements a week that constitute normal regularity.
- How frequent are your bowel movements? Do you have hard stools, excessive straining, painful defecation, and/or a sense of incomplete evacuation after toileting?
- How long have you suffered from constipation? Is it a recent development or a chronic problem? If chronic, has it been present since your birth or early childhood?
- Have you used laxatives for this condition? Are you using them now? If so, which ones do you use, and how frequently? What result have you gotten from these medications?
- Have you ever found blood in your stool? If yes, was it bright or dark red? Any clots? Was the blood streaked on the sides of the stool or was it mixed into the stool?
- Have you used enemas to facilitate defecation? If so, with what results? Do you use any physical maneuvers to facilitate defecation such as digital disimpaction or pressures in the vagina? If so, describe them.
- Do you have a history of sexual and/or physical abuse? Are there any unusual stresses in your life at the present time? Do you have a history of psychological or psychiatric problems, past or current?
- Which medications are you currently taking? Have you recently indulged in illicit drug abuse? If so, which drugs are you using? How often do you take them?
- How much water do you drink every day? How many caffeinated and alcoholic beverages do you drink every day?

- Does anyone else in your family suffer from constipation? If so, which relatives?
- Do you suffer from other medical difficulties such as diabetes, underactive thyroid, neurological problems, or previous abdominal surgeries? If so, what type of treatments are you currently taking?

After a detailed history is taken, a doctor will perform a physical examination to confirm his or her initial impression and to exclude hidden factors not mentioned in the oral history. As a rule, this physical exam is normal in healthy subjects. Problems of obstruction in the colon must be also ruled out by performing a barium enema or an endoscopy. The latter provides direct visualization of the colon wall and allows biopsies to be performed if needed, making it the preferred test.

Many experts also recommend a sigmoidoscopy for younger subjects, or a full colonoscopy for people forty years old and over. A sigmoidoscopy is a limited GI scope in which only the rectum and the lower part of the colon are examined. A colonoscopy is the examination of the entire five-foot-long colon.

My personal preference in most cases is a colonoscopy. A colonoscopy is more reassuring to patients, and helps relieve the inevitable fear of cancer. Plus, preparation for a colonoscopy requires the administration of a complete colonic cleansing, which improves general health and increases the chances of success for other therapeutic measures. Physicians may also order laboratory blood counts for anemia, blood chemistry tests, and thyroid function tests.

Once it is determined that laboratory tests are normal and that there are no obstructions in the colon, a physician will usually prescribe simple measures to combat chronic constipation such as increased fiber and fluid intake, as well as relaxation techniques. If these measures fail, the physician will then order further, more advanced tests such as colonic transit time, anorectal manometry, and electromyography (EMG). The results of these tests vary widely, however. There is a large overlap between normal and abnormal, and frequently results do not correlate with symptoms. These discrepancies have caused some experts to question the usefulness of such advanced tests in general, although most doctors feel that they have their place in patient management.

Hopefully, none of these measures will be necessary. In fact, in most cases of stubborn constipation, the natural methods of diet, herbs, massage, hydration, and exercise get the job done quite effectively without need for further intervention.

chapter fifteen

Overcoming Leaky
Gut Syndrome

There are a number of clinical disorders, especially gastrointestinal disorders, that appear to have so many symptoms and seem to be linked to so many similar ailments that they end up being categorized under the loose and flexible term "syndrome." Leaky gut syndrome is one of these diseases. This rather explicit and uninviting name refers to a series of ornery digestive symptoms caused by increased permeability in the lining of the intestinal tract.

In a healthy individual, the wall of the intestinal tract is designed to absorb food molecules, and to prevent harmful microorganisms and toxic materials from passing out through the bowel wall and into the bloodstream. The intestinal wall also plays a part in immune function, producing a variety of antibodies necessary for destroying invading pathogens.

In today's heavily polluted environment, the gastrointestinal tract of even the healthiest individual is called on to process an overwhelmingly large flow of septic and infectious materials. These materials contain contaminated foods; corrosive chemical substances; an assortment of bacteria, viruses, parasites, and fungi; and metabolic by products produced by these materials such as fat, undigested protein, and toxic wastes.

Subjected to this incessant flow of poisonous matter, the lining of the intestinal tract in certain people slowly begins to lose its integrity. First it weakens. Then it becomes loosened or inflamed. Finally, the porelike junctions along the gastrointestinal tract start to become abnormally large. Soon bulky, partially digested food particles, toxic substances, and infectious microbes start to permeate through the intestinal walls, and to enter the bloodstream. The gut has now become overly porous or, technically speaking, *hyperpermeable*.

Imagine what happens when a besieging enemy attacks the protective walls of a city day after day. Eventually the city's defenses weaken, and the invaders batter a series of holes all along the wall. The enemy then pours into the city, wreaking havoc and taking no prisoners. An analogous event occurs when harmful materials cause fissures in the intestinal conduit. These materials pour through the enlarged openings in the gut and enter the bloodstream, bringing toxicity and infection everywhere they go.

Once compromised in this way, a person becomes vulnerable to a wide range of possible problems—chemicals that poison the system, infectious materials that spread disease, and large, alien bits of matter that disrupt the body's internal workings. A person's intestinal wall, in other words, designed by nature to keep harmful wastes away from the rest of the body, now literally has holes in it. This person's gut has become "leaky."

SYMPTOMS OF LEAKY GUT

The symptoms of leaky gut syndrome vary widely, depending on the type of contaminants the hyperpermeable gut allows in. These symptoms can be metabolic, endocrine based, neurological, and even psychological.

Think of it this way: the leaky gut itself is the medical equivalent of a door. When this door is thrown open, a horde of harmful entities comes into the room. The first entity that enters causes problem X, with its corresponding symptoms. The second entity causes problem Y, and so on. Or these entities may cause no problems at all, at least not for a while. The types of ailments and symptoms ultimately generated by a leaky gut depend to a large extent on the susceptibility and immune capability of the individual under attack. A partial list of possible leaky gut symptoms includes the following:

- Allergic reactions
- Digestive problems
- Fatigue and lack of energy
- Hyperactivity
- Joint problems
- Low-grade fever
- Malaise
- Nausea
- Psychiatric disorders
- Reduced immune response
- Shortness of breath
- Skin disorders

These symptoms, in turn, are related to a number of possible ailments and complications that the leaky gut triggers. These include the complications discussed in the sections below.

Disease

The list of diseases associated with leaky gut syndrome is long and somewhat controversial. Some researchers insist that dermatitis, eczema, acne, and several other skin disorders often have their origins in a hyperpermeable intestinal wall. The same is true for digestive symptoms such as irritable bowel, acute gastroenteritis, chronic diarrhea, indigestion, pancreatic defects, compromised liver function, and several more. Ailments on the leaky gut list include asthma, attention deficit disorder (ADD), autism-like reactions, bowel cancer, celiac disease, chronic fatigue syndrome, cystic fibrosis, food allergies, iron deficiency, rheumatoid arthritis, ulcerative colitis, Crohn's disease, and more.

Dr. Picco and colleagues at the National Institute for Cancer in Genoa, Italy, writing in the journal *Clinical and Experimental Rheumatology* (2000), report instances of increased gut permeability in a number of children suffering from juvenile arthritis. Dr. Vaile and colleagues from Canada studied a number of patients with the connective tissue disorder ankylos-

ing spondylitis. Reporting in the *Journal of Rheumatology* (2000), they ob
served an increase in gut leakiness among subjects with this malady and,
interestingly, in some of the patients' close relatives as well. Dr. Fresko and
colleagues report in the *Annals of the Rheumatic Diseases* (2001) that, according to test results, patients with Behcet's syndrome, a rare malady that
produces ulcers throughout the body, suffer from intestinal permeability
far more frequently than healthy control subjects.

Dr. Carratu and colleagues in Italy, writing in the *Journal of Pediatric
Gastroenterology and Nutrition* (1999), list a high incidence of gut leakiness in patients suffering from diabetes. Similarly, Dr. Schwarz and colleagues, writing in the journal *Wiener Klinische Wochenschrift* (1999),
inform us that the movement of bacteria through a leaky gut amplifies the
spread of inflammation throughout the body of a critically ill patient, and
frequently contributes to multi-organ failure. Dr. D'Eufemia and colleagues studied the role of intestinal leakiness in Italian children with
autism. Their article in the journal *Acta Paediatrica* (1996) reports that an
amazing 43 percent of children suffering from this disease showed abnormal intestinal leakiness, as opposed to *zero percent* of the study's forty control subjects.

The evidence mounts. Dr. Humbert and colleagues in France tell us in
the *Journal of Dermatologic Science* (1991) that psoriasis suffers are far
more likely, statistically speaking, to have intestinal leakiness than healthy
persons. Dr. Person and Dr. Bernard, writing in the *Journal of the American Academy of Dermatology* (2000), claim that such rare and disparate
disorders as Reiter's syndrome, pyoderma gangrenosum, pustular psoriasis, and Behcet's syndrome all share a single common pathogenesis—
leaky intestines.

Again, it is the open-door theory: The more toxins that are released
through the gut into the body, the stronger is the likelihood of disease. A
glaring example of this phenomenon is the leaky gut associated with ulcerative colitis and Crohn's disease. Victims of both of these diseases
often experience a multitude of symptoms including such diverse complications as arthritis, hepatitis, kidney stones, blood clots in the leg veins,
and even cancer.

Food Allergies

In a healthy person, food enters the small intestine and is moved along efficiently until it exits via evacuation. With a leaky gut, certain large-sized food proteins are absorbed *before* they are fully broken down. In response, the body's immune system eyes these proteins suspiciously, quickly classifying them as foreign invaders. The alarm is sounded, and soon an armada of antibodies is manufactured to fight off the supposed intruders. During this flawed immunological reaction, the person's intestinal lining is further loosened and/or inflamed, and is rendered even more porous than before, crippling the patient with a cycle of recurring and seemingly incurable food allergies and leaky gut.

While people of all ages can develop food allergies, this ailment is becoming alarmingly common in infants as well as in older adults. Such reactions can lead to mouth ulcers, constipation, anal itching, and irritable bowel syndrome. Young patients generally develop allergies to eggs, milk, peanuts, and soy. Seafood is another big culprit.

Candida

Candida albicans is a type of fungus or yeast that attacks millions of women annually, producing skin rashes and a persistent form of vaginitis. Looked on for many years as nothing more than a pesky female infection, and still controversial to a certain degree, today many experts believe that if *Candida* is allowed to multiply unchecked, this yeast overgrowth can contribute to a number of serious ailments including allergies, depression, migraine headaches, kidney stones, and severe digestive difficulties.

In many cases, leaky gut syndrome, with its attendant intestinal hyperpermeability, encourages the spread of *Candida*. Once established in the gut, moreover, colonies of *Candida* contribute to increased intestinal inflammation and permeability, leading even further to a diverse group of possible diseases.

Mineral Malabsorption and Deficiency

When a gut becomes leaky, proteins that transport minerals from the digestive tract to the bloodstream start to leak out or are destroyed. As a result, the body no longer absorbs and transports needed amounts of minerals such as calcium, magnesium, zinc, and copper in the proper way, and it suffers accordingly. Even if people eat a balanced diet and take daily mineral supplements, the mechanism in their intestines that absorbs these minerals is compromised by the destruction of these proteins and their transport mechanisms, thus reducing the potency of these mineral supplements considerably.

Malnutrition

People who are chronically malnourished and who suffer a compromised blood flow to their digestive organs show a considerably higher chance of developing leaky gut than those who are well nourished. Because the intestinal mucosa of a malnourished person does not absorb nutrients properly, leaky gut can also make this malnutrition worse. As with many leaky gut reactions, a symptom can be a cause of hyperpermeability, or it can be an effect.

Psychological and Psychiatric Disorders

Many experts insist that mood swings, depression, memory lapses, "foggy" thinking, lack of concentration, ADHD in children, and even severe psychiatric disorders, such as schizophrenia and dementia are all possible complications of a leaky gut.

The origin of these problems, advocates of this theory insist, stems both from the high degree of toxicity generated by gut permeability and from the harmful changes that take place in brain chemistry when a person is afflicted by allergies, toxins, and infection.

For example, Dr. Wood and colleagues from the gastroenterology unit at General Infirmary in Leeds, England, studied intestinal permeability among a group of chronic psychiatric inpatients. Reporting in the *British*

Journal of Psychiatry, Dr. Wood found that a significant proportion of patients showed abnormal intestinal leakiness. Writing in the *Journal of Medical Hypothesis,* Dr. W. M. Davis suggests that accumulations of aluminum in the brain of alcoholics due to increased leakiness of the intestines may be responsible for the amnesia and dementia suffered by so many of his patients. Animal studies with rats, as reported in the journal *Brain, Behavior, and Immunity* (1995), further suggest a relationship between depressed laboratory animals and increased gut permeability. Many other clinical studies show similarly disturbing links between mental disorders and leaky gut.

A Six-Step Plan for Treating Leaky Gut Syndrome the Natural Way

If any of the above scenarios sound familiar, and/or if you think you may be falling victim to this insidious disorder, there are measures you can take right away, this very minute, to get things under control—a six-step plan. Each step is based on natural methods, and each can be self-applied. For people suffering from yeast infections, the dietary information and supplement sections featured below will be especially useful.

Here is a note of caution, however: If you are currently suffering from a serious digestive disorder of any kind, or if you suspect that *Candida* has become a chronic lodger in your body, it is recommended that you apply this six-step plan under the supervision of a nutritionist and/or physician. A health-care professional will handhold you through these various steps, and will have useful suggestions for increasing their effectiveness. Using the services of a professional is not always a prerequisite in cases of leaky gut, but is highly recommended.

Here, in outline form, is how the six-step leaky gut plan works:

1. Perform an overall detoxification of the digestive system.
2. Reduce inflammation and leakiness in the intestinal lining by using natural medications.
3. Reinoculate the gastrointestinal tract with helpful digestive bacteria.

4. Identify possible eating allergies with an elimination diet. If an allergy is detected, remove the offending foods from the menu.
5. Establish a long-term eating plan that reduces the chances of recurrence in the future.
6. Modify lifestyle to complement the benefits gained in the above five steps.

Let's review these steps one at a time in the following sections.

1. Detoxify Your System

The first, and in certain ways most important, aid for a leaky gut is to cleanse your digestive system using detoxification techniques.

Once detox is performed, the medications and eating strategies recommended in the sections that follow will then do their job in a more efficient and effective way. You will feel better after detox, think better, and have more energy. It's a win-win deal.

The information presented in this section is designed to get you started in the art and science of internal cleansing. A more comprehensive overview of detox methodology is presented in Chapter 9. We suggest that you use this chapter in concert with the instructions provided below to achieve maximum results.

Detoxification is a slow process, especially in people who have eaten poorly for many years, and who have lived compromised lifestyles. After a few weeks of applying these methods, you will begin to feel cleaner inside. That is a given. Still, if your body is heavily toxified, the entire process can be a lengthy one. Stick with it, and believe it will work.

Several detoxification techniques that help clean your gut are discussed below.

Fasting

In many cases of leaky gut syndrome—not all, but many—a two- or three-day juice fast is recommended to cleanse the digestive tract, and to rid the system of the toxins that contribute to gut permeability.

There are, of course, numerous forms of juice fasts. One of the most simple and effective is the classic juice fast. Here's how it works.

Drink only vegetable juice for three to four days, preferably juice extracted in a juicer from fresh vegetables such as carrots, celery, parsley, and beets. Also, drink plenty of water along with the juices. If you find that your hunger becomes overpowering, especially around mealtimes, add a soft vegetable to your regimen or perhaps some slices of watermelon.

During the period you are fasting, stay active and exercise frequently to sweat and throw off toxins. Don't worry about your energy level. In a majority of cases, fasting increases vitality and mood rather than depresses it.

Finally, note that before fasting, it is a good idea to check with your doctor. Certain medical conditions do not lend themselves to a prolonged empty stomach. For detailed information on how, when, and why to fast, consult Chapter 9.

Caution: Patients suffering from malnutrition should *never* fast.

Eat Selectively

We will address the question of which foods are best for leaky gut syndrome later in the chapter. The following are foods you should *not* eat, especially if your leaky gut is accompanied by yeast infections:

- Sugars of any kind
- Refined carbohydrates (white flour, saturated fats, hydrogenated oils)
- Fatty and fried foods
- White vinegar
- Fermented products such as pickles or miso, plus foods that contain molds, fungi, or spores such as cheese and dried fruits
- Coffee and tea
- Alcohol (especially fermented drinks like beer and hard cider)
- Carbonated beverages
- Foods that trigger allergies (food allergies are discussed later in the chapter). Foods most likely to trigger allergic reactions include peanuts, chocolate, wheat, dairy foods, corn products, soy-based foods, and eggs.

During the initial cleaning-out period, it is best to go easy on fruits and fruit juices. For people suffering from an overgrowth of *Candida*, fruit sugar and fruit juices should be avoided.

Try also to eat organic foods as frequently as possible, and to avoid highly processed, heavily preserved foods. A number of health-care professionals believe that the chemical preservatives and additives so liberally inserted into a majority of our food today is a major cause of leaky gut syndrome.

High-Fiber Diet

We will talk more about high-fiber diet below. At this point, it should be pointed out that a menu heavy in fruits, vegetables, and grains not only improves bowel function but also acts as a scouring mechanism, removing encrusted wastes and residues that form along the intestinal walls. See the table on page 331 in Chapter 16 for a list of high-fiber foods.

Psyllium Powder

Normally used to restore regularity, the high-fiber content of psyllium powder has a cleansing effect on the bowels, eliminating large amounts of toxic digestive debris that builds up over the years. Take one heaping teaspoon of psyllium powder mixed with a glass of water at least once a day and, if necessary, twice a day. Be sure to help down the first glass of dissolved powder with a second and even third glass of water.

Drink Fresh Water

Drink at least eight glasses of water a day for internal cleansing. Flush, flush, flush. Avoid tap water, and use a high-quality bottled variety instead.

2. Reduce Inflammation in Your Intestinal Lining with Herbs and Supplements

There are a host of natural medications that do the job here. Some of the most effective include the following:

- **Alfalfa**—A powerful tonic for the entire body, a diuretic, and an appetite stimulant, alfalfa specifically cleanses the kidneys, promoting overall body detoxification, and purifies the blood. Take alfalfa as a tea or in capsule form.
- **Antispasmodics**—Chamomile, fennel, peppermint, sage, and wild yam are all antispasmodics, which means they help reduce cramping and muscle spasms in the gastrointestinal tract. They also make tasty teas, and all have a general cleansing effect on the stomach and intestines.
- **Bitters**—Bitter herbs such as wormwood, gentian, dandelion greens, and devil's claw stimulate saliva and digestive-enzyme production, and help the stomach secrete more hydrochloric acid (HCl). Digestion improves as a result, regularity returns, and healing of the leaky intestinal lining is sped up. Bitters also increase the flow of bile and stimulate the liver, quickening the detoxification process. Take your bitter herb of choice in a tea. Or, better, purchase a commercial bitters mixture. Swedish Bitters include an especially useful mix, as do Angostura Bitters.
- **Caprylic acid**—A fatty acid derived from butter, coconuts, and palm oil, and also produced naturally in the body in very small quantities, caprylic acid is reputed as a powerful antifungal agent that effectively fights off *Candida* colonization. Take 500 mg in time-release or enteric-coated form, two or three times a day. For information on ordering caprylic acid, see the Appendix.
- **Colostrum**—Found in mother's milk, both the cow and human variety, colostrum enhances infant immune response and keeps newborns protected from disease. It also contains substances that some people now believe play a beneficial role in healing gut hyperpermeability.

  Colostrum, for example, is known to repair damaged stomach tissue. It enhances nutrient uptake, and acts as a sealant in the mucous layer of the intestines, protecting it against parasites and toxic substances. Growth factors in colostrum likewise exert an anti-inflammatory effect on the leaky gut, speeding up healing, and strengthening the body in general so that it can effectively fight off infection. Colostrum supplements are found in most health-food stores. Or you can order them over the Internet. See the Appendix for details.

- **Cucumber**—Cucumber's watery consistency helps wash away toxins while its medicinal properties reduce inflammation and strengthen the intestinal wall. Cucumber is a cooling herb and is useful against any type of overheating ailment. Take it both as a food and as a medicine for leaky gut.

- **Demulcents**—Demulcent herbs are composed of a cellulose structure that helps protect inflamed intestinal tissue, and sooths the irritations caused by leaky gut. Demulcent herbs include comfrey, flaxseed, marshmallow, licorice, and Irish moss.

- **Fennel**—Dr. Ruberto and colleagues in the journal *Planta Medica* (2000) report that the essential oils in fennel have antioxidant and antibacterial effects on the gut, both of which are helpful for cases of leaky gut. Make a tea from a half ounce of the dried seeds steeped in boiling water. Allow them to cool, then drink cold two to three times a day.

- **Garlic**—Known as "nature's penicillin," garlic has strong antimicrobial properties that destroy harmful bacteria in the gut and clean and detoxify the liver. It also generates an antispasmodic effect on the gastrointestinal tract, strengthening the body's immune response to infection and stimulating the activity of the digestive organs in general, helping them to help themselves. Take several cloves of fresh garlic every day, either directly or in capsule form. Garlic is also a boon to cardiovascular health.

- **Ginger**—This ubiquitous and delicious root helps just about any digestive problem you can think of. Use it as a general stomach tonic, as an anti-inflammatory for the bowels, as a digestive stimulant, and as an aid for leaky gut. Westerners prefer the dried or crystallized root, but the more potent form is prepared the Eastern way by purchasing a stalk of fresh ginger root, peeling, slicing a one-inch piece into several smaller pieces, and boiling for twenty minutes. Add some honey and drink a cup of fresh ginger tea twice a day.

- **Glutamine**—The amino acid l-glutamine promotes protein synthesis and helps heal damage along the intestinal walls caused by a leaky gut. It also acts as an antispasmodic, relieving stomach cramping and relaxing the digestive tract. According to an article in the journal *Gastroenterology Clinics of North America* (1998), "Supplemental use of glutamine either in oral, enteral, or parenteral form stimulates gut mucosal cellular proliferation, and maintains mucosal integrity. It also prevents intestinal hyperpermeability."

  Dr. Bond and colleagues from Belgium studied the effect of glutamine on patients with leaky gut caused by overuse of nonsteroidal anti-inflammatory drugs such as aspirin. According to their article in the journal *Alimentary Pharmacology Therapeutics* (1999), glutamine decreases the permeability caused by anti-inflammatory drugs when taken with these drugs or immediately after. Glutamine, in short, is one of the most essential of all supplements for leaky gut sufferers. Take one to two 500-mg capsules a day.

- **Goldenseal**—A small perennial herb, goldenseal exerts a healing effect on the mucous membranes of the gastrointestinal tract, helping cleanse and heal the intestinal lining. It also bolsters the body's natural immune defenses, helping fight off the ill effects of a leaky gut. Studies by Dr. Rehman and colleagues in San Diego, as reported in the *Journal of Immunology Letters* (1999), confirm that goldenseal enhances immune function by increasing antigen-specific antibody production. Take goldenseal in capsule form or brew it as a tea from a teaspoon added to a cup of boiling water. Drink half a cup twice a day.

- **Milk thistle**—The herb milk thistle is used widely as a hepatic (a liver cleanser) and as a preventive against gallstones. It is also effective in liver cirrhosis, relieves indigestion, improves kidney filtration, speeds up metabolism of fats, improves bowel function, and increases the flow of bile—all useful functions for leaky gut sufferers. Take this wonderful herb in tea or capsule form, or mix a teaspoon of the powder into a glass of water. Drink three times a day. Silymarin, a flavonoid complex made from milk thistle, can also be taken in a dose of 100 mg three times a day. Its healing effects are similar.

- **Slippery elm**—A highly effective demulcent preparation for digestive problems of all kinds, slippery elm soothes inflamed tissues in the digestive tract, speeds the healing of the mucous membranes along the intestinal walls, and, as a bonus, fights constipation. Take it in capsule form, or mix a spoonful of the powder into a glass of water. Drink three to four times a day.

- **Shark liver oil**—Used with increasing frequency for cancer patients, shark liver oil contains essential fatty acids, omega-3 fatty acids, antioxidants, and alkyglycerols to strengthen the immune system. It is now also used by a number of health professionals to treat leaky gut syndrome. Reported benefits include relief of joint pain and skin rashes, rapid detoxification, protection against toxins, increased oxygen transport to cells, and reduction of cholesterol. If your local health-food store does not carry shark oil—many now do—you can order it directly on the Internet. See the Appendix for details.

- **Green tea**—In a study reported at the annual Digestive Disease Week in 2002, Dr. James Watson and colleagues from Canada maintain that components in green tea prevent the disruption of gut-wall barrier and tend to make the gut wall less permeable.

- **Vitamins**—Vitamins that help the gastrointestinal system cleanse and repair itself, and thus heal a leaky gut, include the following:

  - **Vitamin A**—Vitamin A heals and soothes the mucous lining of the intestines. It also promotes the production of IgA and IgM antibodies that protect the gastrointestinal tract from infection. Studies done by Dr. Cui and reported in the *Journal of Nutrition* (2000) confirm that high doses of vitamin A supplements strengthen immune function against a variety of bacterial and parasitic infections.
  - **Vitamin B complex**—A good vitamin B complex supplement tones and protects the entire digestive system. It also speeds up healing in the abdominal regions.
  - **Vitamin C**—Take 500 mg of vitamin C a day to bolster general immunity and speed internal healing.

- **Pantothenic acid**—Pantothenic acid aids digestion and fights stress. Pantothenic acid and biotin (discussed below) are included in most, but not all, vitamin B complex preparations. Check the label. If either nutrient is missing, take it as a separate supplement.
- **Biotin** —Biotin helps process carbohydrate and fat metabolism, improving diabetes symptoms and strengthening hair and nails. When synthesized by bowel bacteria, it is reputed to replenish helpful microflora in the gut, especially the type of bacteria destroyed by medications and antibiotics.

- **Minerals**—Make sure your daily intake of critical minerals such as calcium, magnesium, zinc, potassium, selenium, and iron is adequate. In many cases, taking a single multivitamin/mineral supplement does not provide the full daily calcium requirement, especially if leaky gut is a problem.

3. Reinoculate Your Gastrointestinal Tract with Helpful Digestive Bacteria

One of the most dependable aids in the battle against leaky gut syndrome is to repopulate the gastrointestinal tract with colonies of healthy microflora. These delicate and all-important microorganisms act as the bowel "army and marines," playing a crucial role in digestion, elimination, and bowel cleansing. In most people with leaky gut, colonies of healthy microflora are severely depleted.

Reinoculating the digestive tract with friendly intestinal flora is an easy and pleasurable task. It requires only that you eat foods rich in lactobacteria, live-culture yogurt, and acidophilus products in particular. Concentrated products containing a variety of probiotics are also useful. See Chapters 7 and 8 for details.

4. Identify Food Allergies with an Elimination Diet, Then Reduce or Eliminate the Offending Foods

Since food allergies can be both a cause of leaky gut and a result, it is important to determine whether you are sensitive to certain vegetables, fruits, grains, seeds, seafoods, legumes, and so forth. If so, the next step is to remove these offending foods from your daily diet. In some cases, this step alone is all that is needed to reduce or even eliminate the problems associated with allergic food disorders.

The standard way to test for allergic food response is with an *elimination diet*. Here's how it works:

Begin by eliminating a certain suspect food from your diet for twelve to sixteen days. This part of the diet is known as the *elimination phase*.

At the end of this period, this food is then systematically returned to the diet and reactions are observed. This is the *challenge phase*.

If allergic symptoms improve during the elimination phase and return during the challenge phase, the targeted food is identified as an allergic trigger, and is henceforth to be avoided.

For example, let us say that dairy foods are removed from the diet for twelve to sixteen days. At the end of the elimination phase, specific dairy products are then reintroduced back into the diet. You may, for example, start drinking three glasses of milk every day for three days during reintroduction. If no reaction occurs, milk is crossed off the list as a possible allergen. Butter and cheese or other dairy products, such as yogurt, are then eaten in a similar three-day trial. If the allergy does not return at any point during the challenge phase, dairy products are ruled out as possible allergens.

The same elimination and challenge phases can be instituted with other foods known to cause allergies such as wheat and grains, egg products, sugar, seafood, yeast-based foods, beef, and alcohol. Since some people appear to be allergic to food additives, food colorings and preservatives are also tested in this way.

Elimination diets can be administered and fine-tuned in many ways. You can implement them yourself, though if you are a newcomer to this technique, it is probably better to pursue an elimination diet under the watchful eye of a nutritionist or health-care professional.

5. Establish a Long-Term Eating Plan That Reduces the Chance of Leaky Gut Flare-Ups and Recurrence

Once you know which foods, if any, cause allergies, the next step is to establish an eating plan that is friendly to your digestive tract, and that minimizes the chances of leaky gut flare-up.

The first rule here is to eat a high-fiber diet. A great deal has been said about the digestive benefits of fiber throughout this book, and once again the point is stressed. High fiber is perhaps the number one aid for helping weakened digestive systems and for protecting against intestinal hyper-permeability. See the table on page 331 in Chapter 16 for a list of high-fiber foods.

More specifically, eat a diet that is abundant in vegetables, fruits, and grains, making exceptions, of course, for foods that trigger allergic reactions. Go easy on dairy products, however, even if no allergies are present. Yogurt is usually an exception to this rule. Eat cheese no more than two times a week, and keep your consumption of milk to one glass a day at most. Also, drink plenty of fresh-squeezed vegetable and fruit juices. Try a carrot, celery, and apple juice combination. Or a cabbage and celery combination. Make up your own blends. Fresh-squeezed juices deliver nutrition directly to cells in the intestines. If you have a leaky gut, they help your gut heal faster.

Some people with leaky gut also profit from a raw food diet composed of fruits, vegetables, and grains—say, 70 percent raw foods, 30 percent cooked foods. Raw foods are brimming with enzymes and other nutrients that are often cooked out in the preparation process. Highly recommended in this regard are grains for breakfast, fruits for lunch, and vegetables for dinner.

Should you avoid meat if you suffer from a leaky gut? Controversy swirls over the relationship between meat and leaky gut syndrome, and as yet there is no definitive conclusion. For many people with leaky gut, lean meats and fowl offer no problem whatsoever, while heavier meats like beef cause bloating, and constipation. Some people have no difficulty of any kind with meat, while others cannot tolerate the smallest morsel without experiencing a flare-up.

If you do decide to eat meat, consider eating the organic kind. Organic meats are more expensive than nonorganic, yes, but they are free from the additives that contribute to leaky gut problems, and they help keep the intestinal tract clean of toxins. In the long run, however, each person who is bothered by a leaky gut must find his or her own dietary comfort zone. Certainly if you are suffering from inflammation and leakiness of the intestinal tract, it is prudent to avoid rich, fatty meats that are difficult to digest, and that slow down peristalsis. If you experience no problem eating meat, then, well, no problem.

Foods that come especially recommended for soothing and healing leaky gut include the following:

- **Barley and barley water**—Believed to control *Candida,* aid digestion, and cool the system.
- **Beets and beetroot**—High in fiber and healing phytochemicals.
- **Broccoli**—Good fiber and very gut-friendly.
- **Dandelion greens**—A blood, liver, and kidney tonic. Helps relieve constipation.
- **Mung beans**—Used in the Orient for controlling *Candida.*
- **Papaya**—Improves digestion and soothes inflamed stomach lining.
- **Salmon, tuna, and cod**—The EPA fish oils in all three types of fish are helpful for leaky gut.
- **Sweet potato**—A surprisingly effective blood purifier.

6. Modify Your Lifestyle to Support the First Five Steps

Lifestyle modification for leaky gut syndrome has two aspects: (1) Stop doing certain things that you are now doing, and (2) Do certain things that you are not doing.

Top priority in the first category, the "stop doing" category, is smoking. Stop today, and within the next few weeks you are likely to see improvement both in your leaky gut and in your overall well-being. Cigarette and cigar smoke are especially punishing to the mucosa of the intestinal lining, and regular use makes a bad leaky gut leak more. Quit now.

If you drink to excess, be aware that habitual overuse of alcohol literally burns the inside of the stomach and intestinal lining, and can be one of the major triggers for leaky gut. Cut down now.

If you overeat, or if you habitually eat at irregular hours, these habits can cause trouble in the bowels. Keeping regular hours at the dinner table and eating in moderation will help. Some people find that eating four or five small meals a day at regular hours rather than three large ones at breakfast, lunch, and dinner also helps.

In the "to do" category, regular exercise is high on the list. If you are a couch potato, know that inactivity takes its toll on health, energy level, and mental acuity. The body is built to move, to work, and to remain active. When overly passive, our organs atrophy and lose their pep. Exercise, on the other hand, keeps the mechanism well oiled. Incorporate at least thirty to forty minutes of good aerobic exercise into your schedule at least four times a week if possible. Chances are you will feel better and brighter right away and will notice improvements in your digestion as well.

Finally, the old and familiar advice: Relax. A tense, anxious digestive tract produces excess acids that add to the woes of a leaky gut and, some researchers believe, may even have something to do with causing it.

Take time out of the day to rest and refresh. Go for a walk. Sit in the park. Play a game. Or watch one. Chat with your friends. Watch the birds. Draw a picture. Play with a child. Sing a song. Let go. Unwind. Enjoy.

Feels better already, doesn't it?

chapter sixteen

Herbal, Dietary, and Other Natural Remedies for Common Digestive Ailments

Sir Thomas Browne, a seventeenth-century English writer and physician, once remarked that "there is nothing new in medicine, and everything old." The following time line that recently made the rounds on the Internet brings this point home.

THE HISTORY OF MEDICINE

5000 B.C.	Take roots, herbs, and stones.
2000 B.C.	Sacrifice a goat to the gods.
500	Pray and perform penance.
1200	Do cauterization and bloodletting.
1860	Potions, plasters, tonics, and elixirs.
1920	Prescribe drugs and perform surgery.
1980	Antibiotics, lab tests, high-tech medical devices.
2003	Take roots, herbs, and stones.

The author of this amusing chart is unknown, but the story's intent is clear—what goes around comes around.

Despite the fact that the human race has healed itself for millennia with earth medicines, and despite the fact that many drugs in today's standard pharmacopoeia are derived from plants and minerals, a majority of physicians continue to ignore these gifts of nature as complements to modern therapy. For many years, herbs, minerals, vitamin therapy, diet, and adjunct natural remedies have been looked on as antiquated medicine at best, and as medical quackery at worst.

Today, Western society has once again discovered the curative value of the vegetable and mineral kingdoms. One remarkable statistic tells us that every day more than *30 million Americans* ingest some type of herbal potion or supplement as part of their regular health regimen. In 1970, it was reported that one out of ten persons regularly used herbal medicines. Today, it is estimated that *one out of three* avail themselves of this alternative. Currently, Americans spend $27 billion every year on complementary and alternative medicine, which is approximately as much as they spend on conventional medicine.

How valid and effective is this return to "roots, herbs, and stones"? Certainly, a portion of the natural medicine boom is founded on questionable theory and untested data. In many instances, perhaps more than we care to know, the virtues of herbal remedies are oversold and, like many commercial products, hyped beyond a reasonable doubt.

At the same time, no one wants to throw the baby out with the bathwater. Clearly, there are herbal and mineral substances that really do boost the immune system, calm the nerves, raise the energy level, protect the heart, lower cholesterol, fight free radicals, and contribute to the prevention and cure of digestive ills. Innumerable clinical trials, some of them performed in the United States, most carried out in Europe and Asia, demonstrate that in many instances—not all, but many—the digestive ailments listed in the following sections respond as well (or better) to natural remedies than they do to conventional medicines. What's more, they do this at a lower cost, in less time, and with fewer side effects.

The following sectons describe common gut ailments and the natural remedies that help them.

ALCOHOLIC HANGOVER

Causes and Symptoms

Alcoholic hangover results from the convergence of several unfortunate chemical factors. These include (1) toxins released into the system by the metabolism of alcohol and other impurities (the purer the alcohol, the less the magnitude of hangover), (2) the dehydration that follows, and (3) the consequent depletion of key body nutrients such as vitamin B_6 and vitamin C. Typical hangover symptoms include headache, a flulike malaise, dry mouth, nausea, dizziness, sweating, oversensitivity to light and sound, stomach upset, and diarrhea. Most of us know the drill.

During a hangover, many biochemical changes take place in the balance of a drinker's hormones and neurotransmitters. This imbalance leads to the symptoms described above, as well as to rapid heart rate and an increased burden placed on the cardiovascular system. Sometimes this load is so great that it leads to heart attacks and coronary mortality. While suffering from hangover, drinkers may also undergo a diffuse slowing of brain waves (as registered on an EEG) that lasts for as long as sixteen hours *after* the alcohol is cleared from the body. Physical and mental performance is accordingly impaired. Hangovers, in short, though much joked about, are no laughing matter. Familiarity breeds contempt.

How many drinks does it take to get us drunk and hungover? For a 180-pound man, six drinks do the job nicely. For a 130-pound woman, three to five drinks can lead to inebriation and hangover.

Are there ways for drinkers to avoid the ever-present hangover? A few. One word of advice is to simply drink in moderation—an obvious but effective strategy. Another way is to drink clear liquors such as vodka and white wine rather than "dark" liquors such as whiskey and rum. Brandy, red wine, tequila, and rum are more likely to cause hangovers than white wine, vodka, and gin. In one study, when equal amounts of bourbon and vodka were ingested by subjects, 33 percent of bourbon drinkers suffered hangovers compared to 3 percent of vodka drinkers.

Why the difference? Along with the alcohol itself, dark liquors contain small quantities of toxic substances created during the fermentation process. These toxins include methyl alcohol, aldehydes, histamine, tannins, iron, lead, and cobalt, all of which can make a bad hangover a good deal worse.

Other tricks to lessen hangover (slightly) include not drinking on an empty stomach, avoiding high altitudes when drinking, and not drinking when overtired or sick. More tips are mentioned in the section below.

Herbal and Natural Remedies for Hangovers

The best way to quell a hangover is to rid the body of alcohol as quickly as possible. Herbal potions and other natural remedies that speed up this process include the following:

- **White willow bark**—Similar in its effects to aspirin, white willow bark is easier on the stomach than aspirin and some say faster to chase away hangovers. Extracts are available at most health-food stores. Place a few drops in a glass of water, and drink.
- **Kudzu root**—The powdered root of this legendarily fast-growing plant is reputed to be an excellent medicine not only for hangovers but also for discouraging the drinking habit in general. Take two to three capsules before a night on the town and observe the results. Kudzu root is available at some health-food stores and in all Chinese pharmacies under its botanical name, Pueraria.
- **Lime and cumin**—Place a teaspoon of freshly squeezed lime juice (or bottled lime juice if fresh is not available) in a glass of orange or grapefruit juice. Add a pinch of cumin, and sip throughout the day. This drink is a common Ayurvedic remedy for alcohol poisoning.
- **Vitamin B_1 (thiamine)**—An honored bit of partying wisdom has it that one 5-mg vitamin B_1 tablet—or better, a complete vitamin B complex—makes hangover time shorter and less intense. Try it and see.

Other Natural Remedies for Hangovers

Consider the following traditional cures for hangovers. Use them singly or several at a time.

- Eat bananas, tomatoes, and strawberries.
- Eat dry toast with black coffee or espresso (no sugar).
- Take 2,000 mg of vitamin C.
- Try the homeopathic remedy Nux Vomica, available in most health-food stores. Use in 6X or 12X strength tablets. Follow the dosage recommended on the label.
- Drink one or two glasses of water every hour as a toxin flush.
- Drink half a glass of tomato juice with fresh lemon or lime squeezed into it every hour until the symptoms decrease.
- Get plenty of rest and, if possible, sleep. Before dozing, drink lots of water and eat something salty such as soda crackers. When you wake up, take more water, more salty foods, and an electrolyte replenisher drink such as Gatorade.

Facts to Know About Alcohol and Hangovers

If you are a regular drinker and prone to hangovers, be aware of the following facts:

- Red wine is more likely to cause hangover than white, as mentioned earlier. Wine in general, red or white, is also likely to cause worse hangovers than drinks like vodka, bourbon, or gin. If you are a wine lover, however, don't despair. In moderate amounts, wine aids cardiovascular function and replaces lost stores of iron. It contains B vitamins along with important minerals such as phosphorus, calcium, potassium, and magnesium. So enjoy. Just don't overdo.
- A person's mood affects how drunk and hungover he or she becomes. A depressed, fatigued, stressed-out, anxious, angry, or fearful drinker suffers the negative effects of alcohol more intensely than

drinkers who start out the evening in a genial mood. Drinking to drown your sorrows is a fast way to a bad hangover.

- If you are taking a medical drug of any kind, especially a sedative, antihistamine, or tranquilizer, do not drink alcohol. For certain people, and at certain times, the combination of drugs and alcohol can be harmful and even lethal.

- As mentioned earlier, drinking at high altitudes (such as on an airplane) is more likely to get you drunk (and hungover) than drinking at sea level. Drinking while flying, in fact, produces a double whammy. The alcohol dehydrates you, and the prolonged sitting and inactivity at high altitudes, combined with the alcohol, increase the risk of forming blood clots in your legs. Sometimes these blood clots can be deadly.

- The more slowly you drink, the less likely you are to suffer alcohol's harmful effects. It is estimated that a 150-pound person can stay sober, even in the midst of conviviality, by having no more than one 80-proof drink per hour. At the same time, sobriety is a relative term. Even small amounts of alcohol depress psychomotor function to a variable degree. Significantly, for people who drive or who perform intricate work, alcohol affects complex motor tasks more profoundly than simple repetitive ones.

DIARRHEA

Causes and Symptoms

Though diarrhea is dealt with in other sections of this book, this ailment is so common that further information, especially in relation to natural remedies, rounds out the therapeutic picture.

Diarrhea is medically defined as an abnormal increase in the amount, frequency, and liquidity of bowel movements. Brought on most commonly by decreased absorption or oversecretion of fluids from the bloodstream into the bowels, it can appear suddenly and leave as suddenly—acute diarrhea. Or it can affect a person for weeks, months, and even years—chronic diarrhea.

Many factors and situations can cause diarrhea. These include a flu or cold, overuse of laxatives and antacids (specifically, antacids containing magnesium salts), a prolonged course of antibiotics, parasites (*Giardia,* worms), chronic disease (Crohn's disease, IBS, ulcerative colitis, cancer), bacterial infection, food poisoning (*E. coli, Campylobacter, Salmonella*), food allergies (egg, wheat, soy), lactose intolerance, and sudden emotional upset, to name the most prominent.

Symptoms that may accompany diarrhea include fever, malaise (as with a flu), vomiting and nausea (as with food poisoning), mucus in the stools, chills (a possible infection or inflammatory bowel disease), cramps, bloating, and gas.

All of us get diarrhea at one time or another. Usually it comes and goes with no harm done, and most cases pass in a day or two. But be on the alert. All forms of bloody diarrhea, intense diarrhea that lasts for more than three or four days, and diarrhea associated with fever, chills, weight loss, dizziness, and bleeding should be referred to a physician's care immediately. Be especially wary of prolonged bouts in children under the age of seven. More than a day or so of intense diarrhea in a child may be cause for alarm. Take the child to a physician without delay.

Herbal and Natural Remedies for Diarrhea

Certain diarrhea-curing herbs and potions appear time and again throughout world medical literature. Many of these potions are side-effect free, and most work with gratifying speed and effectiveness, often making conventional over-the-counter medications unnecessary. Next time diarrhea comes, try any of the following:

- **Activated charcoal**—Charcoal absorbs toxins and restores regularity. Take two or three capsules or tablets every morning, afternoon, and night until the diarrhea lessens. It is important to take activated charcoal separately from meals and/or from other medications.
- **Agrimony**—Steep a teaspoon of agrimony in boiling water for ten minutes, then drink a cup three times a day.

- **Blueberry, red raspberry, or blackberry tea**—All three berry potions work well to restore regularity. Steep the dried leaves and berries in boiling water for ten minutes, then drink a cup three times a day. Note that blackberries and blueberries work as well in a jam or jelly as they do in a tea. Since children delight in eating this confection, a spoonful or two is a sly way to make the medicine go down.
- **Carob**—For diarrhea in children, mix a teaspoon of carob powder in two cups of water, boil down to a single cup, allow it to cool, and give it to the child sweetened.
- **Chamomile tea**—Chamomile is an excellent antispasmodic and anti-inflammatory. Drink a cup of freshly brewed chamomile tea every four hours until the diarrhea lessens.

  Or try chamomile mixed with other herbs. Mix the following herbs in equal parts: chamomile flowers, dried peppermint leaves, senna leaves, milfoil, and black birch bark. Place the mixture in two cups of water and boil to a single cup. Cool and drink every four hours.
- **Cinnamon**—Cinnamon is one of the most beloved and most used spices in the world. It is mentioned in the ancient Hindu scriptures, as well in the Bible. In the Middle Ages, it was valued as highly as gold, and the quest for it was one of the motivating factors behind the European exploration in the fifteenth century. Indeed, an argument could be made, oblique perhaps, that America owes its discovery in part to cinnamon. Besides its antibacterial properties, cinnamon is easy on the digestion, and its aroma is captivating. For diarrhea, mix a teaspoon of cinnamon in a cup of hot water and drink every four hours until the condition improves.
- **Garlic**—Steep two cloves of fresh garlic in a cup of hot water for fifteen minutes, and drink a cup every four hours. The antimicrobial qualities in garlic make it especially effective for combating diarrhea caused by bacterial infection.
- **Ginger**—Steep an inch-long piece of peeled fresh ginger in boiling water for ten minutes. Cool and drink frequently throughout the day until the diarrhea improves. The benevolent effects of ginger on digestion are being acknowledged today in high and surprising places.

For example, at the end of my meal at Rain, a stylish New York City restaurant, I was served ginger candy rather than the usual chocolate wafer or mint.

- **L-glutamine**—Take one to two 500-mg capsules a day as an anti-spasmodic. L-glutamine speeds up the replacement of damaged cells in the intestines, and helps relieve the type of intestinal cramping that accompanies diarrhea.
- **Oil of oregano**—For diarrhea that stems from bacterial, viral, or parasitic origins, take two capsules of oil of oregano every six hours. Continue use until the diarrhea lessens.
- **Peppermint oil**—Place fifteen drops of peppermint oil in a cup of warm water, and drink three times a day.
- **Pomegranate**—Though once rare on American supermarket shelves, pomegranate juice is now available at a number of health-food stores. It works quickly and efficiently with cases of simple diarrhea. Drink a glass every three to four hours.
- **Psyllium powder**—Though usually used to relieve constipation, the husks in psyllium powder soak up excess fluid in the bowels, and add needed bulk and solidity to loose stools.
- **Slippery elm bark**—Slippery elm bark tea is soothing to the linings of the stomach and intestines, and helps reduce inflammation. Drink a cup every four hours until the diarrhea lessens. Another way to prepare slippery elm is to mix a half teaspoon of the powdered herb with a cup of boiling water, mix, and eat it frequently as a gruel. Capsules of slippery elm can also be taken, although these tend to be less potent than the tea or gruel.
- **Vitamins and minerals**—The following vitamins and minerals help maintain and revive digestive vigor, and add extra ammunition in the battle against diarrhea: vitamin A, vitamin B_1 (thiamine), vitamin B_3, vitamin E, zinc, and trace minerals.

Assorted Folk Remedies for Diarrhea

The following folk remedies for diarrhea are easy to make and sometimes surprisingly effective:

- Place three tablespoons of flour into a glass of water, mix well, and drink three times a day.
- Cook a pot of rice, drain the water into a separate jar, and drink a glass of the rice water three times a day. Rice water works best on diarrhea when taken hot, like tea.
- Squeeze half a lime (or half a lemon if a lime is not available) into a glass of warm water and drink three times a day.
- Add two teaspoons of apple cider vinegar to a glass of water and drink twice a day.

Dietary Remedies for Diarrhea

Anytime diarrhea strikes, even short, transient bouts of it, a good deal of water and electrolytes is lost from the body. Replace these critical stores of liquids as quickly as possible in the following ways:

- Drink plenty of liquids. Pure water is best. Helpful too are vegetable broths, gelatin, bouillon, and herbal teas (see the herbs under "Herbal and Natural Remedies" on page 319).
- Lost electrolytes can be replenished by taking potassium and sodium supplements, and by hydrating the body with electrolyte replacement drinks such as Gatorade and Pedialyte.
- An easy homemade remedy for dehydration is concocted by adding a half teaspoon of salt, sugar, and baking soda to a glass of water, and sipping slowly. If you have liquid glucose in your medicine chest, substitute it for the sugar.
- Keep your stomach as *inactive* as possible during acute attacks of diarrhea, and avoid fatty, spicy, rich, or fried foods. Also avoid chewy vegetables with tough skins (like potatoes) and/or quantities of seeds,

as well as foods known to generate gas such as carbonated drinks, beans, cabbage, chewing gum, and the synthetic sweetener sorbitol. (See Chapter 13 for a list of gas-producing foods.)

- Broths, herbal teas (peppermint, chamomile, and ginger), carrot juice, ginger ale, white rice, applesauce, and a bit of dry white bread toast and some crackers all help control diarrhea while satisfying your appetite. In cases of intense diarrhea, it is best not to eat at all, especially during the early stages of the attack. Talk to your doctor about this. People who are sensitive to wheat or other foods are advised to avoid these substances entirely until regularity returns.

- The so-called BRAT diet—Bananas, Rice, Applesauce, and Toast taken in equal proportion—is easy on digestion and helps bulk up watery stools. It also provides healthy nutrition, and is easy to get down when you're feeling nauseous. Dr. Ramsook and colleagues in the prestigious journal of *Annals of Emergency Medicine* (2002) report on the effectiveness and ease of this method. Try it next time when diarrhea strikes. Also good for stemming diarrhea are boiled and peeled sweet potatoes with salt and pepper added. (**Caution:** In some people, pepper worsens diarrhea. Use it sparingly.)

- During any attack of diarrhea, avoid liquor and wine. In my office, it is not uncommon to see chronic alcoholics who suffer from loose stools on a daily basis and who have not had a normal bowel movement in years.

- If you are prone to loose bowels, cut back on fruit until your condition improves. The juicier fruits like mangoes and pears contain certain sugars that some people's enzymatic systems cannot easily tolerate. If you do eat fruit during an attack, bananas are the safest option. They have a stabilizing effect on the bowels, and help replace the potassium stores drained out by loose stools. For some people, overuse of vitamin C and too many vitamin C-containing fruits like oranges can also cause diarrhea.

- While it is usually sound policy to avoid dairy foods when suffering from diarrhea (especially if you are lactose intolerant), the exceptions are yogurt and acidophilus products. For many people, these

foods slow the ill effects of diarrhea and, in some cases, cure them
entirely. Yogurt products can also also be eaten by people who are
lactose intolerant. See Chapter 7 for details. Ayurvedic doctors use
cheese whey for a similar purpose, especially for the type of diarrhea
caused by infection. Whey is a known to be an immune-system
booster, an energy producer, and a source of calcium.

- Once regularity returns, concentrate on eating foods that are heavy
  in fiber. Studies show that when fiber is given to people who are
  prone to diarrhea, smooth bulky stools are quickly produced, along
  with increased peristalsis and the rapid restoration of normal bowel
  flora.

Traveler's Diarrhea

When vacationing in exotic places, it is always best to avoid tap water
(bottled is best), uncooked meats and vegetables, ice cubes made from local tap water, spicy foods, and foods that may be contaminated by contact
with spoiled food or dirty hands. Be especially careful of foods sold by
street vendors. Though tempting, these dishes are frequently infected
with diarrhea-causing microorganisms. Be wary too of foods left out in the
open air for long periods of time, and of cooked foods that appear to be
stale and old. (If they look old, they probably are old.) Raw eggs, fish, may-
onnaise, and fresh meats can all easily become contaminated, especially
in parts of the world where hygiene is a low priority.

A recent study presented at the annual Digestive Disease Week conference in 2002 evaluated the effect of milk and calcium on traveler's diarrhea. Dr. Bovee-Oudenhoven of The Netherlands studied two groups of
otherwise healthy subjects who were infected with *E. coli* bacteria. One
group received a low-calcium diet while the other drank milk products
containing 1,400 mg more calcium than the first. On the first day, both
groups reported the same amount of diarrhea. By the second day, most
members of the milk and calcium group no longer showed symptoms,
while it took another twenty-four hours for the low-calcium group to recover. Researchers concluded that milk and calcium supplementation are

definitely helpful for treating traveler's diarrhea. They hypothesized that calcium boosts the number of helpful bacteria in the gut, and speeds up the healing process for diarrhea.

Finally, recent studies suggest that an enzyme known as bromelain, found in pineapple, keeps infectious organisms such as *E. coli* and *V. cholerae* from attaching to the intestinal wall, and from harming chemicals that trigger digestive secretions. In one study, reported in Australia by Dr. Chandler and Dr. Mynott in the journal *Gut* (1998), bromelain supplements successfully reduced the incidence of diarrhea among laboratory animals, and protected them against strains of lethal bacterial disease. The researchers also observed that pigs who ingested bromelain showed significantly increased weight gain compared with untreated pigs. Bromelain supplements are available at health-food stores and should be included in every traveler's baggage.

DIVERTICULOSIS AND DIVERTICULITIS

Causes and Symptoms

When the colon is habitually subjected to overstretching and herniating, it eventually starts to produce dozens and sometimes scores of sacs or pockets along the surface of its inner walls. These herniated sacs are known as diverticula, and the condition they produce is known as *diverticulosis*.

Some of these sacs are approximately the size of a pinhead. Others can be the size of a marble or even larger. While the colon itself is five-feet long, most diverticular sacs form in the sigmoid section, the lower part of the colon.

As a rule, these sacs are harmless. Many people can have them for years and not know they are there. On some occasions, however, fragments of food or feces become trapped in the diverticula, producing perforations in the thin wall of the sac. Infection may then set in, causing a more serious condition known as diverticulitis, a disorder that can, on occasion, become life threatening.

When diverticulosis begins to act up and cause trouble, its main symptoms are a steady, sometimes cramping and intense pain usually felt on the left side of the abdomen. This pain is made worse when pressure is applied to this area. When diverticulosis turns into the more serious diverticulitis, symptoms include pain, fever, nausea, constipation, and chills.

What particular influences contribute to the formation of the diverticula in the gut? Prolonged insults to the gastrointestinal system from laxatives, harsh medications, and frequent use of purgatives can all contribute to the formation of diverticula. Chronic constipation, plus the long-term habit of suppressing intestinal gas, can also be a factor. However, the most common cause of diverticular disease by far is a diet lacking in fiber and heavy on overprocessed, refined foods.

Why is a low-fiber diet a factor? Because lack of fiber in the diet produces small, hard, low-bulk stools that push against the colon wall as they move through the gut, stretching and bubbling the gut wall, slowing down peristalsis, and sapping the vigor of the digestive tract. Over time, the constant pressure exerted by these stools causes stretching and tearing, and soon the diverticula begin to form.

Rare in underdeveloped countries where unprocessed, high-fiber foods are the norm, diverticular disease is largely a Western phenomenon. Currently, it is estimated that one-third of Americans over age forty and more than one-half of Americans over age sixty suffer from this ailment. For reasons not entirely understood, women develop diverticulitis more often than men.

Herbal and Natural Remedies for Diverticular Disease

The conventional medical treatment for diverticulitis calls for bowel rest, stool softeners, a modified eating regimen heavy on fluids, easily digestible foods, and antibiotics.

Once the condition is under control, a high-fiber diet is recommended. As a supplement to this treatment, you can take certain herbs and supplements to speed up recovery after your physician puts you on a healing diet. These include the following:

- **Aloe vera**—A powerful anti-inflammatory, aloe vera coats the inside of the esophagus and stomach, nourishes the mucous lining of the intestines, and neutralizes excess stomach acid. Drink a half cup of the liquid three times a day between meals, or take it in capsule form. Since aloe vera produces constipation in a few people, be sure to wash it down with a carminative (gas-reducing) tea such as mint or lemon balm.

- **Combination herbal tea**—Tea made from the following herbal combination is frequently recommended for constipation: Mix equal parts of licorice root, cascara sagrada, dandelion root, yellowdock, fennel seed, and ginger. Drink one cup of this potion two to three times a day before meals.

    Caution: Do not use cascara for longer than two weeks at a time. If this tea really works for you, substitute burdock root in its place. People with hypertension should avoid using licorice.

- **Docosahexaenoic acid (DHA)**—Docosahexaenoic acid (DHA) is an omega-3 fatty acid that is critical for nervous system function and for the healing of wounds. A deficiency may lead to attention deficit disorder in children, impairment of mental and visual function, depression, and Alzheimer's disease. Because of its healing properties, it is useful for diverticulitis. Preformed DHA can be found in fatty fish and cod liver oil, or it can be taken in commercial supplements. The recommended dose is 200 mg a day.

- **Garlic**—Garlic is a superb digestive, relieving pockets of gas that contribute to the formation and/or expansion of diverticula. It also stimulates peristalsis and encourages the growth of healthy intestinal flora in the bowels, both of which speed the healing of the diverticula. Take it daily in capsule or pill form, or add fresh cloves of garlic to your daily salads and main meals.

- **Glucomannan**—A water-soluble form of dietary fiber, glucomannan is effective for constipation and diabetes, and helps lower cholesterol. Dr. Staiano from Naples, Italy, reports in the *Journal of Pediatrics* (2000) that glucomannan increases stool frequency and reduces laxative and/suppository use among neurologically impaired and constipated children, a group that is notoriously difficult to treat. Dr. Passaretti, writing in the *Italian Journal of Gastroenterology* (1991), suggests that glucomannan makes an ideal therapeutic tool for the chronic constipation and related problems, especially the problems that plague people with diverticulitis. Glucomannan can be purchased in many health-food stores. The suggested dose is 3 to 4 g a day.

- **Eicosapentaenoic acid (EPA)**—Also useful for diverticulitis is eicosapentaenoic acid (EPA), one of several omega-3 fatty acids required by the body. EPA is often deficient in the Western diet. EPA improves cardiovascular health and fitness, benefits hypertension, diabetes, osteoporosis, attention deficit disorder, and rheumatoid arthritis. It even appears to help prevent colon cancer. Our main dietary source of EPA is cold-water fish such as wild salmon. Commercial fish oil supplements may also raise the concentrations of EPA in the body and help fight diverticulitis.

- **Powdered flaxseed**—Purchase flaxseeds directly from a health-food store, then pulp them up in a blender. Eat the powder directly, or sprinkle it over desserts and vegetables—it sticks to the teeth a bit, but it is quite tasty.

    For many years, doctors cautioned patients with diverticular disease against foods such as flaxseed, berries of all kind, popcorn, nuts, and tomatoes, the theory being that the seeds in these foods can easily get caught in the diverticula and cause infection. Today, thinking has changed on this subject, and most physicians consider seeds harmless and, in some cases (as in the above), beneficial for diverticulosis.

- **Psyllium powder**—Used for a wide variety of digestive ailments, the high-fiber content of psyllium powder enlarges stools and decreases their transit time through the bowels, both vital boons for people suffering from diverticular disease. Take one heaping teaspoon of psyllium powder mixed with a glass of water at least once a day and, if necessary, twice a day. Be sure to wash down the mixed powder with a second glass of water.

· **Vitamins and supplements**—Vitamin C, vitamin A, and trace minerals such as copper, magnesium, and zinc are all useful for increasing intestinal strength and preventing diverticular complications.

Other Natural Remedies for Diverticular Disease

· **Increased water intake**—People with diverticular disease are advised to drink eight to ten glasses of water a day. Combined with a high-fiber diet (discussed below), water helps swell the size of stools, helping them slip easily and quickly through the bowels.
· **Thorough mastication**—While the stomach works diligently to break down food into small particles, it does not always succeed, and can always use the help provided by thorough mastication. Small, well-pulped particles of food digest faster, pass through the bowels more quickly, and increase the amount of nutrients that can be extracted. Well-chewed food, moreover, is less likely to get trapped in the diverticular pouches. If possible, chew each bite of food twenty-five times. Eat as slowly as you can, and be careful not to bolt your food.
· **Solar plexus massage**—Place your right palm on your solar plexus in the pit of your stomach. Place your left palm on top of your right palm and massage this area in a firm, clockwise motion for five to ten minutes every day. Regular massage of the upper abdominal area improves bowel function, reduces gas, and tones the digestive system.

Dietary Recommendations for Diverticular Disease

The table on page 331 lists the foods that fit the high-fiber bill. Pile these foods high on your plate at every meal; meanwhile, cut down on highly processed foods, rich foods, junk foods, sugared foods, refined foods, and heavy meats. With diverticulosis, it's high fiber all the way.

Other high-fiber carbohydrates include beans, peas, black-eyed peas, bran cereals, corn, barley, millet, figs, apricots, dates, berries of every variety (especially blackberries and strawberries), plums, apples, pears, bananas, cherries, coconut, almonds, and leafy greens of all kinds.

Note: Foods rich in fiber tend to produce gas. This means that people already prone to flatulence are advised to add fiber to their diets in increments rather than in one fell swoop. If flatulence becomes a problem *after* introducing high quantities of fiber to the diet, cut back and experiment until you establish the balance that best suits your needs.

GASTRITIS

Causes and Symptoms

Gastritis is a general medical term describing any type of inflammation of the mucous membrane stomach lining. Like many other digestive ailments, it has several possible causes. These include the following:

- Bacterial and/or viral infections, specifically infection by *Helicobacter pylori (H. pylori),* the bacteria also responsible for causing peptic ulcer disease and, some experts suspect, stomach cancer. In the United States, 50 percent of people over age sixty are believed to be infected with *H. pylori*
- Food poisoning
- A decrease in the cells that produce essential digestive acids
- Intolerance for certain drugs such as nonsteroidal anti-inflammatory drugs, for example, aspirin and ibuprofen
- Acidic or stimulating foods such as coffee, black tea, vinegar, quinine water, orange juice, pickled vegetables, and hot, spicy foods
- Stomach-lining irritants such as cigarettes and alcohol
- Unknown causes. Occasionally gastritis has no traceable etiology. In such instances, the word "gastritis" is used as a generic umbrella term to describe a basically undiagnosable ailment.

Although there are many types of symptoms caused by gastritis, the most common include belching, bloating, abdominal discomfort (often

❧ High-Fiber Foods ❧

FOOD	AMOUNT OF FIBER
Acorn squash (1 cup)	6 grams
Apple (1 cup)	3 grams
Asparagus (1/2 cup)	1 gram
Broccoli (1/2 cup)	1 gram
Brown rice (1 cup)	3 grams
Brussels sprouts (1/2 cup)	3 grams
Cabbage (1/2 cup)	2 grams
Carrots (1/2 cup)	2 grams
Cauliflower (1/2 cup)	1 gram
Kidney beans (1/2 cups)	3 grams
Lima beans (1/2 cup)	4 grams
Oatmeal (2/3 cup)	3 grams
Peach (1 cup)	1 gram
Potato (1 cup)	2 grams
Raspberries (1 cup)	6 grams
Spinach (1/2 cup)	1 gram
Tangerine (1 cup)	2 grams
Tomato (1 cup)	2 grams
White rice (1 cup)	1 gram
Whole-wheat bread (1 piece)	3 grams
Whole-wheat cereal (1 cup)	2 grams
Zucchini (1 cup)	1 gram

made worse by eating), pain in the lower ribs, nausea, occasional vomiting, a bad taste in the mouth, gas, hiccups, indigestion, loss of appetite, and, in severe cases, bloody vomiting and black stools. The symptoms of gastritis can be either chronic or acute.

Herbal and Natural Remedies for Gastritis

- **Amino acids**—Several amino acids show clinical promise for treating gastritis. In a double-blind trial conducted by Dr. Salim, as reported in the *Canadian Journal of Surgery* (1993), patients taking 200 mg of the amino acid cysteine four times a day report substantial healing from bleeding gastritis caused by nonsteroidal anti-inflammatory drugs such as aspirin. They also report a smaller incidence in the need for surgery. Another amino acid, glutamine, improves blood flow to the stomach, and aids stomach and intestinal-lining repair. Preliminary evidence also suggests that the amino acid arginine protects the stomach lining from digestive irritants and increases blood flow to abdominal areas. All three of these amino acids can be purchased in separate pill or capsule form at any pharmacy or health-food store.

- **Chamomile**—The digestive standby chamomile contains the flavonoid apigenin, a substance that some researchers believe helps sooth inflamed and injured mucous membranes, especially the mucous membranes lining the stomach. Other ingredients in chamomile reduce free-radical activity, a second boon for gastritis sufferers. Dr. Madisch and colleagues, using a placebo-controlled study, report in the journal *Zeitschrift für Gastroenterologie* (2001) that herbal preparations containing chamomile flower are significantly superior in relieving gastritis-related indigestion than that of placebo.

- **Echinacea**—The common American herb echinacea is a digestive aid and an anti-inflammatory, and appears to have a beneficial healing effect on irritated stomach linings. Echinacea also stimulates the immune system, helping the body make needed self-repairs. Dr. Speroni and colleagues from Italy, reporting in the *Journal of Ethnopharmacology* (1993), confirmed echinacea's anti-inflammatory and wound-healing properties. Echinacea works well as a tea and in capsule form.

- **Fennel leaves**—Traditionally used as a dieter's herb, fennel soothes the stomach lining, helps maintain the tone of stomach muscles, and fights infections in the intestinal tract. An article in the journal *Planta Medica* (2000) reports that essential oils obtained form fennel have antioxidant as well as antimicrobial activities. Make a tea from a half ounce of the dried leaves steeped in boiling water. Allow it to cool, then drink cold at least three times a day until the symptoms of gastritis lessen. Some people also drink a tea made from fennel seeds as a gastritis preventive.

• **Gamma-oryzanol**—Several studies in Japan performed by Dr. K. Itaya, as reported in the journal *Nippon Yakurigaku Zasshi* (1976), suggest that supplementation with gamma-oryzanol may help heal gastritis and stomach ulcers. A similar Japanese study, reported by Dr. Ichimaru and colleagues in the journal *Nippon Yakurigaku Zasshi* (1984), asserts that gamma-oryzanol is useful for healing gastritis in mice. An added benefit of gamma-oryzanol is its proven ability to lower cholesterol. Gamma-oryzanol is found in grains and rice bran oil and is available in capsule and tablet forms at most health-food stores. Take 100 mg two to three times a day.

• **Goldenseal**—Another popular American herb, goldenseal generates laxative, tonic, and antiseptic effects. It is particularly healing for mucous membranes, and is a genuine aid for helping repair stomach-lining cells destroyed by gastritis inflammation. Studies by Dr. Rehman and colleagues in San Diego, reporting their findings in the journal *Immunology Letters* (1999), confirm the fact that goldenseal enhances immune function by increasing antigen-specific antibody production. Take goldenseal in capsules form or make a tea from a teaspoon of the herb steeped in a cup of boiling water. Drink half a cup twice a day.

• **Licorice root**—Traditionally used to reduce inflammation and injury to the stomach lining, in test-tube studies, the flavonoid contents of this herb have been found to discourage the growth of the stomach ravaging bacteria *H. pylori*. Though licorice root is a fine overall tonic and extremely helpful for digestion, gastritis, and ulcers, as reported in *Scandinavian Journal of Gastroenterology* (1984), people with hypertension should avoid it. A deglycyrrhizinated form of licorice known as

DGL provides similar healing efficacy with less potential for side effects. Ask for this specific form of licorice when purchasing licorice.

- **Slippery elm and marshmallow root**—Mix a teaspoon of slippery elm powder with a teaspoon of marshmallow root, and take with water two to three times a day. These two herbs mixed together decrease gut inflammation and promote stomach healing. Slippery elm has also been shown to possess significant antioxidant properties.

- **Vitamins and minerals**—Vitamin A, vitamin B complex, and zinc all aid in the repair and regeneration of stomach-lining tissue. B-complex vitamins detoxify the liver and improve digestion. Note that the antioxidant beta-carotene is believed to reduce free-radical damage to the stomach (people with gastritis often test low for supplies of beta-carotene). Experiments in Sweden by Dr. Sjunnesson and colleagues, as reported in the journal *Complementary Medicine* (2001), confirm that a high intake of selenium, beta-carotene, and vitamins A, C, and E all help reduce growth of *Helicobacter pylori* in guinea pigs. Eating foods high in beta-carotene (such as carrots) is also believed to reduce the risk of chronic gastritis.

- **Chinese herbal preparations**—Here are two useful Chinese patent medicines for gastritis, available at any Chinese pharmacy or from mail-order sources (see Appendix).

  - **Aplotaxis-Amomun Pills (Chinese Xiang Sha Liu Jun Wan)**—Good for poor digestion with nausea, burping, nausea, bloat, chronic diarrhea, and both acute and chronic gastritis. The manufacturers recommend that you avoid cold and raw foods while taking this medication.

  - **Gastropathy Capsules, Weiyao (Chinese Wei Yao)**—Excellent for both chronic and acute gastritis, especially when accompanied by a great deal of stomach acidity and stomach pain. This medicine also helps promote tissue regeneration of the stomach mucosa and of stomach muscles.

Dietary Remedies for Gastritis

Gastritis sufferers are advised to avoid hot, fatty, spicy, rich, and irritating foods. Also contraindicated are coffee, black tea, carbonated drinks, tonics, orange juice, caffeine, sugar, and salt. In the beginning stages of treatment, it is also smart to eliminate gas-producing foods from the menu such as broccoli, Brussels sprouts, beans, sprouts, onions, and cabbage. If you suffer from any of form of food allergy, avoid these foods as well; food allergies can exacerbate the symptoms of gastritis.

Meanwhile, during acute attacks, eat more vegetables and bland foods. Some people with gastritis supplement their diets with extracted vegetables juices (carrot, cabbage, and raw potato juice in particular). Others eat only a single food at each sitting for several weeks straight; for example, only cereal for breakfast, only watermelon for lunch, and only tofu for dinner. Eating a single food at a sitting is easy on the digestion, gives the stomach lining time to heal, and helps control weight.

Note, finally, that some health-care professionals recommend that gastritis patients start their dietary modification regimen by fasting for two or three days, or by going on a non-solid food and juice regimen. Fasting and juice fasts clean out the toxins that cause gastritis, allow the digestive tract to rest and recuperate, and give the stomach lining time to repair itself. When the fasting period is over, it is advised that patients eat selectively for two weeks, choosing easily digestible fruits and vegetables. After the second week, when the stomach has had time to recover and the gastritis is under control, patients can return to their normal diet.

Lifestyle Changes for Gastritis

The following lifestyle suggestions all help control and heal common gastritis symptoms:

- If you smoke, quit now. Cigarette smoke is a major irritant to the stomach lining, and can make a bad case of gastritis a whole lot worse. Plus, cigarettes increase your risk for a variety of cancers of the digestive system. Stop while there's time.

- If you are a heavy drinker, speak with your doctor concerning how many drinks a day (if any) are safe for your condition. At least 50 percent of alcoholics are believed to suffer from gastritis.

- *H. pylori* infection, one of the possible causes of gastritis, can be spread from person to person. Wash your hands frequently during the day, before meals, and when touching food. If another person in your home is infected with *H. pylori,* take appropriate precautions.

- Go easy on the aspirin and other nonsteroidal anti-inflammatory drugs. These preparations can irritate the stomach lining and exacerbate gastritis. Excessive use causes bleeding of the mucous membranes. Ask your doctor for advice if you are a regular user of these medications.

- Relax and take it easy. Though there is no proven link between gastritis and emotional upset, we know that stress plays a role in many stomach ailments, and there is no reason to assume that gastritis is an exception. So go easy on yourself. Ease up. Relax your stomach and your mind. There's no downside to it.

Heartburn

Causes and Symptoms

Heartburn, also known in its chronic form as GERD (gastroesophageal reflux disease), is characterized by a burning sensation in the center of the chest that sometimes creeps up to the base of the throat. It is caused by the flow of acidic gastric juice, known as acid reflux, moving up the esophagus rather than remaining in the stomach where it belongs.

Most of us experience a bit of heartburn now and then, especially as we age. Estimates have it that at least 50 million Americans endure this unwelcome visitor at least once a month. Almost 10 percent experience it daily. Persistent cases, though, should never be taken for granted.

Heartburn and acid reflux can be symptoms of *esophagitis,* an inflammation in the lining of the esophagus that requires prompt medical attention. Even without esophagitis, chronic heartburn affects mental and physical well-being, and requires careful medical treatment. Over time, acid reflux can damage the wall of the esophagus. It can cause ulcers, bleeding, narrowing of the esophagus with obstruction to the passage of food, and even cancer. A study in the *New England Journal of Medicine* (1999) reports that, if left untreated, chronic heartburn increases the chances of esophageal cancer, one of the most virulent and least treatable forms, by approximately eight times. If you have suffered from heartburn for more than twenty years without treatment, your risk is increased forty-four times.

But don't be alarmed. A vast majority of heartburn cases are mild, and can be avoided simply by steering clear of certain foods. On the guilty list you will find spicy foods, fatty foods, hot foods (as in chili peppers), rich foods (as in sauces and gravies), fried foods (as in French fries and fried onion rings), carbonated drinks (as in soda), *possibly* smoking, and definitely overeating.

Beware also of alcohol. Alcohol overrelaxes sphincter muscles in the esophagus and stomach, allowing acid reflux to rise, and possibly triggering swallowing difficulties. Certain prescription drugs can also worsen acid reflux. This includes Bentyl, which is taken for spastic colon, and several popular hypertension drugs such as Calan and Inderal.

Symptoms of heartburn include belching, hiccups, a sour taste in the mouth, and a burning sensation in the chest and/or throat that occasionally becomes so intense people think they are having a heart attack. When lying down, the burning and discomfort tend to get worse, and many chronic heartburn sufferers are woken out of a sound sleep every night by this unpleasant sensation.

Herbal and Natural Remedies for Heartburn

Hundreds and probably thousands of herbal and folk remedies have been used through the years to soothe heartburn. Some of the most effective and easily attainable include the following:

- **Aloe vera**—A time-honored anti-inflammatory herb, the juice from this succulent desert plant coats the esophagus, keeping rising stomach acids under control. Drink a half cup of aloe vera juice twice a day between meals. Note that aloe tends to cause diarrhea in a few people. If this is a problem, take the aloe with a carminative (gas-reducing) tea such as mint or lemon balm. Aloe vera should not be used during pregnancy or by patients with kidney disorders.
- **Bitters**—Bitter herbs such as wormwood, gentian, dandelion greens, and devil's claw increase saliva and enzyme production. This action helps the stomach neutralize more hydrochloric acid (HCl), which, in turn, improves heartburn. Take any of these herbs in a tea or, better, purchase a good commercial bitters product. The brand Swedish Bitters, available at many health-food stores, includes an especially useful mix of bitter herbs, as do Angostura Bitters.
- **Chamomile**—This old standby herb once again proves its mettle, its anti-inflammatory properties helping tame reflux stomach acid and quiet digestion. You'll have to drink quite a bit of it to see results though; at least four cups a day between meals is the suggested usage. Chamomile can also be taken in tablets or in a tincture mixed with hot water.
- **Coriander seeds**—This Ayurvedic remedy calls for crushing an ounce of coriander seeds and mixing the pulp with two or three teaspoons of sugar. Add a cup of water, bring to a boil for approximately thirty seconds, then let the tea simmer for ten minutes. Drink a cup in the morning and in the evening before bed.
- **Chewing gum**—Not usually known for its curative powers, chewing gum increases the flow of saliva in heartburn patients, and neutralizes acid reflux. Increased saliva also facilitates the passage of food down the esophagus and into the stomach. Commercial gums containing the digestive enzyme pepsin and introduced by Dr. Edward Beeman some years ago were very popular as a digestive aid. Production of these stopped in 1978.
- **Cumin seeds**—Take an ounce of cumin seeds, soak them in water

for a few minutes, then eat a spoonful or two, three times a day. Cumin is a powerful acid neutralizer.

• **Deglycyrrhizinated licorice** —Known as DGL, this form of licorice has powerful anti-inflammatory properties and leaves a protective coating on the esophagus and intestinal lining. Numerous publications, as reported by Dr. F. Borrelli in *Phytotherapy Research* (2000) and Dr. A. R. Dehpour in *Journal of Pharmacy and Pharmacology* (1994), attest to the anti-ulcerogenic properties of licorice and its derivative compounds. Dr. A. Bennett writes in the *Journal of Pharmacy and Pharmacology* (1980) that a combination of the ulcer medication cimetidine and licorice is better at healing ulcers than either of these substances used alone. DGL has reduced many of the side effects associated with its parent compound, licorice.

• **Ginger root**—Westerners generally seem to prefer dried or crystallized ginger root, though the more potent form is prepared by purchasing a stalk of fresh ginger root, slicing up a one-inch piece, peeling it, then boiling it for twenty minutes. Add some honey to the mixture and drink a cup of fresh ginger tea twice a day.

• **Lemon balm**—Try two to three teaspoons of lemon balm leaves steeped in a tea. Taken three times a day, this tea acts as a carminative (gas reducer) and helps neutralize acid reflux. With honey, it makes a delicious drink.

• **Mustard**—Mustard is a little known and perhaps surprising remedy for heartburn. The next time you have an attack of acid reflux, try eating a half teaspoon of any yellow or gray commercial mustard. As one user described it, "The mustard seems to chase the acid right back into my stomach—and quick!"

• **Pantothenic acid**—For some people, acid is quickly controlled by adding pantothenic acid to the daily vitamin regimen. When taken with thiamine and choline, its effects tend to be even more dramatic. Pantothenic acid is abundant in certain foods including avocados, yogurt, salmon, and sunflower seeds.

• **Rice bran oil**—Rice oil, basically a form of pure gamma-oryzanol (see gamma-oryzanol under "Gastritis" on page 333) is an excellent tonic for the digestive system in general, and a specific against acid reflux in particular. Take approximately 150 mg two times a day on an empty stomach for best results.

• **Turmeric powder**—Purchase a packet of gelatin capsules at a pharmacy or health-food store. Fill the capsules with turmeric powder, and take two capsules each day after breakfast. Or purchase commercial tumeric tablets of 500 mg each. In India, turmeric powder is highly regarded as a remedy against heartburn, breaking down fatty foods and reducing acidity. Turmeric has also been linked to possible prevention for Alzheimer's disease. (In India, where virtually every dish contains turmeric, prevalence of Alzheimer's disease is very low.)

Other Natural Remedies for Heartburn

A majority of heartburn episodes are due simply to eating and drinking the wrong kinds of foods. Stick to the following rules of low-acid eating and your heartburn will be reduced accordingly.

• Avoid fried foods, rich foods, fatty meats (bacon, sausage), too many sweets (especially chocolate and confections made with oil), foods with chili or cayenne pepper added, some creamed foods and soups, acidic foods like tomatoes and citrus, alcoholic beverages, and carbonated drinks.

   Many forms of junk foods and fast foods also generate acid, as do coffee and tea, both the caffeinated and decaffeinated kind. If you drink milk, avoid whole milk, and stick with the 1 or 2 percent variety. For some people, vegetable oils trigger acid reflux, though responses vary. Indeed, as with many digestive disorders, tolerance levels for acid vary widely from person to person. Some people can eat all of the foods mentioned above with impunity. Others pop a few French fries dipped in ketchup and are awake all night. The best way to determine which foods cause heartburn in your system and which are harmless is to observe your own eating patterns. See how different foods affect you, take note, and plan your menu accordingly.

- Rich, high-calorie foods that are heavy in fats slow down the movement of food through the stomach, with increased reflux resulting. For people who suffer from acid stomach, a diet low in fat and high in protein is preferable. Protein generates considerably less acid than fats.

- If you smoke, stop. If you drink, do so in moderation. If you are obese, lose weight. Smoking, drinking, and extra weight all make heartburn worse.

- Do not drink with your meals. Or at least reduce the amount of liquid you take at every meal. The more food and liquid there is in the stomach at any given moment, the greater the chances are of developing heartburn. Take all liquids before meals or an hour after you are finished. For this same reason—that heartburn is more likely to occur on a full stomach than on an empty one—avoid overeating.

- People who take corticosteroid drugs such as prednisone for more than a month often develop heartburn. If you are using these drugs on a long-term basis, consult with your physician concerning the best way to minimize the negative effects.

- Do not eat anything for three hours before you go to bed each night. If you must eat, fill up on bland provisions such as rice or toast, and stay away from any of the acid-forming foods mentioned earlier.

- Drink eight glasses of pure water a day.

- Take a leisurely five- to ten-minute walk after every meal. Relaxed walking stimulates digestion and discourages stomach acids from working their way up to the esophagus. It is customary for people in India to take a short walk every night after dinner.

- Eat four or five small meals a day rather than three large ones. Small meals digest easier and more quickly than large meals, and cause fewer digestive problems.

- If nighttime acid reflux is a concern, try elevating the head of your bed six inches or so. Raise the height of the bed itself; do not simply tuck pillows under your head. Too many pillows actually makes night heartburn worse. Commercially available bed wedges are also available.

- Certain types of ethnic restaurant cuisine tend to cause gas and heartburn galore, especially for people unaccustomed to foreign fare. If you enjoy a particular ethnic cuisine that also has digestive repercussions, choose your menu items carefully when ordering. Avoid acid-causing foods, eat in moderation, then follow up the meal with a cup of tea made from any of the acid-neutralizing herbs mentioned earlier. Indian restaurants often offer customers cardamom seeds after meals, another way of cutting down on heartburn.

IRRITABLE BOWEL SYNDROME (IBS)

Causes and Symptoms

Irritable bowel syndrome (IBS), also known as spastic colon and mucus colitis, is one of the most common of all digestive ailments. It affects 30 to 50 million Americans, most of whom are female. Currently, it accounts for 25 to 40 percent of the referrals made to gastroenterologists.

Determining the precise number of people who actually develop this disorder is difficult, however, as many sufferers never seek medical council. Plus, there's the fact that IBS is one of the least talked about of all diseases, primarily because its symptoms are so embarrassing and difficult to live with. Typical indicators of IBS include the following:

- Constipation in some people, chronic diarrhea in others, and a combination of the two in still others. Regardless of the type, bowel symptoms are associated with abdominal pain often relieved on defecation.
- Flatulence, nausea, pain, bloating, intestinal cramping, mucus in the stool, stabbing pains in the rectum, and indigestion.
- Bowel urgency, incontinence, and, at times, total loss of bowel control are all possible IBS symptoms, though none are sureties.
- In people with IBS who suffer from chronic diarrhea and hemor-

rhoids, anal fissures are common. These fissures are caused by the pressure and friction of constant bowel movements. In people with IBS who suffer from constipation, fissures usually develop due to excessive straining.

- A number of IBS female sufferers often experience painful menstrual periods accompanied by bouts of diarrhea. As a rule, this problem clears up when the menses is over.
- There are a number of IBS symptoms not directly related to bowel function. These include chest pains, headache, fatigue, sleep disorders, and loss of appetite. Some IBS patients also report swollen sensations in their throats between meals, as if a phantom ball or piece of food is lodged. Others experience pain when swallowing.
- Many people with IBS also have coexisting ailments such as fibromyalgia, chronic fatigue syndrome, and migraine headaches.

Concerning the specific etiology of IBS, it belongs to a group of ailments lumped under the title *functional gastrointestinal disorders*. Ailments in this category include chronic constipation, chronic diarrhea, nonulcer dyspepsia, and several others, all of which have one puzzling trait in common: no one can identify the biochemical or structural factors that cause them.

In other words, IBS is diagnosed only when other ailments producing similar gastrointestinal symptoms are all ruled out. Despite the vagueness of its origins, however, there is no lack of possible causes for this difficult disease. On the list of possibilities are emotional triggers such as stress, fatigue, shock, anxiety, and depression. Food allergies, hormonal imbalance, yeast infections, a diet low in fiber and high in refined foods, plus abuse of medications, street drugs, and laxatives are all possible physical factors. In some cases, IBS develops while a patient is convalescing from traveler's diarrhea, a virus, or from surgery. In still other instances, food poisoning or neurological dysfunction in the gut is the cause.

Different people, in other words, come to this disorder through different paths. Its root cause seems to be based simply on the fact that the digestive tract is a vulnerable and delicate organ. Visit continual physical and/or mental abuse on it, and over time, in some way, for some reason, IBS-like symptoms result.

The Rome II Criteria

How do you know if you have IBS, as opposed to a similar digestive malady? A group of medical professionals recently met in Rome to discuss this very question. The answers they came up with were formulated into a protocol known originally as the Rome Criteria, and recently revised and renamed the Rome II Criteria.

The Rome II Criteria tells us that you may have IBS if you have experienced continuous or recurrent abdominal pain that is relieved by evacuation, and is associated with a change in the frequency or consistency of bowel movements. Both pain and disturbance of bowel habits must be present. Finally, in the past year, you must have experienced these symptoms for twelve weeks or more.

It is even more likely that you have IBS if you additionally meet two or more of the following criteria:

- Mucus in the stool
- Bloating in the abdomen
- A change in stool frequency (diarrhea, constipation, alternating bouts of each)
- A change in stool consistency (watery, loose, hard)
- Difficulty passing stool (feelings of incomplete evacuation, sudden urgency, or straining)

Clearly, the Rome II Criteria offers a helpful series of diagnostic guidelines. Note, however, that in the last analysis, the only way to be absolutely certain that you suffer from IBS is by means of a physician's diagnosis, supported with findings from one or more lab tests such as a sigmoidoscopy, colonoscopy, barium enema, small bowel tests X ray, stool, thyroid function tests, lactose intolerance tests, and others.

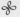

Conventional Treatment for IBS

Conventional drug treatments include anti-cholinergic drugs, antacids, prokinetic agents, and antidepressants. Recently, Lotronex was released as the first drug for IBS, but it was hastily withdrawn because of many medication-induced deaths. Another drug, Zelnorm, is effective only for constipation-type IBS, and only in females, and it costs more than a hundred dollars a month. Its efficacy is only modestly superior to that of a placebo (about 10 percent). In my experience, none of the conventional methods is impressively effective, and most tend to provoke unpleasant side effects. Natural remedies are becoming increasingly popular to treat IBS and supplement conventional medical treatment.

Natural Remedies for IBS

Natural treatment for IBS is often envisioned by clinicians as a four-pronged strategy using the following:

1. Herbs, minerals, and supplements
2. Dietary modifications
3. Lifestyle improvements
4. Psychological evaluation and counseling

Let's have a look at each of these approaches in the sections that follow.

Herbs, Minerals, and Supplements

Herbs, minerals, and nutritional supplements perform two basic functions for IBS sufferers:

1. They act as antispasmodics, reducing the pain of gastrointestinal cramps.
2. They help soothe and relax the gastrointestinal tract. A relaxed digestive system, in turn, heals more quickly.

Herbs for the purpose of healing IBS may be used as dried extracts (capsules, powders, or teas), glycerites (glycerin extracts), or tinctures (alcohol extracts). Unless otherwise indicated, teas should be made with one teaspoon of herb per cup of hot water. Steep covered for five to ten minutes for leaf or flowers, and from ten to twenty minutes for roots. Drink two to four cups a day.

- **Artichoke**—Dr. A. F. Walker and associates from the University of Reading in England studied the effect of artichoke leaf extract (ALE) on the symptoms of irritable bowel syndrome. Reporting their findings in the journal *Phytotherapy Research* (2001), the researchers assert that ALE treatment leads to significant reductions in the severity of symptoms. Both patients and physicians rated it as highly effective. In fact, 96 percent of the patients felt that ALE was at least equal to or better than the conventional treatments they had previously used for their symptoms. ALE is not widely available in retail health-supply stores, but it can be attained from vendors on the Internet. See the Appendix for information.

- **Clown's mustard**—The herb clown's mustard, also known as candytuft or bitter candytuft, is a wild flower that grows in Europe and the United States. Recently, it has been the subject of much gastrointestinal research, especially in Germany. Dr. M. T. Khayyal, writing in the journal *Arzneimittelforschung* (2001), reports on its ulcer healing and prevention properties. It also appears to be useful for improving a variety of IBS symptoms. See the Appendix for sources.

- **Enteric-coated peppermint oil**—Peppermint oil has been clinically shown in many studies to reduce spasms in the colon, relieve pain, and improve the symptoms of IBS in general. Dr. J. H. Liu, writing in the *Journal of Gastroenterology* (1997), has documented its efficacy on the basis of a randomized controlled trial. In one clinical evaluation, eighteen out of nineteen test subjects using peppermint oil reported lessened pain and substantial symptom relief from IBS-related complications. Peppermint oil is also reputed to fight off the yeast infection candidiasis, which some health-care professionals

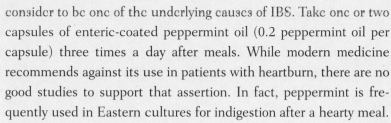

consider to be one of the underlying causes of IBS. Take one or two capsules of enteric-coated peppermint oil (0.2 peppermint oil per capsule) three times a day after meals. While modern medicine recommends against its use in patients with heartburn, there are no good studies to support that assertion. In fact, peppermint is frequently used in Eastern cultures for indigestion after a hearty meal.

- **Fennel seed**—Fennel seed is a powerful herbal antispasmodic; eat a teaspoon of the seeds several times a day to relieve bloating, gas, and spasms in the gastrointestinal tract. A tea made from fennel seed and a one-inch piece of chopped fresh ginger root makes an excellent general digestive aid for IBS sufferers.

- **Goldenseal**—A common multiuse American herb, goldenseal has a healing effect on the mucous membranes of the gut, reduces swelling, relaxes intestinal muscles, and helps repair damaged tissue. Take the capsules or make it into a tea. Drink half a cup twice a day.

- **L-glutamine**—For diarrhea relief and regularity, L-glutamine is a powerful antispasmodic, helping relieve intestinal cramping and restoring normal bowel activity. Take two 500-mg capsules every morning until symptoms improve.

- **Magnesium**—Magnesium salts are commonly prescribed as cathartics to relieve constipation, associated cramps, and spasms of the gastrointestinal tract. It is specifically helpful for people with IBS who suffer from constipation (use of magnesium with diarrhea can be counterproductive and is not recommended). Magnesium dose needs to be individualized according to need by a health-care professional. Magnesium should not be used by patients with renal failure.

- **Omega-3 fatty acids**—Derived from fish (cod liver oil) and flaxseed oil, omega-3 fatty acids reduce inflammation in the gastrointestinal areas, repair digestive tissue, and provide the added bonus of buttressing cardiovascular health. Omega-3 fatty acid supplements are available at any health-food store.

- **Rice bran oil**—Rice bran oil or gamma-oryzanol has a protective effect on the mucous lining of the stomach, and helps reduce IBS symptoms. For more information, see gamma-oryzanol under "Gastritis" on page 333.

- **5-HTP**—5-HTP is a food supplement that is a precursor to the neurotransmitter serotonin. There is some clinical evidence to show that 5-HTP not only aids in getting a good night's sleep, but improves IBS forms of constipation. See Chapter 4 for more information on 5-HTP.

Dietary Modifications

- **Fiber supplements**—It is generally felt that a diet composed primarily of refined, low-fiber foods contributes to the development of IBS. Conversely, diets rich in fiber help relieve IBS symptoms, and are often prescribed. Whether patients have IBS-diarrhea type, IBS-constipation type, or alternating types (constipation *and* diarrhea), they can also expect a recommendation of fiber supplementation from their physicians at the very beginning of treatment. Isabgol, a commercial form of psyllium sold in health-food stores, is probably the most effective. Psyllium seed powder and flaxseeds, both world-class sources of fiber, are also known to regularize gut motility. For people with diarrhea, these products provide bulk and form to the IBS sufferer's stool by absorbing excess water.

- **Improved diet**—There is no "standard" diet for IBS. A regimen of careful eating is advised.

  A diet consisting of 60 percent fresh vegetables and fruits, both the raw and cooked variety, is recommended. Avoid fatty foods, fried and spicy foods, and junk foods, and cut back on dairy products. Yogurt is an exception, however. It can usually be eaten in quantity by people with IBS.

  Also, increase your daily intake of water and fresh-squeezed juices, but, for the time being, avoid sugar-based drinks, carbonated drinks, coffee, and black tea. If you have an allergy to wheat, eat breads and cereals made from oats, barley, rice, rye, corn, and rice bran.

- **Supporting "good" intestinal bacteria**—Intestinal infection can initiate and perpetuate IBS. There is much evidence to show that increased amounts of helpful intestinal bacteria such as *Lactobacillus acidophilus* and *Bifidobacterium bifidum,* both found in soured-milk products like yogurt and probiotics, inhibit these harmful pathogens from growing on the mucous lining of the intestine and prevent gas-producing bacteria from proliferating. In the process, they reduce symptoms of IBS including flatulence, diarrhea, and bloating. See Chapters 7 and 8 for details and instruction.

· **Food allergies**—There is increasing clinical evidence to show that, in some cases, food allergies trigger IBS. Many patients show immediate improvement when an elimination diet (discussed below) is used, and offending foods are identified and removed from the diet. One recent study demonstrated that as many as two-thirds of test subjects suffering from IBS were allergic to at least one food, and several were allergic to many.

Dr. R. Nanda has documented in the journal *Gut* (1989) that almost half of the patients he studied with IBS respond to dietary exclusion or dietary elimination plans. Food allergies are notoriously complicated, and if you think you suffer from one or more, it is best to have your condition reviewed by a qualified health-care professional.

· **Elimination diet**—A typical elimination diet consists of several discrete steps:

1. A specified food is removed from the diet.
2. The patient's reactions to this selective style of eating are observed. Do the IBS symptoms get better while the person is not eating this food? Worse? Do they remain the same?
3. The food is reintroduced back into the diet, and the patient's reactions are observed again. If the patient's symptoms improved, do they worsen again when the food is reintroduced? Do they remain the same?

Since many people are allergic to wheat, for example, a typical elimination diet might remove wheat products from the menu for, let us say, three weeks. After the three-week period is complete, these wheat products are reintroduced.

If improvement was shown when the patient stopped eating wheat, and if allergic symptoms now return when the wheat is reintroduced, this offers strong evidence that the subject is indeed allergic to wheat. From now on, he or she avoids this food. In this way, offending foods can be identified, isolated, and eliminated from the diet.

Dr. Richard McCallum, a digestive-disease expert and former chief of gastroenterology at the University of Kansas and the University of Virginia, stated at a 2002 consultants' conference in New York City that he frequently recommends elimination diet programs for patients with IBS. He is convinced that these diets help some patients, even though the allergy theory of IBS is not scientifically validated.

Lifestyle Improvements

Harmful personal habits such as smoking, obesity, overeating, alcohol abuse, lack of exercise, and drug dependence all wreak havoc on the digestive system and, in many cases, contribute to the seriousness of symptoms in irritable bowel syndrome. For people suffering from this ailment, the following advice is given by physicians and specialists alike:

- Exercise at least three times a week. Aerobics, sports, dance, walking, swimming, jogging, yoga, and tai chi are all beneficial. Stay active—that's the key.
- Some people find that heat treatment with hot-water bottles, hot packs, or electric heating pads applied to the abdomen lessons IBS symptoms.
- If you smoke, stop now. Smoking makes every digestive disease worse.
- If you drink heavily, cut down. Too much alcohol exacerbates IBS symptoms and, in some cases, triggers them.
- Check with your doctor concerning your weight. If you are overweight, and definitely if you are obese, seek guidance. Losing weight can help.

- Try not to overeat. When you do eat, eat slowly.
- Avoid stress. Many medical professionals consider stress and anxiety to be principal components of the biopsychosocial model for the causation of IBS. Sometimes, simply getting away from the daily routine, avoiding crisis and confrontational situations, and taking it easy and relaxing are all that's needed to calm and even banish the symptoms of IBS.

Psychological Evaluation and Counseling

IBS is an ailment of the mind and emotions, as well as the body. Frequently, it is both. What helps in this regard? We know that many IBS sufferers experience reduction of IBS-related diarrhea, constipation, and pain simply by attending psychotherapy sessions. Relaxation therapy is also highly recommended, along with group therapy. Stress management, hypnosis, and biofeedback have all been used with some success in treating this difficult ailment. In general, IBS patients find that if they learn to deal with their mental tensions and with pent-up fears, to not sweat the small stuff and meet life's challenges head-on, improvements soon follow.

MOTION SICKNESS

Causes and Symptoms

When we sit in the backseat of a bumpy car, when we sway to and fro on a boat at sea, when we bounce up and down on a horse and a carriage, motion sickness often follows. What's going on?

The explanation you are most likely to hear—actually, no one knows for sure what causes this ailment—is that during a rough ride, the fluid in our semicircular canals, that part of the inner ear responsible for balance, receives so many conflicting signals—up, down, sideways, forward, reverse—that it becomes disoriented, short-circuits, and triggers the agonies of motion sickness.

Though the symptoms of this unpleasant illness seem to strike from all directions, they are basically centered in two parts of the body—the head and the gut. Typical symptoms are dizziness, disorientation, headache, pallor, salivation, sweating, malaise, nausea, queasy stomach, burping, hiccups, and sometimes intense vomiting. The body usually cures itself in a few hours; for some people, however, the agonies of sea sickness continue for hours and even for days.

One easy chemical fix is to take an antihistamine before setting out on a bumpy journey. Antihistamines tend to make people drowsy, however, not a good bet if someone is at the wheel. Other over-the-counter motion sickness medications produce similar reactions. Meanwhile, for many people, natural remedies work just as well.

Herbal and Natural Remedies for Motion Sickness

- **Activated charcoal**—Charcoal absorbs stomach juices and calms the digestive system during travel uproar. Take two to four capsules or tablets of charcoal a half hour before leaving on your trip. **Note:** Charcoal neutralizes and absorbs other nutrients, chemicals, and digestive juices. Take all food and medications a few hours before or after use.
- **Chinese patent medication**—Travelers in the know, especially with a tendency to be those bothered by motion sickness, take a bottle of Ren Dan (also called Benevolence Pills) with them when they travel. A powerful inhibitor of seasickness and motion sickness, Ren Dan helps avoid (and sometimes cures) diarrhea, dizziness, and vomiting. It is also an excellent specific for helping users adjust to the climate of a new location. Take this medication approximately a half hour before setting out on a journey. Follow the instructions included in the box for dosage. See the Appendix for sources.
- **Combination elixir**—Add a half teaspoon of baking soda, sugar (or glucose syrup), and salt to a glass of water. Sip this potion frequently while traveling.
- **Ginger**—Once again, ginger to the rescue. Studies by Dr. R. Schmid, reported in the *Journal of Travel Medicine* (1994), document that ingesting fresh ginger while traveling is a more effective remedy against motion sickness than Scopolamine or related over-the-counter med-

ications. You can take ginger in fresh or capsule form; chew it in soft, crystallized candy form; or ingest the powder. For most people on the bumpy road, ginger really works. Chewing it is often all that is needed to stem the queasy feelings.

- **Herbal formula for motion sickness**—Combine the following ingredients: One-inch piece fresh peeled ginger, two inch slices licorice root, two teaspoons fresh or dried peppermint leaves, one teaspoon dried valerian root, a dash of cayenne pepper, and two cups of water.

   Place the combined ingredients in a pot and bring to a boil. Simmer for twenty minutes, or until the liquid boils down to approximately one cup. Drink this potion a half hour before leaving on your trip, and take some with you in a thermos as backup.

- **Peppermint oil**—Put two or three drops of peppermint oil into a cup of boiling water, and drink a half hour before leaving. During your trip, take the oil along, and sniff it periodically. Peppermint tea is also useful.

Other Natural Remedies for Motion Sickness

Over the years, travelers have developed the following simple tricks for coping with motion sickness:

- Always avoid dehydration. Drink several glasses of water or fruit juice before leaving. Drink plenty of water while traveling. Avoid drinking alcohol at least twenty-four hours before leaving on your trip.
- Stop eating three hours before you leave.
- Purchase a "sea band" bracelet at any pharmacy. Many people prone to motion sickness swear by this inexpensive and easy-to-use device.
- Massage the crease lines along both your wrists, emphasizing pressure on the center of each wrist.
- Apply circular self-massage to your solar plexus for five minutes. Wait five minutes, then massage again.

• When traveling in a car or bus, be sure to sit in the front seat. If flying, sit in an aisle seat, preferably one located over the wings. If on a ship, position yourself in the middle of the ship, as near to the waterline as possible. When in a moving vehicle, gaze at a distant point and keep your focus glued to this spot. Do not look around or side to side more than you have to. If you are riding in a car, fix your gaze on a distant object ahead on the road. If you are in a boat, fix your gaze on the horizon. If you are in a plane, stare out the window at a spot on the ground below.

Nausea

Causes and Symptoms

Basically a symptom, not a disease, nausea accompanies digestive ailments with such frequency that it often seems like a disorder unto itself, and just as often acts that way. It can also be annoyingly persistent. Just when you think it's gone, back it comes again. And again. And again.

Nauseous feelings are difficult to describe, though common to just about everyone's experience. They are characterized by a sick, queasy sensation in the stomach and throat, often accompanied by a feeling that one is about to vomit. In many cases, this vomiting does not come, a mixed blessing for those who feel that if they could *just* get it up and out, all would be well.

Nausea can be triggered by a spectrum of ailments ranging from colds and flu, to motion sickness, pregnancy, parasites, food allergies, food poisoning, gastrointestinal disease, and many others. Certainly, we all know the feeling. But what to do when it strikes?

Herbal Remedies for Nausea

Herbs that counteract nausea and relieve vomiting are known as antiemetics. The following preparations fall under this category:

- **Barley water**—Boil a small handful of pearl (hulled) barley for an hour. Remove the barley and preserve the water. Mix a half cup of the barley water with a half cup of warm milk, and drink. Barley water makes a soothing elixir for any intestinal disruption including nausea, vomiting, and indigestion. Then, when you're feeling better, eat the barley.
- **Ginger**—For nausea, the dried powder is best. Take a teaspoon with a cup of hot water and wait several minutes. If no improvement follows, take another half teaspoon of the ginger. If the powdered variety is not handy, peel a half-inch piece of fresh ginger, boil it in two cups of water for twenty minutes, and drink. Do not add a sweetener. You can also take ginger tea or powder with other antinausea herbs like peppermint. According to an article in the medical journal *Lancet* (1998), ginger is more effective at curing nausea than most conventional medications. A survey of obstetricians conducted by Dr. M. L. Power and colleagues, and reported in the journal *Primary Care Update Obstetricians and Gynecologists* (2001), shows that a majority of the surveyed professionals recommend ginger as one of the top choices for nausea during pregnancy. Interestingly, female physicians were more likely to prescribe ginger than their male counterparts.
- **Mint and peppermint**—During bouts of nausea, a quick cup of mint or peppermint tea often stops nausea in its tracks. When treating nausea with mint tea, it is best not to add a sweetener. A drop of peppermint oil added to hot water or a glass of juice produces a similar healing effect.

Other Natural Remedies for Nausea

- **Bland food to the rescue**—Although eating may be the last thing on your mind when you're nauseous, bland foods coat the intestinal lining and help settle the stomach. Starches are especially good in this regard. Try bananas and rice, and be sure to drink the water the rice is boiled in. Applesauce is also helpful, and if you are suffering from heartburn along with nausea, a plain piece of toast is a powerful acid reflux absorber.

- **Acupressure**—Dr. E. Werntoft writes in the *Journal of Reproductive Medicine* (2001) that acupressure is superior to placebo in providing relief of nausea and vomiting during pregnancy. The moment nausea appears, press the following acupressure points:

  1. With palms facing up, press the point along the crease of the inner wrist in line with (and at the base) of the thumb. Press firmly on this spot for twenty seconds, pause for a moment, then press for another twenty seconds. Apply to both wrists.

  2. Starting at the base of the knee, place your hand on your shinbone and measure down one hand's width. From this point on the shinbone, measure the width of one thumb toward the outside of the leg (the side with the big toe). Press firmly on this point for twenty seconds, pause for several moments, then press again for another twenty seconds. Press this same point on both legs.

- **Chinese patent medications**—If you suffer from occasional nausea, there are several excellent over-the-counter Chinese herbal medicines that help. Chinese patent medicines are inexpensive, time tested, and often amazingly—and quickly—effective. Two Chinese products you should consider trying for nausea and digestive problems in general are the following:

  - **Six Gentlemen Tea Pill (Xiang Sha Liu Jun Wan)**—A classic Chinese herbal formula, which means it is more than 400 years old, Six Gentlemen Tea is highly effective for treating nausea, indigestion, overeating, diarrhea, and morning sickness.
  - **Po Chai Pills (Protect and Benefit Pill)**—Po Chai is an effective over-the-counter herbal for nausea, vomiting, and bloating. Travelers often bring several bottles with them to protect against "tourist's stomach."

If you live near an urban area with a Chinatown, you can purchase these medications at any Chinese pharmacy. If not, check the Appendix for the addresses of companies that sell Chinese herbs and patent medications.

- **Newspaper print**—Sniff a page of newspaper four or five times in a row. Ridiculous, perhaps, but this simple trick is a time-honored quick fix for queasy stomachs. What makes it work? Word has it that there is a chemical in printer's newspaper ink that quiets stomach rumblings. What the heck, try it.

appendix

Resources

Artichoke Leaf Extract

Artichoke leaf extract can be ordered online from:
    www.naturalhealthconsult.com
    www.b-natural-online.com
    www.lef.org/prod_hp/php1067.html

Ayurvedic Medicine

Supplies for Ayurvedic medicine can be purchased online from:
    http://www.herbscancure.com/
    http://www.indiamart.com/bioremedies/
    http://www.webindia.com/rnrajan/profile.htm
    http://dir.indiamart.com/indianexporters/ayur.html
    http://www.allayurveda.com/
    http://www.nutritiondynamics.com/products/Herbs_&_Homeopathic/
        Ayurvedic/main.html
    http://www.indianherbalremedies.com/herbs.asp

Consult this website for links and general information on Ayurveda:
    http://www.compulink.co.uk/~mandrake/ayurveda.htm

Sources for Safi Indian Ayurvedic medicine include:
  http://trade.Indiamart.com
  www.crownhealthcareproducts.com

Bentonite Clay
To order bentonite clay online, visit:
  www.aimforbetterhealth.com
  www.curezone.com/cleanse/bowel/bentonite.asp

Butyrate Enemas
Butyrate enemas can be ordered from the pharmacies listed below. A doctor's
  prescription is needed.
Lloyd Center Pharmacy, phone: 800-358-8974
Key Pharmacy, phone: 800-878-1322

Caprylic Acid
Caprylic acid is available online from:
  www.thewayup.com/products/0139/htm
  www.lifelinknet.com
  http://1001herbs.com/caprylic_acid/

Clown's Mustard
The potion containing clown's mustard is called Iberogast. You may find it at:
  iHerb Ltd.
  1435 South Shamrock Avenue
  Monrovia, CA 91018
  Phone: 623-358-5678
  www.iherb.com

Colostrum
A good-quality colostrum is available online from:
  www.globalhealthtrax.com

Detoxification and Fasting
Helpful products for people who want to detox can be ordered from:
  Blessings from Nature
  North Wickham Road 12-409
  Melbourne, FL 32940

Phone. 800 49 DETOX
www.cleanout.com

For cleansing and fasting products, visit the following websites:
http://dmoz.org/Health/Alternative/Fasting_and_Cleansing/
http://dmoz.org/Recreation/Drugs/Suppliers_and_Shops/Detox_Products/
http://www.paradise-health.com/
http://www.greatestherbsonearth.com/nsp_cleansing_fasting.htm

Helpful links to fasting sites can be found at:
http://www.thebigholistic.com/info/hydrotherapy/hydrotherapylinks.htm

Digestive Aids
General aids can be purchased online from:
http://www.joellessacredgrove.com/Herbs/a-herbs.html
http://www.lef.org/protocols/abstracts/abstr-044b.html

Diverticulosis
Information and resources can be found at:
http://www.niddk.nih.gov/health/digest/pubs/divert/divert.htm
http://www.nlm.nih.gov/medlineplus/ency/article/000257.htm
http://www.focusondigestion.com/script/main/art.asp?li=MNI&arti-
clekey=347

Gastritis
Information and resources can be found at:
http://www.niddk.nih.gov/health/digest/summary/gastritis/gastritis.htm
http://www.laurushealth.com/Library/HealthGuide/IllnessConditions/
topic.asp?hwid=nord119

Heartburn
Information and resources can be found at:
http://www.gerd.com/
http://www.helpheartburn.com/
http://www.aboutgerd.org/week.html

Herbs
Medicinal herbs can be purchased at health-food stores and online from:

www.herbsnow.com
http://www.viable-herbal.com/herbology/herbs19.htm
http://jbje.tripod.com/esthetopia/id20.html
http://www.teatreeplace.com/links/herbalremedies.html
http://www.cotswoldherbs.co.uk/
http://www.denes.com/universal/health/health.html   (especially for pets)
http://www.greatestherbsonearth.com

For lists of medicinal herbs and descriptions of their healing qualities, see the
following:
http://www.geocities.com/nashville/rodeo/3276/herb.html
http://www.joellessacredgrove.com/Herbs/a-herbs.html
http://www.all-natural.com/herbnutr.html

A useful herb-seller's database is offered online at:
http://earthnotes.tripod.com/where.htm

Web pages with links to sites for Chinese herbs include:
http://gancao.net/aculinks/phpHoo2.php3?viewCat=73
www.starprana.com/natural/
www.fragrant.demon.co.uk/tcm.html

Hydrocolators
Hydrocolators can be purchased at many pharmacies or ordered online at:
www.wholebodyhealing.com/store

Intestinal Gas
For general information see:
http://www.niddk.nih.gov/health/digest/pubs/gas/gas.htm

Commercial herb mixtures that help combat intestinal gas can be ordered online from:
http://www.atlantis1.com/Health/default.htm   (order CCleansing Powder)
http://www.soulhealer.com/intestnl.htm
http://www.soulhealer.com/366-2.htm   (for activated charcoal)
http://www.curezone.com/diseases/parasites/parasitescleanse.asp   (especially for parasites)
http://www.bodyandfitness.com/Information/Herbal/Research/fennel.htm

Irritable Bowel Syndrome

Information and resources can be found at:

    http://www.healthcyclopedia.com/irritable_bowel_syndrome.html
    http://www.panix.com/~ibs/   (links)

Leaky Gut Syndrome

Information and resources can be found at:

    http://www.health-n-energy.com/leakygut.htm
    http://www.gsdl.com/news/1999/19990227/
    http://osiris.sunderland.ac.uk/autism/gut.htm
    http://www.accessnable.com.au/handbook/leakygut.htm
    http://www.lovelyhealth.com/Leaky_Gut_Syndrome.htm
    http://www.denmar.net/hs9.html

Orange Peel Extract

Orange peel extract can be ordered from:

    www.seacoastvitamins.com
    Phone: 800-555-6792

www.bnatural-online.com

Probiotics

    Allergy Research
    NutriCology
    30806 Santana Street
    Hayward, CA 94544
    Phone: 800-545-9960
    Fax: 510-487-8682
    www.nutricology.com

PB8

    Tsang Nutrition
    3 Raymond Street
    Dudley, MA 01571
    Phone: 508-943-8472
    Fax: 240-536-4474
    http://tsangenterprise.com

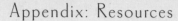

FindSupplements
695 Shenandoah Avenue
San Marcos, CA 92078
Fax: 253-390-4053
www.findsupplements.com

Natural Factors
Vitavita
Phone: 888-584-2377
www.vitavita.com

D'Adamo
Suzanne's Natural Foods
3106 South Connecticut
Joplin, MO 64804
Phone: 417-781-0909
www.suzannes.com

Natren
Natren, Inc.
3105 Willow Lane
Westlake Village, CA 91361
Phone: 800-992-3323
www.natren.com

NutraCea
NutraCea
El Dorado Hills, CA 95762
www.nutrastar.com

Custom Probiotic
www.customprobiotics.com

Relaxation
Books on stress and relaxation include:
Lucinda Bassett, *From Panic to Power,* HarperInformation, 1996
Herbert Benson with Miriam Z. Klipper, *The Relaxation Response,* William
  Morrow, 2000

Martha Davis, Ph.D, et al., *The Relaxation and Stress Workbook,* New Harbinger, 2000

Christina Feldman, *Principles of Meditation,* Thorsons, 1999

Susan Lark, *Dr. Susan Lark's Anxiety and Stress Self-Help Book,* Celestial Arts, 2000

Sources of books on health and relaxation can be found on the Web at:
http://www.thebigholistic.com/info/hydrotherapy/hydrotherapylinks.htm
http://www.isma.org.uk/booklist.htm
http://www.mindtools.com/smpage.html
http://www.womenshealth.com/orderitems/stress_item.html (especially for women)
http://www.vhl.org/bookstore/wellness.htm
www.relax7.com/5htm
http://www.cxam_ta.ac.uk/accelerated6.htm
www.smd-services.com/information/pdfs/anxiety_disorders_bibliography_2002.pdf

Relaxation tapes and videos can be ordered online from:
http://mshafer.com/books_audiotapes.html
http://www.healthynewage.com/stressless.html
http://www.wholeperson.com/wpa/v/rv/rv.htm
http://www.worldofhealth.co.uk/html/medical_conditions/med_medical_stress.htm
http://www.epinions.com/Movies-Sports_Recreation-keyword-Instructional/pp_~2

St. John's Wort
A website dedicated exclusively to the use of St. John's wort in fighting depression:
http://www.all-natural.com/nat-proz.html

Shark Liver Oil
Shark liver oil can be ordered online from:
www.lovelyhealth.com/prodSLO.htm

Two good books on shark liver oil and its uses are:
Peter T. Pugliese, M.D., with John Heinerman, Ph.D., *Devour Disease with Shark Liver Oil,* Bertram, 1999

Neil Solomon, M.D., and Richard Passwater, Ph.D., *Shark Liver Oil: Nature's Amazing Healer,* Kensington, 1997

Yoga

For general information, contacts, and books on the practice and philosophy of yoga, see any of the following websites:

http://www.santosha.com/philosophy/yoga-philosophy.html

http://www.himalayaninstitute.org/

http://www.kaliraytriyoga.com/yoga_philosophy.htm

http://dmoz.org/Society/Religion_and_Spirituality/Yoga/

http://www.suite101.com/welcome.cfm/yoga

http://www.focalpointyoga.com/why_practice_yoga.htm

Videos demonstrating yoga techniques can be purchased online at:

http://www.fourgates.com/yogavideo.asp

http://www.martialartsgear.com/Yoga/Yoga_Mats_And_Videos/
    Yoga_Mats_And_Videos.shtml

http://www.yoga-videos.net/

http://www.yoga-insideout.com/

http://www.lightenupyoga.com/freedom_fr_back_pain_video.html

http://www.yogakitty.com/yogavideos.html

Exercise and meditation products (including mats, clothes, exercise equipment, books, meditation cushions) can be purchased online at any of the following sites:

http://yoga shop-for.com

http://www.bheka.com/StoreFront.bok

http://www.lakeshoreyoga.com/home.htm?pagesix.htm~mainFrame

http://www.kensingtonyoga.com/equipmentclothes.htm

http://www.sunandmoonoriginals.com/

http://www.halfmoonyogaprops.com/

http://www.matsmatsmats.com/yoga/yoga-mats.html

http://www.fourgates.com/yoga.asp

http://www.aboutyoga.com/

For links to interesting yoga sites on the Web, go to:

http://www1.fitnessmall.com/yoga.html

http://home.earthlink.net/~mayfair224/stores.htm
http://www.bindu.freeserve.co.uk/viniyoga/links.htm
http://www.worldofalternatives.com/UKHomeopathy/links/yogaequip.html
http://www.storesonline.com/site/383826/page/60623
http://dmoz.org/Society/Religion_and_Spirituality/Yoga/

Yogurt
A good dry starter culture for making yogurt can be purchased from:
    Charles Hansen Laboratory
    9015 West Maple Street
    Milwaukee, WI 53215

Precision stainless-steel thermometers for measuring the heat of milk can be ordered from:
    Western Instruments
    614 Frelinghuysen Avenue
    Newark, NJ 07114

index